Medical Management of
Type 1
Diabetes

SIXTH EDITION

Edited by
Francine R. Kaufman, MD

American
Diabetes
Association.

Director, Book Publishing, Abe Ogden; *Managing Editor*, Greg Guthrie; *Acquisitions Editor*, Victor Van Beuren; *Production Manager*, Melissa Sprott; *Composition and Project Management*, Cenveo; *Cover Design*, Jody Billert; *Printer*, Victor Graphics.

Printed in the United States of America
1 3 5 7 9 10 8 6 4 2

♾ The paper in this publication meets the requirements of the ANSI Standard Z39.48-1992 (permanence of paper).

ADA titles may be purchased for business or promotional use or for special sales. To purchase more than 50 copies of this book at a discount, or for custom editions of this book with your logo, contact the American Diabetes Association at the address below, at booksales@diabetes.org, or by calling 703-299-2046.

American Diabetes Association
1701 North Beauregard Street
Alexandria, Virginia 22311

DOI: 10.2337/9781580404563

Library of Congress Cataloging-in-Publication Data

Medical management of type 1 diabetes.—6th ed. / Francine R. Kaufman, editor.
   p. ; cm.
Medical management of type one diabetes
Includes bibliographical references and index.
ISBN 978-1-58040-456-3 (alk. paper)
I. Kaufman, Francine Ratner. II. American Diabetes Association. III. Title: Medical management of type one diabetes.
[DNLM: 1. Diabetes Mellitus, Type 1. WK 810]

616.4'6206—dc23
            2012009322

Contents

Psychosocial Factors Affecting Adherence,
Quality of Life, and Well-Being: Helping Patients Cope   181

Complications   203

A Word About This Guide

This is the sixth edition of *Medical Management of Type 1 Diabetes*. Originally written as the *Physician's Guide to Insulin-Dependent* (type 1) *Diabetes: Diagnosis and Treatment*, this book has been repeatedly revised to provide the reader with the latest information on type 1 diabetes. This is just one of the many books for clinicians published by the American Diabetes Association. Other titles include *Intensive Diabetes Management, Medical Management of Type 2 Diabetes, Medical Management of Pregnancy Complicated by Diabetes*, and *Therapy for Diabetes Mellitus and Related Disorders*. This book has had an impressive list of previous editors, Mark A. Sperling, MD; Julio V. Santiago, MD (whose many contributions to the field of diabetes will never be forgotten); Jay S. Skyler, MD; Bruce W. Bode, MD; as well as many prestigious contributors who brought forward the necessary information to advance the field and improve the outcomes of people with type 1 diabetes throughout the world.

I am particularly honored to be the editor since the fifth edition and to have the opportunity to build on the work of so many others. The goal of *Medical Management of Type 1 Diabetes* is to continue focusing on key areas, including important clinical trials and the latest ADA Standards of Care. The first section is on Diagnosis and Classification/Pathogenesis of diabetes, and discusses the latest molecular advances and strategies to influence the type 1 process. The Diabetes Standards and Education section elucidates treatment goals and the importance of key areas in diabetes self-management education. Tools of Therapy includes insulin regimens, new agents to treat type 1 diabetes, advances in glucose monitoring, and the contribution of lifestyle. The section on Special Situations deals with the salient issues on treating and preventing DKA and hypoglycemia, as well as management of pregnancy and surgery. Psychosocial Factors focuses on understanding barriers and improving adherence, taking into account age, developmental factors, stress, and emotional/behavior disorders. Complications lays out the latest strategies to screen, treat, and prevent the organ system damage associated with diabetes.

This comprehensive guide to the clinical care of the patient with type 1 diabetes across the age spectrum, reveals that patients benefit from the effective management of their blood glucose levels, adherence to healthy lifestyle principles, such as proper nutrition and regular exercise/activity, control of blood pressure and blood lipid levels, and involvement with a proactive health care team. By continuing to update this book, the American Diabetes Association is promoting quality care for all people with type 1 diabetes.

FRANCINE R. KAUFMAN, MD
Editor

Contributors to the Sixth Edition

EDITOR

Francine R. Kaufman, MD
Children's Hospital Los Angeles
Los Angeles, California

CONTRIBUTORS

Paulina N. Duker, MPH, APRN, BC-ADM, CDE
American Diabetes Association
Alexandria, VA

Stephanie A. Dunbar, MPH, RD
American Diabetes Association
Alexandria, VA

M. Sue Kirkman, MD
American Diabetes Association
Alexandria, VA

Acknowledgments

The American Diabetes Association gratefully acknowledges the contributions of the following health care professionals and members of the Association's Professional Section to previous editions of this work:

Bruce W. Bode, MD; Lloyd P. Aiello, MD, PhD; Jerry D. Cavallerano, OD, PhD; Paul C. Davidson, MD, FACE; Sandy Gillespie, MS, RD, LD, CDE; Charlotte Hayes, MMSc, MS, RD, CDE; Lois Jovanovic, MD; Philip A. Lowe, MD; Stephen Pastan, MD; David G. Robertson, MD; Ronald J. Sigal, MD, MPH, FRCPC; R. Dennis Steed, MD, FACE, CDE; and Deborah Young-Hyman, PhD.

The Editor thanks the reviewers who aided in the review and critique of this book, including M. Sue Kirkman, MD; Stephanie A. Dunbar, MPH, RD; and Paulina N. Duker, MPH, APRN, BC-ADM, CDE.

Diagnosis and Classification/ Pathogenesis

Highlights

Diagnosis and Classification

Pathogenesis

Highlights
Diagnosis and Classification/
Pathogenesis

DIAGNOSIS AND CLASSIFICATION

■ Diabetes encompasses a wide clinical spectrum. The vast majority of cases of diabetes fall into two broad etiopathogenetic categories:

- type 1 diabetes, the cause of which is an absolute deficiency of insulin secretion
- type 2 diabetes, the cause of which is a combination of resistance to insulin action and an inadequate compensatory insulin secretory response

■ Indications for diagnostic testing include

- positive screening test results
- obvious signs and symptoms of diabetes (polydipsia, polyuria, polyphagia, weight loss)
- an incomplete clinical picture, such as glucosuria or equivocal elevation of random plasma glucose level or A1C.

■ When diabetes is fully evolved, fasting plasma glucose levels are ≥126 mg/dL (>7.0 mmol/L), random plasma glucose levels are ≥200 mg/dL (>11.1 mmol/L), and A1C is ≥6.5% (A1C elevation may not occur in the presence of certain hemoglobinopathies). Type 1 diabetes generally presents with unequivocal hyperglycemia, although natural history studies, such as the Diabetes Prevention Trial - Type 1 (DPT-1) and the multinational TrialNet study, have shown onset can be indolent and early diabetes can be relatively asymptomatic.

■ Approximately 1.89 per 1,000 children and youth have diabetes. Over 80% of those children under the age of 10 years, and the majority of children between the ages of 10 and 19 years have type 1 diabetes. Incidence is similar in males and females. The percentages of type 1 diabetes are highest in non-Hispanic white youth, intermediate in Hispanics and African Americans, and markedly less common in Asian Pacific Islanders and American Indians. Type 1 diabetes has been increasing 3–4% per year in children and youth, and even more in young children under the age of 5 years. It is estimated that in 2007 about 16,000 youths developed type 1 diabetes and 3,800 developed type 2 diabetes.

■ At presentation, patients with type 1 diabetes can be any age and often have experienced significant weight loss, polyuria, and polydipsia before presentation. The oral glucose tolerance test is rarely needed to diagnose type 1 diabetes. Delayed diagnosis is a serious, sometimes fatal, problem, especially among younger children.

■ Approximately 25% of children who present with newly diagnosed type 1 diabetes are ill with diabetic ketoacidosis, those <2 years of age are at highest risk, and may die from rapid metabolic decompensation and/or delayed diagnosis due to lack of suspicion of diabetes.

■ Type 1 diabetes can develop at any age and is sometimes mistaken for type 2 diabetes among adults who may have a more gradual course of onset, including those with latent autoimmune diabetes, which is referred to as LADA.

PATHOGENESIS

■ The primary defect in type 1 diabetes is inadequate insulin secretion by pancreatic β-cells.

■ Genetic predisposition, which can be determined by the presence of certain genetic alleles (HLA-DR/DQ alleles can be either predisposing or protective), clearly plays a role in the development of type 1 diabetes. However, a host of environmental triggers, including infectious agents and food antigens, may be involved in initiating the autoimmune process, which is initially detected by the presence of autoantibodies to islet cell components (GAD65 or GADA, ICA512 or IA-2A, zinc transporter 8 or ZnT8A, and insulin autoantibodies or IAA). This is followed over months to years by the progressive loss of insulin secretion due to β-cell destruction, particularly in those with persistent, multiple autoantibodies.

■ Fasting hyperglycemia occurs when β-cell mass is reduced by 80–90%. Typical symptoms of diabetes, i.e., polyuria, polydipsia, and weight loss, appear once hyperglycemia exceeds the renal threshold of ~180 mg/dL (~10.0 mmol/L) glucose.

■ After diagnosis and correction of acute metabolic abnormalities, some individuals experience a "remission or honeymoon phase," a temporary period when there is preservation of endogenous insulin secretion as determined by C-peptide levels, the need for exogenous insulin is diminished, glycemic control is improved, and glycemic variability reduced. Multiple interventions have been tried to preserve β-cells, but none has been shown to be effective in reversing the auto-destructive process.

■ Within 5–10 years after clinical presentation, β-cell loss is complete; at this point, insulin deficiency is absolute, C-peptide secretion is lost, and circulating islet cell antibodies might not be detected.

Diagnosis and Classification/Pathogenesis

DIAGNOSIS AND CLASSIFICATION

Diabetes is a chronic disorder that is *1)* characterized by hyperglycemia; *2)* associated with major abnormalities in carbohydrate, fat, and protein metabolism; and *3)* accompanied by a marked propensity to develop relatively specific forms of renal, ocular, neurologic, and premature cardiovascular diseases. Diabetes encompasses a wide clinical spectrum. The vast majority of cases of diabetes fall into two broad etiopathogenetic categories:

- type 1 diabetes, the cause of which is an absolute deficiency of insulin secretion
- type 2 diabetes, the cause of which is a combination of resistance to insulin action and an inadequate compensatory insulin secretory response

Diabetes may also occur because of specific genetic defects and secondary to a number of conditions, such as pregnancy, and syndromes, as well as diseases of the pancreas, several endocrinopathies, and use of certain drugs.

Although type 1 diabetes accounts for ~5–10% of all diagnosed cases of diabetes, its immediate risks and stringent acute treatment requirements demand rapid recognition, early diagnosis, and effective management. This chapter explores characteristics that differentiate type 1 diabetes from other forms of diabetes, discusses criteria for correct diagnosis, and illustrates various clinical presentations.

CRITERIA FOR DIAGNOSIS

The criteria for diagnosing diabetes is a fasting plasma glucose concentration ≥126 mg/dL (7.0 mmol/L), a random plasma glucose level ≥200 mg/dL (11.1 mmol/L) and/or A1C ≥6.5% in the presence of the signs and/or symptoms of diabetes. If the signs and/or symptoms are absent, plasma glucose concentrations must be repeated on more than one occasion to diagnose diabetes. An oral glucose tolerance test (OGTT) is rarely needed, and its use is contraindicated (Table 1.1) in the face of dehydration and acidosis.

The clinical signs and/or symptoms that accompany diabetes are due to persistent hyperglycemia and include polyuria, polydipsia, fatigue, polyphagia, weight loss, and blurred vision. If there is ketosis or ketoacidosis, abdominal pain, vomiting, dehydration, and altered level of consciousness can occur. In the young child or infant, these signs or symptoms are frequently missed until the child presents

Table 1.1   Criteria for Diagnosis of Diabetes in Nonpregnant Adults

Diagnosis of diabetes in nonpregnant adults should be restricted to those who have one of the following:

- Symptoms of diabetes plus casual plasma glucose concentration greater than or equal to 200 mg/dL (11.1 mmol/L). The classic symptoms of diabetes include polyuria, polydipsia, and unexplained weight loss. Casual refers to any time of day without regard to time since last meal.

or

- Fasting plasma glucose greater than or equal to 126 mg/dL (7.0 mmol/L). Fasting is defined as no caloric intake for at least 8 h.

or

- 2-h plasma glucose greater than or equal to 200 mg/dL (11.1 mmol/L) during an oral glucose tolerance test (OGTT).* The test should be performed using a glucose load containing the equivalent of 75 g anhydrous glucose dissolved in water.

or

- A1C ≥6.5%

In the absence of unequivocal hyperglycemia with acute metabolic decompensation, these criteria should be confirmed by repeat testing on a different day.

*An OGTT is rarely needed to diagnose type 1 diabetes and is not recommended for routine clinical use.

as significantly ill due to ketoacidosis associated with dehydration, acidosis, and/or develops a severe candidal diaper rash.

An elevated glycated hemoglobin (A1C) confirms the presence of significant preexisting hyperglycemia (barring the presence of a hemoglobin variant). Pre-diabetes (previously known as impaired glucose tolerance or impaired fasting glucose) as distinguished from diabetes, refers to abnormal plasma glucose values that do not meet the established criteria to diagnose diabetes. Pre-diabetes may be seen in the development of type 1 diabetes as the result of the autoimmune destruction of the β-cell mass, but is rarely detected clinically outside of research protocols in which high-risk relatives undergo screening and close follow-up.

RISK OF DEVELOPING TYPE 1 DIABETES

Although type 1 diabetes is much less common in the general population than type 2 diabetes, type 1 diabetes is by no means rare among children and young adults. Data derived from the SEARCH study in the US showed that 0.78 per 1,000 children under the age of 10 have diabetes. Type 1 accounts for more than 80% of these cases. In youths 10–19 years of age, 2.80 per 1,000 have diabetes: 85.1% of white youths of this age-group have type 1, while the percentage is lower among other ethnic/racial groups—53.9% in Hispanic youth, 42.2% in non-Hispanic blacks, 30.3% in Asian/Pacific Islanders, and 13.8% in American Indian youth.

Type 1 diabetes has been increasing 3–4% per year in youths, and even more in young children under the age of 5 years. This makes diabetes one of the most common childhood diseases, with a much higher incidence rate than other chronic childhood diseases, such as cystic fibrosis, juvenile rheumatoid arthritis, nephrotic syndrome, muscular dystrophy, or leukemia. About 160,000 people under age 20, and 400,000 people over 20 years of age, have type 1 diabetes.

The annual incidence of type 1 diabetes decreases after age 20. In those over 20 years old, incidence is similar in men and women, and it is lower in African Americans, Hispanics, Asian Americans, and American Indians than in whites, as is found in the younger age range.

Type 1 diabetes has strong HLA (human leukocyte antigen) associations. There is linkage to the DQA and DQB genes, and diabetes risk is also influenced by the DR genes. HLA-DR/DQ alleles can either be predisposing or protective, and the general population and family members can be assessed for risk by genetic evaluation. Most whites with type 1 carry HLA-DR3 or HLA-DR4 alleles, in blacks it is HLA-DR7, and in Japanese it is HLA-DR9. The statistical risk of a family member developing type 1 diabetes is linked to the genetic similarities of the family members. For example, when one identical twin develops diabetes, the risk to the other twin is 25–50%. This is in contrast to a 0.4% risk in the general population, a 15% risk in HLA-identical siblings, and a 1% risk in HLA-nonidentical siblings. Without knowing HLA type, in general, the risk for type 1 diabetes in a first-degree family member is ~5%.

DISTINGUISHING TYPE 1 DIABETES FROM OTHER FORMS

Type 1 Diabetes

Type 1 diabetes can develop at any age. Although more cases are diagnosed before the patient is 20 years old, it also occurs in older individuals. Because patients with type 1 diabetes are insulinopenic, insulin therapy is essential to prevent rapid and severe dehydration, catabolism, ketoacidosis, and death (Table 1.2). Patients who are diagnosed with symptoms are usually lean and have experienced significant weight loss, polyuria, polydipsia, and fatigue before presentation. Some patients are diagnosed without any or with more subtle symptoms and they may be overweight, reflecting the secular trend of increasing obesity amongst adults and children. At presentation, there is often significant elevation of A1C levels, providing evidence of weeks, if not months, of hyperglycemia. In addition, 85–90% have circulating autoantibodies directed against one or more islet cell components (GADA, IA-2A, ZnT8A and IAA). C-peptide levels, which fall to undetectable levels over time, may be in the low normal range at diagnosis. Profound insulinopenia occurs even though the pancreas from patients with long standing type 1 diabetes shows that most retain some islet tissue (1–2%), while others have a pattern of lobular destruction with destroyed and normal-appearing islets.

Type 2 Diabetes

In contrast, patients with type 2 diabetes are less likely to develop ketoacidosis unless severely stressed physiologically, are generally but not always obese,

Table 1.2 Distinguishing Characteristics of the Major Types of Diabetes

Clinical Classes

Type 1 diabetes

β-Cell destruction, usually leading to absolute insulin deficiency

Type 2 diabetes

Ranging from predominantly insulin resistance with relative insulin deficiency to predominantly an insulin secretory defect with insulin resistance

Secondary and other types of diabetes

Gestational diabetes mellitus

Distinguishing Characteristics

Type 1 diabetes patients may be of any age, are occasionally but not usually obese, and often have abrupt onset of signs and symptoms with insulinopenia before age 20. They often present with ketosis in conjunction with hyperglycemia and are eventually dependent on insulin therapy to prevent ketoacidosis and to sustain life.

Type 2 diabetes patients usually are >30 years old at diagnosis, are obese, and have relatively few classic symptoms. They are not typically prone to ketoacidosis except during periods of stress. Although not dependent on exogenous insulin for survival, they may require it for adequate control of hyperglycemia.

Forms of diabetes not easily classified as type 1 or type 2, such as ketosis-prone diabetes in otherwise phenotypically type 2 individuals, or gradual-onset antibody-positive diabetes in adults, referred to as LADA, are increasingly being recognized.

Patients with secondary and other types of diabetes have certain associated conditions or syndromes (see Table 1.3).

Patients with gestational diabetes mellitus have onset or discovery of glucose intolerance during pregnancy.

may be asymptomatic or only mildly symptomatic, and usually have a family history of diabetes. Type 2 diabetes is said to generally present after age 30, but an increasing number of obese adolescents and young adults have been developing type 2 diabetes, especially among African Americans, American Indians/Native Alaskans, Hispanics, and Asian/Pacific Islanders. Note that some of these patients present in ketoacidosis, or with hyperosmolar nonketotic coma, both of which can be fatal. The discrimination between type 2 and type 1 diabetes is becoming increasingly difficult in many cases, as patients with a type 2 phenotype may present in ketoacidosis but later become insulin-independent. Conversely, more type 1 patients are overweight or obese at the time of presentation.

Patients with type 2 diabetes are not absolutely dependent on exogenous insulin for survival, although insulin therapy is often used to lower blood glucose levels, since there appears to be progressive β-cell failure in type 2 diabetes as well (Table 1.2).

Not Quite Type 1 or Type 2 Diabetes

Some patients are difficult to categorize as having type 1 or type 2 diabetes. The routinely available laboratory tests that help differentiate between the two types are serum C-peptide levels and measurements of autoantibodies to islet cell components; however, even these tests can be problematic. Although almost all patients with longstanding type 1 diabetes will have C-peptide values below the lower limit of normal for that assay method, with most being undetectable, at diagnosis, C-peptide may be in the normal range while there is still a viable β-cell mass. Approximately 15% of patients with clinical type 1 diabetes do not have autoantibodies at the time of diagnosis, and 10–15% of youth with clinical type 2 diabetes do have autoantibodies. Although not routinely used in the clinical arena, markers of insulin resistance, such as adiponectin—which is elevated in type 1 and decreased in type 2—and lipoprotein concentrations, may help differentiate between diabetes types.

With absent availability of measurement of autoantibodies or C-peptide, if a patient is <20 years old, not obese, and has signs and symptoms of diabetes and an elevated fasting plasma glucose, the physician should assume type 1 diabetes and treat with insulin. The presence of moderate ketonuria with hyperglycemia in an otherwise unstressed individual strongly supports a diagnosis of type 1 diabetes, whereas the absence or modest ketonuria is of no diagnostic value.

Clinicians should also be aware that in some cases, typically adults, patients presenting with type 2 diabetes subsequently may be discovered to have type 1 diabetes. In these individuals, autoantibodies to islet cell components may indicate the eventual need for insulin therapy. These patients are usually lean, and their insulin requirements increase as they develop manifestations of complete insulin deficiency. The condition is referred to as LADA and studies suggest that genes associated with type 1 and type 2 coexist in patients felt to have LADA.

In contrast, occasionally some adolescents and young adults who present with typical signs and symptoms of type 1 diabetes, particularly ketosis, later require no or only intermittent insulin treatment. This occurs mainly in African Americans. Table 1.3 illustrates specific conditions often associated with other forms of diabetes and glucose intolerance. Further studies are required to determine the pathophysiology of these conditions.

Genetic Defects Presenting with Childhood Onset

Several forms of diabetes are associated with monogenetic defects in β-cell function. These forms of diabetes are frequently characterized by onset of mild hyperglycemia at an early age, generally before age 25. They were formerly referred to as maturity-onset diabetes of the young (MODY), and they are characterized by impaired insulin secretion with minimal or no defects in insulin action. They are inherited in an autosomal-dominant pattern. Abnormalities at six genetic loci on different chromosomes have been identified to date resulting in mutations on:

- chromosome 12, HNF-1α (hepatic nuclear factor, MODY3)
- chromosome 7p, glucokinase (MODY2)

- chromosome 20q, HNF-4α gene (MODY1)
- chromosome 13, in the insulin promoter factor-1 gene (IPF-1, MODY4)
- chromosome 17, HNF-1β (MODY5)
- chromosome 2, NeuroD1 (MODY6)

Neonatal diabetes (NDM) is a monogenic form of diabetes that occurs in the first 6 months of life. Incident rates are 1 in 100,000–500,000 live births. Low birth weight and failure to thrive may be associated with NDM, and 50% of cases are the permanent form of NDM (PNDM). The others are transient but diabetes can recur later in life. The most common forms of PNDM are due to Kir6.2 (KCNJ11) and SUR1 (sulfonylurea receptor 1) defects (ABCC8), which can be treated with oral sulfonlyureas, as can MODY 1, 3, and 4.

Table 1.3 Other Specific Types of Diabetes

Genetic Defects of β-Cell Function

Examples: Kir6.2 (KCNJ11), SUR1 (ABCC8) (permanent neonatal diabetes, PNDM); chromosome 12, HNF-1α (hepatic nuclear factor, MODY3); chromosome 7p, glucokinase (MODY2); chromosome 20q, HNF-4α gene (MODY1); chromosome 13, in the insulin pro-motor factor-1 gene (IPF-1, MODY4); chromosome 17, HNF-1β (MODY5); chromosome 2, *Neuro*D1 (MODY6)

Genetic Defects in Insulin Action

Examples: type A insulin resistance, leprechaunism, Rabson-Mendenhall syndrome, lipoatrophic diabetes

Diseases of the Exocrine Pancreas

Examples: pancreatitis, trauma or pancreatectomy, neoplasia, cystic fibrosis, hemo-chromatosis, fibrocalculous pancreatopathy

Endocrinopathies

Examples: acromegaly, Cushing's syndrome, glucagonoma, pheochromocytoma, hyper-thyroidism, somatostatinoma, aldosteronoma

Drug- or Chemical-Induced Diabetes

Examples: Vacor, pentamidine, nicotinic acid, glucocorticoids, diazoxide, interferon-α, tacrolimus, second-generation antipsychotics

Infections

Examples: congenital rubella, cytomegalovirus

Uncommon Forms of Immune-Mediated Diabetes

Examples: "stiff man" syndrome, anti-insulin receptor antibodies

Genetic Syndromes Sometimes Associated with Diabetes

Examples: Down's syndrome, Klinefelter's syndrome, Turner's syndrome, Wolfram's syndrome, Friedreich's ataxia, Huntington's chorea, Lawrence-Moon-Bardet-Biedl syndrome, myotonic dystrophy, porphyria, Prader-Willi syndrome

Point mutations in mitochondrial DNA have been found to be associated with diabetes and deafness. In Wolfram Syndrome (referred to as DIDMOAD), diabetes and deafness are also associated with diabetes insipidus and optic atrophy. There also are unusual causes of diabetes that result from genetically determined abnormalities of insulin action. Leprechaunism and the Rabson-Mendenhall syndrome are two pediatric syndromes that have mutations in the insulin receptor gene with subsequent alterations in insulin receptor function and extreme insulin resistance. The former has characteristic facial features and is usually fatal in infancy, whereas the latter is associated with abnormalities of teeth and nails and pineal gland hyperplasia.

CLINICAL PRESENTATION OF TYPE 1 DIABETES

The presentation of type 1 diabetes covers a broad range, from mild nonspecific symptoms or no symptoms to coma. In children, establishing the correct diagnosis is often delayed because the presenting symptoms are ascribed to another process. For example, vomiting and lethargy may be felt to be due to gastroenteritis. Because adequate urine output continues as the result of osmotic diuresis, the child is not considered to be dehydrated and in need of medical care. Polyuria may be incorrectly attributed to urinary tract infection or enuresis; anorexia rather than polyphagia may occur; and fatigue, irritability, weight loss, deterioration of school performance, and secondary enuresis are ascribed to emotional problems. In some cases, "failure to thrive" may be an overlooked indication of diabetes in a young child.

Approximately 75% of cases are diagnosed within 1 month of the onset of symptoms; 25% of patients with previously undiagnosed type 1 diabetes present in diabetic ketoacidosis (DKA). Delayed diagnosis continues to be a serious and occasionally fatal problem, especially among poor and younger children. DKA rates approach 40% in children under 3 years of age and 60% in children under 2 years at diagnosis. The symptoms of polyuria are less obvious in the young child and are frequently missed until metabolic decompensation has occurred. These very young children frequently present with severe dehydration, metabolic acidosis, and a clinical history that is inconsistent with the severity of their clinical appearance (e.g., absence of diarrhea or significant vomiting). Because of the delay in the diagnosis of the younger child, the frequency of coma as a presenting feature is considerably greater in children <2 years of age than in older children, adolescents, and adults. In young adults, the presentation is often less acute, although an absolute requirement for insulin becomes evident with time.

CONCLUSION

Patients with type 1 diabetes are dependent on insulin for as long as they live. Any lean individual <20 years of age with typical signs and symptoms of hyperglycemia accompanied by weight loss should be assumed to have type 1 diabetes. A high index of suspicion is needed to diagnose diabetes in very young children or elderly patients.

BIBLIOGRAPHY

American Diabetes Association: Care of children and adolescents with type 1 diabetes mellitus (Position Statement). *Diabetes Care* 28: 186–212, 2005

The DIAMOND Project Group: Incidence and trends of childhood type 1 diabetes worldwide 1990–1999. *Diabet Med* 23:857–866, 2006

Expert Committee on the Diagnosis and Classification of Diabetes Mellitus: Report of the Expert Committee on the Diagnosis and Classification of Diabetes Mellitus. *Diabetes Care* 26 (Suppl. 1):S5–S20, 2003

Lindstrom T, Frystykt J, Hedman CA, Flyvbjerg A, Arnqvist HJ: Elevated circulating adiponectin in type 1 diabetes is associated with long diabetes duration. *Clin Endocrinol* 65:776–782, 2006

Michels AW, et al.: Immune intervention in type 1 diabetes. *Seminars in Immunology* 23:214–219, 2011

The National Diabetes Information Clearinghouse: Monogenic Forms of Diabetes: Neonatal Diabetes Mellitus and Maturity-onset Diabetes of the Young. www.diabetes.niddk.nih.gov/dm/pubs/mody

Rewers A, et al.: Presence of diabetic ketoacidosis at diagnosis of diabetes mellitus in youth: the SEARCH for Diabetes in Youth Study, *Pediatrics* 2007–1105

Rosenbloom AL, Silverstein JK: *Type 2 Diabetes in Children and Adolescents.* Alexandria, VA, American Diabetes Association, 2003

SEARCH for Diabetes in Youth Study Group: The burden of diabetes mellitus among U.S. youth: prevalence estimates from the SEARCH for Diabetes in Youth Study. *Pediatrics* 118:1510–1518, 2006

Vaziri-Sani F.: A novel triple mix radiobinding assay for the three ZnT8 (ZnT8-RWQ) autoantibody variants in children with newly diagnosed diabetes. *J Immun Methods* 371:25–37, 2011

PATHOGENESIS

The primary defect in type 1 diabetes is decreased insulin secretion by pancreatic β-cells. This single defect accounts for the hyperglycemia, polyuria, polydipsia, weight loss, dehydration, electrolyte disturbance, and ketoacidosis observed in patients presenting for the first time with type 1 diabetes. The capacity of normal pancreatic β-cells to secrete insulin is far in excess of that normally needed to control carbohydrate, fat, and protein metabolism. As a result, clinical onset is preceded by an extensive asymptomatic period during which β-cells are inexorably destroyed. The evolving process of β-cell destruction reaches a point where insufficient insulin is secreted to maintain normal plasma glucose concentrations, which causes the broadly predictable abnormalities in carbohydrate, fat, and protein metabolism characterizing the uncontrolled diabetic condition.

Most patients with type 1 diabetes have immune-mediated diabetes. This form of diabetes results from a cellular-mediated autoimmune destruction of the β-cells of the pancreas. Most of the discussion in this section deals with this form of type 1 diabetes—immune-mediated diabetes. However, some forms of type 1 diabetes have no evidence of autoimmunity or other known etiology and are labeled "idiopathic." Some of these patients have permanent insulinopenia and are prone to ketoacidosis. Although only a minority of patients with type 1 diabetes fall into the idiopathic category, of those who do, most are of African or Asian origin. Individuals with this form of diabetes often suffer from episodic ketoacidosis and exhibit varying degrees of insulin deficiency between episodes. This form of diabetes is strongly inherited, lacks immunological evidence for β-cell autoimmunity, and is not HLA associated. A requirement for insulin replacement therapy in affected patients may come and go.

PATHOPHYSIOLOGY OF THE CLINICAL ONSET OF TYPE 1 DIABETES

Insulin is the primary hormone that suppresses hepatic glucose production, lipolysis, and proteolysis. It increases the transport of glucose into adipocytes and myocytes and stimulates glycogen synthesis. In the presence of adequate plasma amino acids, insulin maintains or perhaps stimulates whole-body protein anabolism. As such, insulin is the primary hormone of anabolism of meal-derived nutrients (Table 1.4).

In the postabsorptive state, the plasma concentration of glucose is maintained in a narrow range (80–95 mg/dL [4.4–5.3 mmol/L]) by precise regulation of hepatic glucose release and peripheral glucose utilization.

Basal plasma insulin concentrations maintain hepatic glucose release at a rate of 1.9–2.1 mg/kg/min (10–12 μmol/l/kg/min). This is of critical importance to provide adequate glucose for the brain, which accounts for nearly 50% of total glucose utilization under these conditions. With prolonged fasting, the plasma insulin concentration decreases even further, permitting increased mobilization of free fatty acids (FFAs). The resulting increase in circulating FFA concentration drives hepatic ketogenesis, which results in ketosis. Increased availability of plasma FFAs, β-hydroxybutyrate, and acetoacetate provides alternative metabolic

Table 1.4 Physiological Effects of High- Versus Low-Insulin States

	High-Insulin (Fed) State	Low-Insulin (Fasted) State
Liver	Glucose uptake	Glucose production
	Glycogen synthesis	Glycogenolysis
	Lipogenesis	Absent lipogenesis
	Absent ketogenesis	Ketogenesis
	Absent gluconeogenesis	Gluconeogenesis
Muscle	Glucose uptake	Absent glucose uptake
	Glucose oxidation	Fatty acid, ketone oxidation
	Glycogen synthesis	Glycogenolysis
	Sustained protein synthesis	Proteolysis and amino acid release
Adipose tissue	Glucose uptake	Absent glucose uptake
	Lipid synthesis	Lipolysis and fatty acid release
	Triglyceride uptake	Absent triglyceride uptake

fuels to glucose and reduces the rates of glucose utilization by peripheral tissues and brain.

After ingestion of a mixed meal, nearly 85% of ingested glucose enters the systemic circulation. The increasing arterial glucose concentration stimulates the secretion of insulin into the portal vein. About half of the secreted insulin is extracted by the liver, which signals the suppression of hepatic glucose release. The unextracted insulin enters the systemic circulation, where it stimulates glucose uptake, primarily by muscle, and decreases lipolysis and proteolysis. This facilitates a continuous entry of glucose into the systemic circulation by permitting a switch from endogenous glucose production to exogenous glucose. As dietary glucose entry decreases with the absorption of the meal-derived carbohydrate, plasma glucose decreases, as does the secretion and plasma concentration of insulin. When plasma glucose reaches or even falls slightly below basal concentrations, hepatic glucose production is again increased by both the decrease in plasma insulin and an increase in plasma glucagon concentration (Table 1.4).

Amylin, a glucoregulatory hormone, is produced in the pancreatic β-cell and co-secreted with insulin. Amylin regulates postprandial glucose concentrations by slowing gastric emptying, suppressing postprandial glucagon secretion, and reducing food intake. Amylin complements the effects of insulin, and both act together to regulate postmeal glucose concentrations. Type 1 diabetes is an amylin-deficient state.

PROGRESSION OF METABOLIC ABNORMALITIES DURING ONSET

The insulin secretory reserves of the normal pancreas are considerable. Therefore, individuals destined to develop type 1 diabetes go through a variable interval of months to years of autoimmune β-cell destruction before abnormalities in insulin secretion or glucose metabolism can be detected (Fig. 1.1). During this time period, amylin secretion is also diminished and then lost.

The earliest detectable abnormality in insulin secretion is a progressive reduction of the immediate (first-phase) plasma insulin response during intravenous

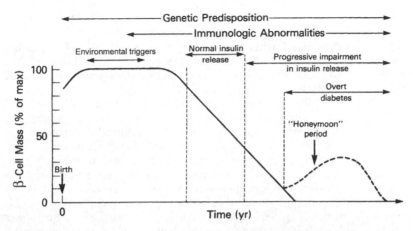

Figure 1.1 Proposed scheme of natural history of type 1 diabetes. Timing of trigger in relation to immunologic abnormalities is unknown. Note that overt diabetes is not apparent until insulin secretory reserves are <10–20% of normal.

glucose tolerance testing. This impairment alone has little deleterious effect on overall glucose homeostasis: fasting plasma glucose concentrations remain normal, and the response to an OGTT is virtually unimpaired. At this stage of the disease, most affected individuals have circulating autoantibodies to islet cell components, islet cell antibodies (ICAs), including antibodies to their own insulin (IAA) and to other islet cell antigens (e.g., glutamic acid decarboxylase [GADA], islet tyrosine phosphatases [IA-2A], and zinc transporter 8 [ZnT8A]). These are markers of an ongoing autoimmune process that eventuates in type 1 diabetes. There is variability to the autoantibody pattern, in the years prior to diagnosis, IA-2A titers increase, but then decrease after diagnosis, while GADA titers persist. Insulin autoantibodies, IAA, are more prevalent in young children. The presence and then persistence of two or more autoantibodies is highly predictive and has replaced assessment of first-phase insulin secretion to determine risk of developing type 1 diabetes (Fig. 1.1). Greater than 70% of those who have 2 or more autoantibodies will develop diabetes over a 7 year observation period.

CLINICAL ONSET OF DIABETIC SYMPTOMS AND METABOLIC DECOMPENSATION

When ongoing destruction has reduced β-cell mass by 80–90%, the individual's insulin secretory capacity becomes insufficient to normally regulate hepatic glucose production (Fig. 1.1). Initially, only postprandial hyperglycemia occurs, reflecting a failure to adequately suppress hepatic glucose production during meal absorption together with some decrease in peripheral glucose utilization. This may also be exacerbated by amylin deficiency. As insulin secretion is further compromised, progressive fasting hyperglycemia occurs as a result of increased basal hepatic glucose production and decreased glucose uptake by peripheral tissue.

Hyperglycemia per se may further compromise glucose utilization by reducing the number and/or activity of glucose transporters available on both insulin-dependent and non-insulin-dependent tissues, a phenomenon known as "glucose toxicity."

When the plasma glucose concentration exceeds the renal threshold of ~180 mg/dL (10.0 mmol/L), glucosuria results in an osmotic diuresis, generating the classic symptoms of polyuria and a compensatory polydipsia. If untreated, the symptoms usually progress as the hyperglycemia and glucosuria increase. With evolving insulin deficiency, weight loss occurs as body fat and protein stores are reduced because of increased rates of lipolysis and proteolysis, and calories are lost in the urine. With the superimposed metabolic abnormalities of diabetes itself or with a minor viral or bacterial infection, plasma concentrations of glucagon, growth hormone, epinephrine, and cortisol increase. These hormones antagonize insulin's effect, further promoting hepatic glucose production (by stimulating both glycogenolysis and gluconeogenesis), lipolysis, ketogenesis, and proteolysis. As long as fluid intake is sufficient to offset the fluid losses resulting from the combined diuresis of both glucosuria and ketonuria, some individuals can remain compensated for weeks, if not months. Should the individual be unable to consume adequate amounts of fluid as a result of nausea from the ketosis or because of an intercurrent illness, rapid and severe losses of both intra- and extracellular fluid and electrolytes can ensue and, in the course of hours, lead to a clinical presentation of severe ketoacidosis.

Remission or Honeymoon Phase

At initial presentation with symptomatic hyperglycemia and/or ketosis, circulating insulin concentrations are low, and there is no significant β-cell response to any of the usual insulin secretagogues. Initially, exogenous insulin requirements are relatively large, due not only to the reduced insulin secretion but also to insulin resistance and counterregulatory hormone elevation.

After the correction of the hyperglycemia, metabolic acidosis, and ketosis, endogenous insulin secretion improves from the residual, albeit small, β-cell population (Fig. 1.1). During this time, exogenous insulin requirements may decrease dramatically. During the remission or honeymoon period, which may last for up to 1 year or longer, good metabolic control may be easily achieved with either conventional or intensive insulin therapy. The need for increasing exogenous insulin replacement is inevitable and should always be anticipated. Evidence from the Diabetes Control and Complications Trial follow-up cohort suggests that intensive insulin therapy from early diagnosis prolongs C-peptide secretion and thus creates less major hypoglycemia and less microvascular complications 10 years after diagnosis. As a result, intensive insulin therapy with strict attention to diet and self-monitoring of blood glucose should be initiated at diagnosis and maintained. Having DKA at presentation of diabetes adversely affects the remission phase duration.

Finally, within 5 years for children and 10 years after clinical presentation regardless of age at presentation, β-cell destruction is essentially complete. At this point, insulin deficiency is usually absolute.

Attempts to Preserve the β-Cell Mass

A number of therapies have been and are being tested to prevent the total destruction of the β-cell mass, both prior to and after the diagnosis of type 1 diabetes. The outcome measure is the C-peptide response to a standardized mixed meal tolerance test. These trials can be divided into those that are immune suppressive, those that are attempting immunoregulation, and those involving intense metabolic control. Early therapeutic attempts centered mainly on general immune suppression. Although effective in small pilot studies in prolonging the honeymoon period or delaying the onset of overt type 1 diabetes, none resulted in permanent remission. Two large, multicenter intervention trials involving either low-dose parenteral insulin therapy (Diabetes Prevention Trial 1 [DPT-1]) or nicotinamide (ENDIT Trial) as immunoregulatory agents in the pre–type 1 diabetes state showed no benefit in delaying or preventing the onset of type 1 diabetes. A second arm of the DPT-1 using oral insulin in those deemed to be of moderate risk (25–50% risk) of developing diabetes showed that a subset of subjects with insulin autoantibodies had a several-year delay in progression to diabetes, and this is being evaluated now in the multinational TrialNet consortia that was developed after DPT-1. Other prevention studies have looked at environmental therapies such as using supplemental vitamin D, omega fatty acids, or altering complex dietary protein exposure using hydrolyzed formula compared to cow's milk.

TrialNet has completed studies on a number of agents at the diagnosis of type 1 diabetes, including mycophenalate mofetil (an inhibitor of purine synthesis) plus daclizumab (anti-CD25), which showed no benefit, and rituximab (an anti–β-cell antibody), and abatacept (CTLA-4 Ig, T-cell costimulation modulation), which both showed an attenuation in loss of C-peptide over the first year of disease due to an initial response followed by a decline in c-peptide that mirrored the control group. Studies of anti-CD3 monoclonal antibodies at onset of type 1 have found some preservation of C-peptide for at least 1 year, but may be associated with acute cytokine release and transient activation of Epstein-Barr virus infection. Ongoing larger studies are still underway to determine the duration of therapeutic effect and safety. Additional interventions being evaluated include GAD-Alum, anti-thymocyte globulin, BCG, insulin peptide B:9-23, heat shock protein DiaPep277, α-1 antitrypsin, closed-loop insulin delivery, and others.

These intervention trials offer an opportunity to preserve a significant mass of β-cells and potentially prevent or delay overt diabetes and modify its course. Potential therapeutic modalities must be approached with caution and should be utilized only in conjunction with carefully defined scientific studies. Individuals at risk for diabetes because of family history and those newly diagnosed should be informed about available clinical trials designed to attempt to interdict the type 1 process.

GENETICS AND IMMUNOLOGY OF TYPE 1 DIABETES

Type 1 diabetes is a genetically influenced and immunologically mediated disease with a prolonged asymptomatic phase (pre–type 1 diabetes), which

Table 1.5 Approximate Familial Risk of Type 1 Diabetes

Relationship to Proband	Risk (%)
Sibling	5–10
Identical twin	25–50
HLA	
Identical	15
Haploidentical	6
Nonidentical	1
Father	6
Mother	3
Offspring of father	12
Offspring of mother	6
General population	0.3–0.4

Modified from Muir A, Schatz DA, Maclaren NK: The pathogenesis, prediction, and prevention of insulin-dependent diabetes mellitus. *Endocrin Metab Clin North Am* 21:199–219, 1992.

eventually results in progressive β-cell destruction, insulin deficiency, and overt clinical symptoms. The identity of the initiating event(s) remains speculative. Viruses, food antigens, and intestinal microbes have been proposed as environmental triggers of β-cell autoimmunity.

The familial predisposition to type 1 diabetes has long been known. A specific mode of genetic transmission has not been established. Predisposition to type 1 diabetes is inherited as a heterogeneous multigenic trait with low penetrance and gender biases. There is a higher concordance rate for type 1 diabetes in monozygotic twins (25–50%) than in dizygotic twins (6%). The empirical risk of type 1 diabetes is increased in first-degree relatives of probands with the disease (Table 1.5). There is an even greater risk for offspring of fathers with diabetes who were diagnosed at a young age; however, the age of onset of diabetes in the mother does not seem to affect the risk for her children.

About 40–50% of the genetic predisposition to type 1 diabetes is conferred by genes on the short arm of chromosome 6, either within or in close proximity to the Class II HLA region of the major histocompatibility complex (MHC). At least 11 other loci have been suggested to be involved, with the largest contribution (about 10% of the genetic predisposition) being accounted for by the flanking region of the insulin gene on chromosome 11, INS-VNTR. Shorter forms of a variable number tandem repeated in the insulin promoter are associated with susceptibility, while longer forms are associated with protection. Other genes associated with T-cell activation and regulation have been identified; cytotoxic T lymphocyte antigen-4 (CTLA-4) and protein tyrosine phosphatase N22 (PTPN22) and multiple genes in the interleukin (IL-2) and IL-2 receptor (IL-2R) pathways. HLA, CTLA-4, and PTPN22 are associated with other autoimmune diseases.

The Class II MHC DR and DQ molecules are comprised of an α- and a β-chain, which present processed antigens to T-cells. The relationship between type 1 diabetes and specific MHC Class II region alleles is complex. There is a strong positive relationship with HLA-DR3 and -DR4 and a strong negative

Figure 1.2 Development of auto-islet autoantibodies among DR3/4-DQ8 siblings of patients with type 1 diabetes in the DAISY (Diabetes Autoimmunity Study in the Young) study with extreme risk for those sharing two HLA major histocompatibility complex (MHC) haplotypes with sibling proband. Figure was adapted from Aly T et al.: Extreme genetic risk for type 1A diabetes. *PNAS* 103:14074–14079, 2006.

relationship with -DR2. Indeed, more than 90% of whites with type 1 diabetes are HLA-DR3 and/or -DR4, while 30% of children who develop type 1 are heterozygote DR3/DR4. Within families, the risk for diabetes is highest for those who are DR3/DR4 heterozygotes and who have inherited identical HLA haplotypes as their sibling with diabetes (Fig. 1.2). There is an even stronger relationship of type 1 diabetes when DQ loci (DQα and DQβ) are considered together with DR loci, i.e., the predisposition to type 1 diabetes in whites is associated with HLA-DR3, DQB1*0201, and with HLA-DR4, DQB1*0302, with the strongest association being the DQα-DQβ combination DQA1*0501-DQB1*0302. Other DQ alleles appear to confer protection from type 1 diabetes, e.g., DQA1*0201-DQB1*0602 provides protection even in the presence of DQ susceptibility alleles. This suggests that protection is dominant over susceptibility. Because Class II MHC genes regulate the immune response, the susceptibility and protective alleles could be involved differentially in antigen presentation of peptides that establish and maintain tolerance or influence the immune response.

Autoantibodies and Autoantigens

The identification of circulating autoantibodies to islet cell components in those who have developed diabetes and subsequently in nondiabetic first-degree relatives has made it possible to detect the preclinical disease. Numerous circulating autoantibodies have been identified, including cytoplasmic ICAs detected by immunofluorescence, insulin autoantibodies (IAAs), auto-antibodies directed against the enzyme GAD (GADA), autoantibodies against islet tyrosine phosphatase (IA-2A and IA2β), zinc transporter 8 A (ZnT8A) and several others. Most (>90%) newly diagnosed patients with type 1 diabetes have one or another of these circulating antibodies as do 3.5–4% of unaffected first-degree relatives. This latter group of antibody-positive individuals is at increased risk for developing type 1 diabetes. The presence of two or more antibodies is highly predictive of increased risk of type 1 diabetes within 5 years.

These autoantibodies generally are not thought to mediate β-cell destruction by humoral mechanisms. Rather, it is likely that as β-cells are destroyed, multiple antigens are exposed to the immune system, with generation of antibodies directed against these components. Thus, these autoantibodies are markers of immune activity or of β-cell damage and herald the disease process several years before overt clinical hyperglycemia. As β-cell function is lost and "total" diabetes evolves, ZnT8A, and IA-2 autoantibodies tend to decrease in titer and/or disappear, while GADA tends to persist.

Many patients with type 1 diabetes have nonpancreatic organ-specific autoantibodies (e.g., toward thyroid, gastric parietal cells, and, less often, adrenal cells). Hashimoto's thyroiditis is the most common autoimmune disorder associated with type 1 diabetes. Celiac disease is also relatively common and associated with expression of autoantibodies to endomysium and tissue transglutaminase. The range of organ involvement with autoimmune disorders varies from none to severe polyglandular failure.

Screening and Intervention Trials

Humoral autoantibodies allow for the identification of individuals who are at high risk for developing type 1 diabetes, such as those with prior transient hyperglycemia, and they play a role in experimental therapeutic trials directed at the preservation of islet cell function. Screening for immunologic markers of type 1 diabetes in any population outside the context of defined research studies is discouraged. Screening of high-risk individuals (e.g., first-degree relatives of someone with type 1 diabetes) should be encouraged, provided that individuals who screen positive are referred to centers participating in cooperative intervention studies or other scientific investigations using appropriate techniques. All subjects who are screened but do not enter a study should be counseled about their risk of developing diabetes, and follow-up should be offered.

Cell-Mediated Immunologic Dysfunction

The existence of insulitis (lymphocytic infiltration of the pancreas by mononuclear cells) has been known for decades and was the earliest evidence for the autoimmune nature of type 1 diabetes. There is evidence of a role for both T- and β-cells as well as lymphokines in the pathophysiology of the β-cell destruction in both human and animal models. However, type 1 diabetes in most animal models is considered a cell-mediated disease because adoptive transfer occurs with T-cells but not with autoantibody transfer. Although therapies directed against T-cells might be more successful, strategies to deplete β-cells and/or autoantibodies might have a role in preventing diabetes.

Environmental Triggers

The concordance rate of diabetes of identical twins suggests that environmental factors may be important in the pathogenesis of type 1 diabetes. Viral infections, e.g., enteroviruses such as Coxsackie B4, rotavirus, and congenital rubella, have been inconsistently implicated as triggers for the immunologic process. The gut microflora play a pathophysiological role through a variety of potential mechanisms including a chronic low-grade inflammation and altered intestinal barrier function. Exposure to substances toxic to the β-cells accounts for only a very small number of cases. Prolonged breast-feeding is reported to lower the incidence rates for type 1 diabetes. Highly hydrolyzed milk formula may decrease β-cell autoimmunity to an even greater extent than cow's milk due to the adverse effect of early exposure to complex dietary proteins. Early gluten exposure has been implicated since a gluten-free diet dramatically decreases type 1 diabetes in animal models. Little direct evidence exists to link any specific factor(s) to triggering autoimmune destruction of the β-cells in type 1 diabetes in humans.

CONCLUSION

Individuals who are genetically or otherwise predisposed to develop type 1 diabetes eventually demonstrate near total failure of insulin secretion as the result of an immunologically mediated progressive destruction of β-cell mass. The emergence of insulinopenia is associated with several intracellular abnormalities in both liver and muscle tissue, leading to excessive hepatic glucose production, decreased muscle glucose uptake, frank glucose intolerance, and, if untreated, ketoacidosis. Because insulin deficiency is primary, patients are dependent on exogenous insulin for life.

BIBLIOGRAPHY

Aly et al.: Extreme genetic risk for type 1A diabetes. *Proc Natl Acad Sci U S A* 103:14074–14079, 2006

American Diabetes Association: Prevention of type 1 diabetes mellitus (Position Statement). *Diabetes Care* 26 (Suppl. 1):S140, 2003

American Diabetes Association: Report of the Expert Committee on the Diagnosis and Classification of Diabetes Mellitus. *Diabetes Care* 26 (Suppl. 1):S5–S20, 2003

Atkinson MA, Maclaren NK: The pathogenesis of insulin-dependent diabetes mellitus. *N Engl J Med* 331:1428–1436, 1994

Bach JF: Insulin-dependent diabetes mellitus as an autoimmune disease. *Endocr Rev* 15:516–542, 1994

Eisenbarth G: Update in type 1 diabetes. *JCEM* 92:2403–2407, 2007

Genuth SM: Diabetic ketoacidosis and hyperglycemic hyperosmolar coma. *Curr Ther Endocrinol Metab* 6:438–447, 1997

Harjutsalo V, Reunanen A, Tuomilehto J: Differential transmission of type 1 diabetes from diabetic fathers and mothers to their offspring. *Diabetes* 55:1517–1524, 2006

Knip M et al.: Dietary intervention in infancy and later signs of beta-cell autoimmunity. *N Engl J Med* 363:1900–1908, 2010

Long SA.: Defects in Il-2R signaling contribute to diminished maintenance of FOXP3 expression in CD4(+) CD25(+) regulatory T-cells of type 1 diabetic subjects. *Diabetes* 59:407–415, 2010

Nepom GT: Immunogenetics and IDDM. *Diabetes Reviews* 1:93–103, 1993

Palmer JP: Predicting IDDM: use of humoral markers: autoantigens of IDDM. *Diabetes Reviews* 1:104–116, 1993

Rabinovitch A: Immunoregulatory and cytokine imbalances in the pathogenesis of IDDM: therapeutic intervention by immunostimulation? *Diabetes* 43:613–621, 1994

Rossini AA, Greiner DL, Friedman HP, Mordes JP: Immunopathogenesis of diabetes mellitus. *Diabetes Reviews* 1:43–75, 1993

Schatz DA, et al.: Type 1 Diabetes, *Endocrinol Metab Clin N Am* 39:527–539, 2010

Skyler JS, Marks JB: Immune intervention in type I diabetes mellitus. *Diabetes Reviews* 1:15–42, 1993

Sosenko JM et al.: A Longitudinal study of GAD65 and ICA512 autoantibodies during the progression to type 1 diabetes in Diabetes Prevention Trial–Type 1 (DPT-1) participants. *Diabetes Care* Oct 12, 2011 online version

Thai AC, Eisenbarth GS: Natural history of IDDM: autoantigens of IDDM. *Diabetes Reviews* 1:1–14, 1993

Type 1 Diabetes Study Group: Effects of insulin in relatives of patients with type 1 diabetes. *N Engl J Med* 346:1685–1691, 2002

Writing Team for the Diabetes Control and Complications Trial/Epidemiology of Diabetes Interventions and Complications Research Group: Effect of intensive therapy on the microvascular complications of type 1 diabetes mellitus. *JAMA* 287:2563–2569, 2002

Diabetes Standards and Education

Highlights

Philosophy and Goals

Patient Self-Management Education

Highlights
Diabetes Standards
and Education

PHILOSOPHY AND GOALS

■ The main influencers of what treatment regimen a patient will adopt and likelihood of achieving treatment goals are
- the diabetes management team's ability to assess the optimal, individualized regimen for patient/family
- the patient's self-care attitudes and abilities
- diabetes team-patient/family alignment of goals and ability to work collaboratively

■ The primary goals of treatment are to
- achieve optimal glycemic goals with a flexible, individualized diabetes management plan
- avoid severe hypoglycemia, symptomatic hyperglycemia, and ketoacidosis
- avoid long term microcirculatory and macrovascular complications
- promote and maintain day-to-day clinical and psychological well-being
- promote normal growth and development in children

■ Results from the Diabetes Control and Complications Trial (DCCT) demonstrated a link between poor glycemic control and development of diabetic complications. The Epidemiology of Diabetes Interventions and Complications (EDIC) Trial confirmed the importance of the establishment of optimal glycemic control as early as possible.

■ The physician and patient must set treatment goals together with the diabetes management team and family. Glycemic goals should be set as close to optimal as possible given the patient's abilities and presence of risk factors.

■ Initial and long-term clinical goals are presented in Clinical Goals. They focus on
- metabolic stabilization
- restoration and maintenance of desirable body weight
- elimination of hyperglycemic symptoms and minimization of severe hypoglycemia

PATIENT SELF-MANAGEMENT EDUCATION

■ The goal of diabetes self-management education is to provide patients with the knowledge, skills, and motivation to incorporate diabetes self-management in their daily lives and to engage in active collaboration with the health care team. The process includes:

- teaching of information needed for diabetes self-management
- training in skills needed for treatment procedures
- guidance and empowerment of the patient, incorporating his or her experiences and preferences, in devising methods to fit the treatment regimen into the individual's lifestyle
- counseling on reconciling diabetes care and the individual's view of quality of life through the identification of strategies needed for behavior change

■ Diabetes self-management education is a planned process that includes

- assessment to identify the patient's individual education needs
- planning specific education strategies
- implementation and documentation of education
- evaluation of learning
- reassessment(s) for new needs over time and across the life span

To be effective, diabetes self-management patient education must be individualized, should be provided in the context of a team approach to diabetes care, and needs to continue across the life span of the individual with diabetes. When indicated, family members and caregivers will be included.

■ Newly diagnosed patients with type 1 diabetes need to learn the basic skills that will enable them to implement their treatment regimen at home. Initial education should focus on teaching survival skills, with more in-depth information and additional topics added after the patient has had time to adjust to diabetes self-care. Written patient guidelines for detecting and treating hypoglycemia and for managing mild illnesses reinforce self-management skills that are not routinely needed and should be part of survival skills education.

■ Patient education is essential for management of type 1 diabetes. Therefore, physicians who treat type 1 diabetes patients need to provide diabetes self-management training opportunities for these patients. Physicians can incorporate diabetes patient education in their clinical practice by

- hiring diabetes educators
- developing a team relationship with diabetes educators working in the community
- referring patients to diabetes education programs recognized by the American Diabetes Association as meeting the National Standards for Diabetes Self-Management Education
- becoming knowledgeable about other diabetes education resources in their communities

Diabetes Standards and Education

PHILOSOPHY AND GOALS

Type 1 diabetes is a chronic disease in which the goal of treatment has been well defined—to achieve the best glycemic control that is possible with the least associated risk of hypoglycemia. The diabetes management team must work with the patient to determine which treatment strategies will best achieve the desired outcomes. The diabetes management team comprises a consortium that includes the endocrinologist or diabetes specialist, nurse, dietitian, social worker, mental health professional, pharmacist, and other health care specialists. The diabetes management team interfaces with the primary care provider, who helps coordinate care and establishes the patient's medical home. Three factors that strongly influence treatment are

- the diabetes management team's ability to assess the optimal, individualized regimen for patient/family
- the patient/family's self-care attitudes and abilities
- diabetes team-patient/family alignment of goals and ability to work collaboratively

The primary goals of treatment are *1*) to promote and maintain day-to-day clinical and psychological well-being; *2*) to avoid severe hypoglycemia, symptomatic hyperglycemia, and ketoacidosis; *3*) to avoid long-term microcirculatory and macrovascular complications, and *4*) to promote normal growth and development in children. The secondary goal of treatment is patient empowerment and the successful facilitation of the necessary behavior change to achieve the best possible glycemic control to prevent, delay, or arrest long-term diabetes complications while minimizing hypoglycemia and excess weight gain or disordered eating. The primary goals are clearly achievable at variable degrees of cost, inconvenience, and risk; the secondary goal, although more difficult, should be attainable by most patients.

GLYCEMIC CONTROL AND COMPLICATIONS: A SUMMARY OF EVIDENCE

Evidence relating hyperglycemia and/or other metabolic consequences of insulin deficiency to the development of vascular complications comes from animal studies, older epidemiologic studies of European and North American patients with type 1 diabetes, and from more recent controlled clinical trials from Scandinavia and North America.

Animal Studies

Strong experimental support for an association between metabolic abnormalities and vascular complications is found in animal studies. Animals that are rendered insulin deficient and hyperglycemic develop pathologic changes resembling early human retinopathy, nephropathy, and neuropathy. These changes can be prevented or ameliorated and, in some instances, reversed by early intensive insulin treatment, by curing diabetes via pancreas or islet transplantation, or by transplanting the affected organ into a nondiabetic animal.

Other Causes of Diabetes

Microvascular disease also develops in some patients with diabetes resulting from removal or destruction of the islets caused by pancreatectomy, chronic pancreatitis, or toxicity (e.g., from the rodenticide Vacor). These observations further support the theory that loss of insulin secretion or some consequent metabolic derangement is responsible for microvascular abnormalities in patients with immune-mediated type 1 diabetes. Genetic predisposition may influence the development of microvascular, neuropathic, and other complications; however, hyperglycemia is a prerequisite to development of these complications.

Kidney Transplantation Observations

Normal kidneys transplanted into recipients with type 1 diabetes begin to show pathologic changes resembling diabetic nephropathy after several years. Normal kidneys transplanted into patients with successful whole-pancreas transplantation have less glomerulopathy than kidneys transplanted into patients treated with conventional therapy. These observations point to a causative role for the diabetic metabolic milieu.

DYSGLYCEMIA AND COMPLICATIONS FROM POPULATION-BASED DATA

In data from 1,066 individuals aged >40 years from the 2005–2006 National Health and Nutrition Examination Survey, the relationship between fasting plasma glucose (FPG), A1C, and retinopathy have shown that retinal lesions do not develop before there is an elevation of measures of glycemia. This data on a specific and early clinical complication of diabetes points to the causative role of even minimal hyperglycemia.

Epidemiologic Studies

Several epidemiologic studies in patients with type 1 diabetes suggest that the higher the glucose level, the greater the incidence of microvascular disease.

Prospective Clinical Trials

The Diabetes Control and Complications Trial (DCCT) examined whether intensive treatment with the goal of maintaining glucose concentrations close to the normal range could decrease the frequency and severity of diabetes complications. Investigators studied 1,441 patients with type 1 diabetes—726 with no retinopathy and 715 with mild retinopathy at baseline. Patients were randomly assigned to intensive therapy administered with insulin pumps or multiple injections of insulin guided by blood glucose monitoring or to conventional therapy with one or two insulin injections per day. The patients were followed a mean of 6.5 years. Results showed that in the primary intervention cohort, intensive therapy reduced the mean risk of developing retinopathy by 76%. In the secondary intervention group, intensive therapy slowed the progression of retinopathy by 54% and reduced the development of proliferative retinopathy by 47%. In both groups combined, intensive therapy reduced the occurrence of microalbuminuria (>40 mg/24 h) by 39% and albuminuria (>300 mg/24 h) by 54%. Clinical neuropathy was reduced by 60%. The most important adverse effect was a threefold increase in severe hypoglycemia. Comparable results were seen in the Stockholm Diabetes Intervention Study after 5 and 8 years.

After completion of the DCCT, most of the participants were enrolled in a long-term observational study titled the Epidemiology of Diabetes Interventions and Complications (EDIC) study. The difference in the median A1C values between the conventional therapy and intensive therapy groups during the 6.5 years of the DCCT (average of 9.1% and 7.2%, respectively) narrowed during follow-up (median at 4 years of 8.2% and 7.9%, respectively). Despite this small difference in glycemic control between the two groups at 4 years of follow-up, the reduction in the risk of progressive retinopathy and nephropathy that resulted from intensive therapy persisted in EDIC study. EDIC study results at 6 years of follow-up of these two groups showed a significant difference in the progression of the carotid intima-media thickness, a measure of atherosclerosis. From DCCT through EDIC, and after an average of 17 years of follow-up, the number of CVD events in the conventional group was more than double that of intensive-therapy subjects and intensive therapy reduced the risk of any CVD event by 42% and the risk of nonfatal myocardial infarction (MI), stroke, or death by 57%. However, the effect of group assignment was not as significant when comparing the original adolescent versus adult DCCT cohorts. At EDIC year 10, it was the mean A1C level during the DCCT that accounted for 79% of the observed difference between adults and adolescents rather than original treatment assignment.

Data available from DCCT and from the observational study of type 1 patients from Allegheny County, Pennsylvania (Pittsburgh Epidemiology of Diabetes Complications Experience (EDC)), conducted from 1983–2005 have shown the diabetes complication rates 30 years after the diagnosis. In the DCCT conventional treatment group, cumulative incidence rates of proliferative retinopathy, nephropathy, and cardiovascular disease were 50%, 25%, and 14%, respectively. They were 47%, 17%, and 14%, respectively, in the EDC cohort and 21%, 9%, and 9%, respectively, in the DCCT intensive therapy group; in addition, less than 1% became blind, required kidney replacement therapy, or had an amputation.

These follow-up findings strongly support the implementation of intensive therapy and lowering of A1C as early as is safely possible, and the maintenance of such therapy for as long as possible, with the expectation that a prolonged period of near-normal blood glucose levels will result in an even greater reduction in the risk of both microvascular and macrovascular complications in patients with type 1 diabetes.

GOALS OF TREATMENT

The physician and patient, with the diabetes management team and family, must set treatment goals together. Although this concept seems obvious, overlooking this often leads to failure of the treatment plan. The physician convinced of the importance of stringent glycemic control in every case will be frustrated by a patient who does not understand the need for, or is unable to accept the goal or methods used to achieve, glycemic control. Conversely, the patient who wants blood glucose levels to be normal all the time and is truly willing to work for it will be frustrated by a physician who lacks the time, facilities, or training to help achieve this goal or who is unable to guide the patient to achieve this safely.

A good diabetes management team–patient treatment match requires open communication and appropriate patient education. At the tightest end of the treatment spectrum, the patient must have a sophisticated and practical understanding of physiology and pharmacology when striving to maintain normal glucose levels when, for example, exercising strenuously. At the looser end, knowledge may be more rudimentary, but patients must at least know that to avoid diabetic ketoacidosis (DKA), they may have to take extra insulin on sick days when appetite is poor and common sense seems to dictate the reverse. Treatment must always be individualized. Success in achieving small incremental steps is more likely to lead to a greater improvement over the long run.

The physician and other team members should avoid seeming autocratic, moralistic, or judgmental. They should work with the patient to try to understand why goals are not met and empathize with the challenges faced by the patient in paying daily attention to the never-ending demands of diabetes self-care combined with other aspects of the patient's life. It is paramount to work with the patient to identify obstacles to the treatment plan so the patient can actively participate in addressing them. It is important to encourage the best incremental steps that are achievable without demanding the impossible, unsafe, or impractical.

Setting individual patient glycemic targets should take into account the results of prospective randomized clinical trials, most notably the DCCT. This trial conclusively demonstrated that, in patients with type 1 diabetes, the risk of development or progression of retinopathy, nephropathy, and neuropathy is reduced 50–75% by intensive treatment regimens when compared with conventional treatment regimens. These benefits were observed with an average glycated hemoglobin (A1C) of 7.2% in intensively treated groups of patients compared with an A1C of 9.0% in conventionally treated groups of patients. The reduction in risk of these complications correlated continuously with the reduction in A1C produced by intensive treatment. This relationship implies that complete normalization of glycemic levels may prevent complications. The nondiabetic reference range for A1C in the DCCT was 4.0–6.0%.

Table 2.1 Summary of Glycemic Recommendations for Many Nonpregnant Adults with Diabetes

A1C	<7.0%*
Preprandial capillary plasma glucose	70–130 mg/dL* (3.9–7.2 mmol/L)
Peak postprandial capillary plasma glucose†	<180 mg/dL* (<10.0 mmol/L)
• Goals should be individualized based on*	
• duration of diabetes	
• age/life expectancy	
• comorbid conditions	
• known CVD or advanced microvascular complications	
• hypoglycemia unawareness	
• individual patient considerations	
• More- or less-stringent glycemic goals may be appropriate for individual patients	
• Postprandial glucose may be targeted if A1C goals are not met despite reaching preprandial glucose goals	

†Postprandial glucose measurements should be made 1–2 h after the beginning of the meal, generally peak levels in patients with diabetes.

Self-monitoring of blood glucose (SMBG) targets in the DCCT were 70–120 mg/dL (3.9–6.7 mmol/L) before meals and at bedtime and <180 mg/dL (<10.0 mmol/L) when measured 1.5–2.0 h postprandially. Intensive insulin therapy (at that time, a combination of human regular and human intermediate-acting insulins, or pump therapy with human regular) was associated with a three-fold increased risk of severe hypoglycemia.

Targets for children (e.g., 100–180 mg/dL before meals for infants to pre-schoolers, 90–180 mg/dL for school-age children, and 90–130 mg/dL for adolescents) are higher because of innate hypoglycemia unawareness and the detrimental effect of hypoglycemia on the developing brain. Targets should be further adjusted in any patient with a history of recurrent severe hypoglycemia or hypoglycemia unawareness (e.g., 90–130 mg/dL [5.0–7.2 mmol/L] before meals and 100–140 mg/dL [5.6–7.8 mmol/L] at bedtime). Since the DCCT, the introduction of insulin analogs, enhanced provider experience, the widespread use of multiple daily injections and insulin pumps giving smaller more frequent doses of insulin and use of continuous glucose monitoring (CGM) appear to have decreased severe hypoglycemia rates found in the DCCT while also decreasing A1C values.

Individual treatment goals should take into account the patient's capacity to understand and carry out the treatment regimen, the patient's risk for severe hypoglycemia, and other patient factors that may increase risk or decrease benefit, e.g., very young or old age, end-stage renal disease, advanced cardiovascular or cerebrovascular disease, or other coexisting diseases that will materially affect quality of life or shorten life expectancy.

The desired outcome of glycemic control in type 1 diabetes is to lower glycated hemoglobin (A1C or an equivalent measure of chronic glycemia) so as to achieve maximum prevention of complications with regard for patient safety.

CLINICAL GOALS

Initial Goals

For the new-onset acutely decompensated patient or the previously diagnosed patient in poor control, goals should include

- eliminating ketosis
- returning to desirable body weight range by reversing water and extracellular electrolyte losses and replenishing lean body mass (protein and intracellular electrolytes)
- eliminating obvious consequences of hyperglycemia, e.g., gross polyuria and polydipsia, vaginitis or balanitis, recurrent infections, and visual blurring due to reversible refractive changes
- avoiding cerebral edema in cases of DKA

Additional Goals

Once the initial goals have been achieved, additional goals should include

- near-normalization of blood glucose values and A1C with avoidance of severe hypoglycemia
- preventing symptoms of hyperglycemia, such as excessive thirst and urinary frequency, and disturbed sleep, school, work, social, or recreational activities
- preventing spontaneous and illness-induced ketosis
- maintaining weight within a desirable range
- stimulating catch-up growth and sexual maturation in children with poor glycemic control
- maintaining normal growth rate in children and adolescents
- maintaining maximum exercise tolerance and stamina
- maintaining a sense of psychosocial well-being and normal initiative in self-care
- minimizing self-treatable hypoglycemia and avoiding severe hypoglycemic events resulting in seizures, accidents (e.g., while driving), and coma
- avoiding hospitalization
- for women, achieving normal fertility and pregnancy outcome
- sustaining normal family and marital relationships and sex life
- preventing diabetes-dictated or diabetes-oriented lifestyle (i.e., diabetes controlling the patient rather than vice versa)
- for youth, planning for and achieving transition to adult diabetes care

In addition to the educational and clinical goals discussed above, patients and the diabetes management team should individualize glycemic control goals. It is desirable to aim for near-normalization of blood glucose, if this can be achieved without significant serious side effects (Table 2.2). All patients should be given the opportunity to pursue these goals using a flexible, individualized diabetes management program, based on an assessment of potential risks and benefits.

Table 2.2 Plasma Blood Glucose and A1C Goals for Type 1 Diabetes by Age Group

Values by age (years)	Plasma blood glucose goal range (mg/dL)		A1C	Rationale
	Before meals	After meals		
Infants through pre-school age (0–6)	100–180	110–200	<8.5% (but >7.5%)	High risk of hypoglycemia
School age (6–12)	90–180	100–180	<8%	Risk of hypoglycemia and relatively low risk of complications prior to puberty
Adolescents and young adults (13–19)	90–130	90–150	<7.5%	• Risk of severe hypoglycemia • Developmental and psychological issues • A lower goal (<7.0%) is reasonable if it can be achieved without excessive hypoglycemia

Key concepts in setting glycemia goals:
• Goals should be individualized and lower goals may be reasonable based on benefit-risk assessment.
• Blood glucose goals should be higher than those listed above in children with frequent hypoglycemia or hypoglycemia unawareness.
• Postprandial blood glucose values should be measured when there is a discrepancy between preprandial blood glucose values and A1C levels.

Assessment of A1C

During diabetes visits, glycemic control is assessed by results of glycohemoglobin tests. Many different types of glycohemoglobin assay methods were available in the past, differing considerably with respect to the glycated components measured, interferences, and nondiabetic range. Glycated hemoglobin A_{1c} (A1C) has become the preferred standard for assessing glycemic control, and in 1996, the National Glycohemoglobin Standardization Program (NGSP) was formed to standardize the A1C test to DCCT values. Since then, A1C measurements in North America have been almost universally standardized to the DCCT assay range.

The International Federation of Clinical Chemistry (IFCC) developed a standard for A1C that results in a measurement of concentration (mmol A1C/mol HbA) rather than percent and a reference range that is different than the DCCT standard. A consensus between the IFCC and world diabetes organizations, including the American Diabetes Association, suggests that in medical journals and in the clinical arena, A1C results will be reported in both ways: the IFCC concentration and the DCCT-standardized A1C (as percent). Mmol/mol is the Systeme International (SI) unit. In the US, most lab reports do not use SI units, so it is unclear whether clinically these units will become more common. Although small studies had suggested this to be the case for type 1 populations, a multicenter study in subjects with type 1, type 2, and no diabetes; of multiple ethnic groups; and on multiple types of diabetes therapies confirmed that there is a close association of A1C with the mean blood glucose over the prior 2–3 months across the entire study population. This has led some laboratories in the US to report, on request, both A1C as a percentage and estimated average glucose (eAG).

In the past, when data compiled from diabetes specialty clinics in North America and Europe were analyzed, patients with type 1 diabetes have shown median A1C values (DCCT standard) of 8.0–9.0%. These correspond to mean blood glucose levels of ~200 mg/dL (~11.1 mmol/L). Adolescents with type 1 diabetes generally average 0.5–1.0% higher values and a blood glucose that is 20–40 mg/dL (1.1–2.2 mmol/L) higher than adults. Hemoglobin variants have the potential to cause falsely low or high A1C readings, especially with older assays. In 2008, only ~5% of assays done in labs in the US give spurious results with Hb, AS, or AC. A list of assays and whether or not they are accurate in patients with hemoglobin variants can be found on the NGSP website (*http://www.ngsp.org/prog/index.html*).

Assessment and Goals of Glycemic Control

In addition to A1C, during diabetes visits, individual glucose values from SMBG and CGM can be obtained from log books, uploading glucose meters and CGM devices, or glancing through the stored data on the meter and CGM screens. Diabetes control is assessed by the patient at home via SMBG, CGM, home A1C testing, and urine or blood ketones.

The premeal SMBG and CGM goal for optimal treatment is similar to the 70–120 mg/dL (3.9–6.7 mmol/L) goal used in the DCCT. Over the course of that study, >75% of morning (fasting) glucose levels were >120 mg/dL (>6.7 mmol/L). In practice, most pre-breakfast glucose levels will be between 80 and 160 mg/dL (4.4 and 8.9 mmol/L) in patients with A1C values <7.0%.

The following levels of glycemic control are appropriate for patients with type 1 diabetes.

- In all pregnant women and women attempting to conceive, seek "stringent" biochemical goals of intensive treatment (A1C <6.0%; preprandial, HS, and overnight blood glucose 60–99 mg/dL [3.3–5.4 mmol/L]; and peak postprandial blood glucose 100–129 mg/dL [5.4–7.1 mmol/L]) by methods detailed below (see Pregnancy, page 161).
- In nonpregnant patients who are well informed about the risks and potential benefits of intensive insulin therapy and are motivated and suitably educable, seek an optimal level of control (<7.0% A1C, or in selected patients as close to normal as possible), if achievable without significant

serious side effects. This is accomplished with average blood glucose levels of 110–150 mg/dL (6.1–8.3 mmol/L). Day-to-day fluctuations in blood glucose level are unavoidable, and both patients and providers should focus on patterns. If the patient does not sense or respond to hypoglycemia or has frequent hypoglycemia, goals should be set higher to reduce the risk of severe hypoglycemia.

Results of Optimal Control

At an optimal level of control, patients are entirely asymptomatic and may perceive a very good or excellent sense of well-being, energy, and exercise capacity and less disease-related anxiety compared with maintenance at poor control. They may also express a greater sense of control over the management of the disease if they use a flexible, individualized management program. However, they may experience increased mild self-treated and also severe hypoglycemic episodes. Some patients may feel excessively burdened by the required frequent monitoring, insulin administration methods, and constant dietary adherence. Negotiation (and renegotiation) of mutually acceptable goals will reduce the chances that patients will abandon reasonable self-care. In fact, treatment of type 1 diabetes always involves a negotiated therapeutic alliance between patient (and family) and the diabetes management team.

CONCLUSION

For patients with type 1 diabetes, the long-term benefits of optimal diabetes management appear extremely promising. A flexible, individualized diabetes management program utilizing the principles of intensive insulin therapy should be encouraged in almost all type 1 diabetes patients from onset. These benefits must be balanced in each patient against actual risks and costs. The diabetes management team together with the patient should set treatment goals on the basis of their own best judgment regarding individual patient capabilities and understanding.

BIBLIOGRAPHY

American Diabetes Association: Standards of medical care for patients with diabetes mellitus (Position Statement). *Diabetes Care* 26 (Suppl. 1):S33–S50, 2003

American Diabetes Association: Tests of glycemia with diabetes (Position Statement). *Diabetes Care* 26 (Suppl. 1):S106–S108, 2003

DCCT/EDIC Research Group: Intensive diabetes therapy and carotid intima-media thickness in type 1 diabetes. *N Engl J Med* 348:2294–2303, 2003

DCCT/EDIC Research Group: Retinopathy and nephropathy in patients with type 1 diabetes four years after a trial of intensive therapy. *N Engl J Med* 342:381–389, 2000

DCCT Research Group: The effect of intensive treatment of diabetes on the development and progression of long-term complications in insulin-dependent diabetes mellitus. *N Engl J Med* 329:977–986, 1993

DCCT Research Group: The relationship of glycemic exposure (HbA$_{1c}$) to the risk of development and progression of retinopathy in the Diabetes Control and Complications Trial. *Diabetes* 44:968–993, 1995

Klein R: Hyperglycemia and microvascular and macrovascular disease in diabetes. *Diabetes Care* 18:258–268, 2005

Nathan D, Cleary P, Backlund JY, Genuth SM, Lachin SM, Orchard TJ, Raskin P, Zinman B: Intensive diabetes treatment and cardiovascular disease in patients with type 1 diabetes. *N Engl J Med* 353:2643–2653, 2005

National Cholesterol Education Program (NCEP) Expert Panel on Detection, Evaluation, and Treatment of High Blood Cholesterol in Adults (Adult Treatment Panel III): Executive summary of the Third Report of the National Cholesterol Education Program (NCEP) Expert Panel on Detection, Evaluation, and Treatment of High Blood Cholesterol in Adults (Adult Treatment Panel III). *JAMA* 285:2486–2497, 2001

Pirart J: Diabetes mellitus and its degenerative complications: a prospective study of 4,400 patients observed between 1947 and 1973. *Diabetes Care* 1:168–188, 252–263, 1978

Reichard P, Nilsson BY, Rosenqvist U: The effect of long-term intensified insulin treatment on the development of microvascular complications of diabetes mellitus. *N Engl J Med* 329:304–309, 1993

Rohlfing CL, Wiedmeyer HM, Little RR, England JD, Tennill A, Goldstein DE: Defining the relationship between plasma glucose and HbA$_{1c}$: analysis of glucose profiles and HbA$_{1c}$ in the Diabetes Control and Complications Trial. *Diabetes Care* 25:275–278, 2002

Santiago JV: Lessons from the Diabetes Control and Complications Trial. *Diabetes* 42:1549–1554, 1993

Silverstein J, Klingensmith G, Copeland K, Plotnick L, Kaufman FR, Laffel L, Deeb L, Grey M, Anderson B, Clark N: Care of children and adolescents with type 1 diabetes mellitus: a statement of the American Diabetes Association. *Diabetes Care* 28:186–212, 2005

Skyler JS: Tactics in type 1 diabetes. *Endocrinol Metab Clin North Am* 26:647–657, 1997

PATIENT SELF-MANAGEMENT EDUCATION

Diabetes management is a team effort. Physicians, nurses, dietitians, pharmacists, and other health care professionals contribute their expertise to the design of therapeutic regimens that will enable patients to achieve the best possible metabolic control. The patient is at the center of the team and, supported by his or her family, has responsibility for day-to-day implementation of the treatment plan. In the case of children, the caregivers take on this responsibility. Therapy will be most effective if the patient understands the regimen, is not ambivalent about the value, and has mastered the skills to do required tasks correctly. Therefore, the clinical management of diabetes relies heavily on patient self-management.

The importance of patient education is underscored by the DCCT, which demonstrated that intensive treatment of diabetes, with great demands in patient self-management, can prevent or delay the long-term complications of diabetes. Because intensive therapy brings an increased risk of hypoglycemia, patient education is critical in providing safety. In addition, diabetes self-management training has been shown to improve A1C with as much as a 0.76% reduction immediately after education is delivered. The effect of diabetes education on A1C is directly correlated to the amount of contact time spent between the educator and the patient; 23.6 hours of educator contact has been shown to decrease A1C by 1%, an amount known to be associated with a dramatic reduction in microvascular disease.

This section provides an overview of diabetes patient education, including information on the principles, process, content, and guidelines for incorporating education into clinical practice. Several terms, "including diabetes self-management education" and "diabetes self-management training," are used to describe patient education in diabetes. They will be used interchangeably in this manual. However, for reimbursement purposes, "diabetes self-management training" is the preferred terminology.

GENERAL PRINCIPLES

The goal of diabetes self-management education is to provide patients with the knowledge, skills, and motivation to incorporate ongoing diabetes self-care into their daily lives and to actively collaborate with the diabetes health care team in managing the disease. To meet this goal, diabetes education must include teaching patients the new information they need to know about the diabetes disease process, training them in the various skills they need for their prescribed treatment plan and procedures, assisting them in developing strategies to fit the regimen into their lifestyle, and helping them reconcile diabetes care with their quality of life so they are motivated to manage their disease. To accomplish this, diabetes self-management education should be responsive to the unique and individual needs of the patient and equally accessible to all patients regardless of economic, social, and environmental circumstances.

Table 2.3 Process of Diabetes Self-Management Education

Assessment	Gathering information, both subjective and objective, to Identify a patient's individual education needs
Planning	Designing education for the patient based on the assessment, including topics, goals for education, and selection of teaching/learning strategies
Implementation	Providing the planned education in an environment that supports learning
Documentation	Documenting the educational activities to inform other members of the diabetes management team and to record the care provided
Evaluation	Measuring the impact of education by testing knowledge and skills and by evaluating behavioral and metabolic outcomes
Reassessment	Periodically reviewing clinical and nonclinical information about the patient to identify new needs and re-educate as needed

Ideally, a diabetes management team should be involved in patient education. In the Diabetes Attitudes, Wishes and Needs (DAWN) study, a survey conducted among patients, nurses, and physicians, it was found that nurses provide better education, spend more time with patients, are better listeners, and get to know patients better than physicians. In addition, patients had better outcomes when they had access to a nurse, but less than 50% of patients surveyed said they had such access. Many physicians do not have a diabetes education team available in their practice setting. They need to refer patients, if possible, to a diabetes education program or to diabetes educators. Physicians can develop a team approach by collaborating with diabetes educators working in diabetes education programs. The American Diabetes Association's Education Recognition Program identifies diabetes education programs that meet the National Standards for Diabetes Self-Management Education through a Medicare-approved accreditation process. A list of active ADA Recognized programs is available on the Association's website and can be accessed at *www .diabetes.org/findaprogram.*

Diabetes self-management education is a planned process that requires resources, including time, materials, space, and professional expertise (Table 2.3). The knowledge and skills patients need to implement their treatment regimen and sustain a lifetime of living with diabetes cannot be acquired during a quick interaction on the day of diagnosis or in a single instructional session in a physician's office or any other setting. Moreover, patient education is an ongoing component of diabetes care, not a one-time encounter. Despite this emphasis on diabetes education, self-management programs have been found to be underutilized in a number of studies, with relatively fewer patients having ongoing contact with educators.

For the newly diagnosed patient, a staged approach to education should be used, with the initial teaching focused on the critical information or "survival skills" that will enable the individual, or caregiver, to implement the regimen at

Table 2.4 Basic Education at Diagnosis: Survival Skills

Topics and the critical knowledge and skills patients need to manage their diabetes at home include:

General facts	Explain the need for daily insulin injections and that treatment of diabetes involves insulin, diet, exercise, and SMBG
Medications	Measure insulin dosage accurately, inject correctly, and understand timing of injections and how to handle insulin and supplies
Nutrition	Explain the relationship of food, insulin, and blood glucose and the amount of food, type of food, and times to eat to maximize blood glucose control
Exercise	Explain the relationships of exercise, food, and insulin and how to prevent hypoglycemia from exercise
Monitoring	Perform accurate SMBG and urine or blood ketone tests
Hyperglycemia and hypoglycemia	Differentiate the signs and symptoms of high and low blood glucose levels and know what actions to take for each situation; know when to seek immediate medical assistance for intercurrent illness, hyperglycemia, or ketonuria
Use of the health care system	Identify how to obtain insulin supplies, whom to call for professional advice, and how to get help in an emergency

home (Table 2.4). Once the patient is comfortable with the fundamental components of the regimen, teaching can be expanded to provide more in-depth information and to introduce additional topics. Continuing education across the life span provides opportunities for learning new management techniques; for making adjustments in the regimen to accommodate lifestyle changes, growth, and aging; to consider adding new therapies or technologies; and to sustain positive clinical and quality-of-life outcomes achieved.

To be effective, diabetes self-management education must be individualized. Teaching methods, however, need not be limited to individual instruction. Group classes and self-study methods can supplement individual instruction and offer advantages in meeting different learning styles and in efficient use of teaching time. Information from all sources must be consistent, whether provided by different health professionals or from diverse instructional materials. Therefore, all members of the diabetes management team need to be aware of the content of the education program.

SELF-MANAGEMENT EDUCATION PROCESS

Diabetes self-management education is a systematic process that starts with an assessment of individual educational needs to guide the planning of teaching/learning strategies, followed by implementation of the plan and documentation of the process, and concluding with evaluation of learning as evidenced by behavior change and health outcomes. Although terms may be different, the process mimics the traditional steps clinicians use to diagnose and treat patients. Understanding the commonalities of patient education and medical care facilitates integration of education into the clinical management of diabetes.

There are guiding principles for diabetes education. These principles are supported by numerous studies and include:

1. Diabetes education is effective in improving clinical outcomes and quality of life,
2. Diabetes self-management education has evolved from didactic presentations to theoretically based empowerment models,
3. There is no one best methodology, and effective programs have incorporated behavioral and psychosocial strategies, culture and age-specific programming, and individual and group sessions,
4. Ongoing support is important for sustained benefit, and
5. Behavioral goal-setting is an effective strategy to support self-management behaviors

Assessment

The first step in the educational process is an assessment to obtain clinical, psychosocial, and educability data to determine an individual education plan. Information obtained in this assessment can guide both treatment and education decisions. For example, if assessment shows that the individual has limited learning skills, treatment with a simple insulin regimen versus a complex algorithm of dose adjustments would be appropriate, with educational strategies including selection of pictorial instructional materials, return demonstration, and a plan for evaluating accurate performance at home.

The education assessment also focuses on the three key areas of the learning process: cognitive/knowledge, psychomotor/skills, and affective/attitude. To develop teaching strategies, the educator needs to evaluate each patient to determine specific knowledge that needs to be acquired; skills that need to be mastered; and personal attitudes toward diabetes, health care, and life skills and experiences that will predict the behavior change potential since most aspects of diabetes self-care and management require behavior changes.

As a general framework, the educational assessment should include

- demographic information: age, gender, level of education, occupation, and family status; and for children, this information must be obtained about parents or caregivers
- medical history: height; weight; BMI; blood pressure; blood glucose values (A1C, fasting, plasma glucose, and self-monitoring results); blood lipid values; medications (prescribed and over-the-counter); allergies; other medical problems; general health status, including smoking, alcohol consumption, sexual activity, and use of social drugs; health service or resource utilization; and for children, developmental capabilities, prior growth records and pubertal stage
- diabetes history: type of diabetes; duration of diabetes; current treatment plan, including medication, diet, exercise, monitoring, and problems with

adherence; acute and chronic complications; family history; previous diabetes education; and for children, diabetes management plan at school or childcare

■ dietary habits: meal times and locations, snacking patterns, food preferences, resources for food preparation, patterns suggestive of disordered eating, and previous diet instructions (note that medical nutrition therapy includes a more detailed history; see Nutrition, page 98)

■ physical activity: work/school activity, recreational activity

■ social history: information on household, extended family, social network, cultural factors, religious practices, health beliefs, and current health practices

■ economic profile: income, health insurance, transportation resources, and neighborhood environment

■ lifestyle: activities of daily living, including work, school, and leisure time; for children, information on after-school, weekend, and summer activities

■ psychosocial status: feelings about diabetes, personal relationships (with spouse, partner, parents, family, peers), developmental stages in life-cycle, history of sleep or eating disorders, stress, anxiety, or depression; health goals

■ education factors: functional health literacy, computational skills, readiness to learn, preferred learning methods, visual acuity, hearing loss, dexterity; life experiences; and for children, developmental stage

■ knowledge and skill level in each of the nine content areas of the National Standards for Diabetes Self-Management Education

Additional information will be required to develop educational plans to meet the idiosyncratic needs of individual patients. However, the extent and completeness of the assessment will be determined by the patient as he or she presents for education. For example, a newly diagnosed patient overwhelmed by the diagnosis may not be ready to digest the need for acquiring all these data before a session. The ultimate goal is to completely assess the patient over time. Parts of the complete assessment can be deferred until the patient is fully able to participate and provide helpful and the most beneficial information for education planning. Assessment should therefore be dynamic, ongoing, and dictated by patient readiness, in order to obtain the most beneficial information to guide education. Also, as with nutrition, each member of the diabetes management team will use a more extensive assessment specific to their area of expertise.

Patient autonomy should be supported by understanding the patients' diabetes-related priorities and needs, acknowledging patients' feelings and experiences, facilitating meaningful self-management choices, offering relevant information, and avoiding controlling patients' behavior.

Planning Educational Strategies

The assessment identifies the topics that need to be included in the education plan and teaching methods that would be most effective. From this analysis, educational goals are developed for each patient. The educational goals must correspond with therapeutic goals established by the diabetes management team and diabetes management goals set by the patient. If the diabetes management team is focused on normalization of blood glucose and the patient is focused on making a minimum number of lifestyle changes, teaching will not be effective until there is agreement. Once goals are established, measurable behavioral objectives are developed with the patient to clearly identify steps that will be used to achieve these goals.

The education plan delineates what is to be taught when, how, where, and by whom. There are numerous teaching strategies that can be used with a patient (Table 2.5). For a newly diagnosed patient, the plan would specify topics that need to be covered immediately to provide the patient with the "survival skills" necessary to manage his or her diabetes at home (Table 2.4). Teaching methods could include

- one-on-one sessions with the dietitian to develop a meal plan
- one-on-one sessions with the diabetes educator to learn insulin injection and monitoring techniques
- observation of patient injection and monitoring skills by staff nurses
- a videotape describing pathophysiology
- Internet education modules

The plan would include methods for evaluating learning accomplished in the initial phase, steps to reinforce what has been taught, and resources for obtaining in-depth education within a reasonable time frame.

Implementation

Teaching can take place in a classroom, at bedside, in an office, in the home, in the cafeteria, in a community facility, or in a number of other settings. Whatever space is used, it is critical that the environment support learning and reinforce the importance of the educational process as part of diabetes care. There should be adequate lighting and furnishings and minimal distractions. Education sessions should be scheduled at specific times. Scheduling will help ensure that teaching and learning take place and help establish the concept that education is a specific part of diabetes care. The same measures used to reinforce routine clinical appointments should be used, including written information giving the appointment time, location (with directions if needed), and the name(s), telephone number(s), or Internet addresses of the educator(s).

Documentation

Documentation of education is as important as documentation of treatment procedures. It provides a means of communication among the diabetes management team as well as substantiating the provision of educational care. Documentation can also provide a reference for reinforcing educational and behavioral objectives necessary to accomplish treatment goals by other members of the diabetes team.

Table 2.5 Teaching Strategies

Methods

- Individual instruction: education can be tailored to individual learning needs and focused on specific details of patient's self-management plan; can also accommodate patient-specific learning barriers like vision problems or cognitive challenges
- Group classes: efficient use of educator time, patients benefit from social support and peer learning
- Self-study: flexible, allows patient to pace learning, educator should monitor and evaluate progress
- Can be mastery-based

Techniques

- Short lecture: effective for presenting new information
- Discussion: allows patient to personalize information, ask questions, disclose feelings, and share experiences
- Skills training: provides "hands on" learning; educator demonstrates, patient practices then performs a return demonstration and receives feedback from educator
- Problem-solving: allows patients to integrate information on several topics, such as diet, insulin, and exercise, and to test their knowledge in hypothetical situations
- Role-playing: can be used to reinforce learning (patient plays educator role), to practice social skills (explaining diabetes to friends), and to explore personal problems (family stress)
- Case studies: provide an objective approach to learning that can be used for planning, for problem-solving, and to help patients identify errors they are making in their diabetes self-management
- Self-assessment: blood glucose records, food diaries, and exercise logs can be used to help patients recognize problems in their diabetes self-management and often to identify solutions
- Contracting/goal-setting: used to get patient buy-in on the specifics of changing behavior. Patient-driven, plan for reevaluating contracts or goals to assess degree of achievement, acknowledge successes, and reinforce needed information. AADE-7 is a framework for contracting/goal-setting
- Demonstrate projects: dining out, cooking classes, supermarket trips offer practical ways to apply complex information

Materials

- Printed materials: can be used to reinforce teaching, for self-study, and as an information resource for future needs (e.g., sick-day guidelines)
- Audio and visual aides: slides, films, overheads, audiotapes and videotapes, food models and labels, sample diabetes products, and dolls and puppets are effective in enhancing learning
- Interactive learning programs: available in printed, audio, visual, and computer formats; allow individuals to learn at their own pace, with frequent evaluation to provide feedback on learning
- Games: crossword puzzles, board games, and group games introduce fun into the educational process while enhancing participant learning
- A case study with questions to evaluate learning and problem-solving skills
- Conversation maps: very effective in stimulating "conversation" and directing teaching to patient-expressed needs

Documentation can be included in progress notes in the patient's medical chart or electronic medical record, maintained in education charts or an electronic database, or written in correspondence and reports. Whatever method of documentation is used, a permanent record of a patient's educational experience must be maintained.

Evaluation

The effectiveness of the educational plan is evaluated in several ways. First, assessment of learning will provide measures of knowledge gained, skills acquired, and changes in attitudes. This type of evaluation often is included in the implementation process to allow for reinforcement in areas where the patient exhibits weaknesses. It is typically done in the short run, in the immediate post-education phase. Periodic reassessments will provide measures of lapses in knowledge, skills, or attitudes that can be remedied with a refresher course. Another evaluation procedure measures changes in behavior. This evaluation takes place some time after education (1–3 months) to measure whether the short-term attitude changes and behavior modifications are maintained and have resulted in sustained behavior change. The behavioral objectives developed during the planning phase may be used, or a different set of objectives can be set at the completion of education as an outgrowth of the learning process. A third approach evaluates the effectiveness of education by examining treatment goals, such as lower A1C, improvement in quality of life evidenced by minimal hypoglycemia, or absence of ketoacidosis. All forms of evaluation yield an assessment of additional educational needs of the patient.

CONTENT OF DIABETES SELF-MANAGEMENT EDUCATION

Topics to be included in diabetes patient education are numerous and vary according to type of diabetes, patient age, and other individual characteristics. The National Standards for Diabetes Self-Management Education specify that programs should be equipped to provide information in nine core content areas. The suggested topics are listed below with basic teaching points for type 1 diabetes:

■ **Describing the diabetes disease process and treatments:** Type 1 diabetes is a chronic metabolic disorder in which the body no longer produces insulin required to use food for energy. The loss of insulin production is due to an autoimmune process that results from an interaction of genes and environmental triggers. Lack of insulin can be life-threatening. Daily insulin injections are essential and need to be balanced with meals and physical activity to manage diabetes. Understanding the interactions among the three (food, insulin, and activity) and their impact on blood glucose levels is important in making self-management decisions. Self-monitoring values provide information that can be used to make adjustments in one or more of the three therapeutic agents.

■ **Incorporating nutritional management into lifestyle:** Food is an important part of diabetes treatment and health. The amount, type, and timing of meals and snacks must be balanced with insulin and exercise to maintain good blood glucose control. Meal planning should be individualized to reflect food preferences and daily schedules, provide optimum nutrition, maintain a healthy weight, and make diabetes self-care as effective as possible.

■ **Incorporating physical activity into lifestyle:** Physical activity is recommended for health and diabetes management. Physical activity can affect blood glucose levels and other health parameters like blood pressure, weight, and stress, usually by lowering them. Exercise for purposes of diabetes education can be characterized as any tolerable increase in baseline activity. Planning for exercise can prevent hypoglycemia that may occur during or after exercise.

■ **Using medication(s) safely and for maximum therapeutic effectiveness:** Insulin must be taken daily as prescribed. It is important to know the type and amount of insulin to be taken and times to administer insulin and to understand the action and duration of the prescribed insulin. Correct techniques for drawing up and injecting insulin with a syringe or pen device are critical to ensure that the dose is accurate. There are different types of insulin regimens, from fixed 2–3 injections, to basal bolus therapy with multiple daily injections or insulin pump therapy. Family members, close friends, coaches, teachers, co-workers, and others who closely interact with the diabetes patient on insulin need to know how to administer glucagon in the event of severe hypoglycemia.

■ **Monitoring blood glucose and other parameters and interpreting and using the results for self-management decision-making:** Proper technique is crucial to achieve reliable results. Blood glucose monitoring results can be used to assess the effectiveness of the treatment regimen, identify low blood glucose levels requiring treatment to prevent hypoglycemia, indicate high blood glucose levels possibly associated with illness, show the effect of different meals and activities on blood glucose, and guide decisions on when to contact health care providers. Proper technique is crucial to achieve reliable results. The downloading of meter data can help with data management. CGM has an additional role in showing trends and patterns and alerting at set or predictive thresholds. Urine or blood testing for ketones is required during times of physical or emotional stress and may be necessary during pregnancy.

■ **Preventing, detecting, and treating acute complications (hypoglycemia, hyperglycemia, and illness):** Hypoglycemia comes on quickly. Therefore, it is important to recognize the signs and symptoms of hypoglycemia and to know how to prevent and treat it (Table 2.6). Hyperglycemia that cannot be explained by diet or another aspect of the regimen (e.g., decrease in exercise or inadequate insulin delivery or amount) may indicate illness. Patients with type 1 diabetes can develop DKA when ill. Therefore, guidelines for sick days need to be followed carefully (Table 2.7). Family members, friends, coworkers, and teachers need to know how to respond in case of emergencies.

Table 2.6 Sample Patient Guidelines for Treating Mild Hypoglycemia: 15/15 Rule

If blood glucose falls below 70 mg/dL:

■ Eat 15 g carbohydrate, preferably in the form of glucose products
■ Wait 15 min—retest, and if blood glucose remains <70 mg/dL, treat with another 15 g carbohydrate
■ Repeat testing and treating until blood glucose returns to normal range
■ If >1 h to next meal, add additional 15 g carbohydrate to maintain blood glucose in normal range

Sources of carbohydrate

Glucose products (preferred):
Glucose tablets	4–5 g/tablet
Glucose gel	15 g/dose
Insta-glucose gel	24 g tube/one-dose tube

Food/beverages (use if above not available), 15-g portions:
Graham crackers	3
Saltine crackers	6
Raisins	2 Tbsp
Syrup or honey	1 Tbsp
Juice (apple/orange)	1/2 cup
Soft drink (regular)	1/2 cup
Skim milk	1 cup
Ginger ale	3/4 cup

Note: Severe hypoglycemia needs to be treated by someone knowledgeable about diabetes. Guidelines should be available in schools and work sites. If the patient cannot swallow well, glucagon must be used instead of oral treatment.

■ **Preventing, detecting, treating, and rehabilitation of chronic complications:** Chronic complications are a serious concern in diabetes. Steps that can reduce the risk of complications include maintaining blood glucose levels as near to normal as feasible, not smoking, having annual eye exams, controlling blood pressure and blood lipid levels, assessing urine microalbumin excretion, and taking preventive care of feet.

■ **Developing personal strategies to address psychosocial issues:** Fear, anger, and denial are common responses to the diagnosis of diabetes and other stages of the disease process. The day-by-day demands of diabetes management can be frustrating. Stress may cause problems with blood glucose control. Coping skills, stress reduction techniques, and professional counseling can help the patient handle the psychosocial impact of diabetes. Type 1 diabetes affects the whole family. Family members, friends, coworkers, and teachers need to know about diabetes and how to support the regimen. Adolescents must not be left to manage diabetes without some degree of parental supervision. Camps and support

Table 2.7 Sample Patient Guidelines for Sick-Day Management

Illness can make diabetes more difficult to manage. Even when you do not feel well, you must take your insulin, test blood glucose and urine or blood ketones, drink fluids, and eat if you can. Eating food is less important. You will need ketone strips and fluids that can be a source of glucose and electrolytes. Therefore, planning ahead for sick days is important. The following guidelines will help you during mild illnesses.

Monitoring

Blood glucose and urine (or blood) ketones need to be tested frequently during illness, often every 2–4 h. Test for ketones if you have unexplainable high blood glucose values >250 mg/dL or if you feel ill, even if blood glucose values are normal. Write down the values and call a member of your diabetes management team when premeal blood glucose values stay >250 mg/dL and/or when you measure moderate or large ketones.

Insulin

Never stop taking insulin even if vomiting and unable to eat. Your body often needs more insulin during illness. Therefore, your health care professional may ask you to take additional insulin (a correction bolus) according to results of blood glucose monitoring.

Food and fluid intake

Use small meals and eat more frequently when you are ill. Soft foods or liquids are often tolerated best. Eating about 10–15 g carbohydrate every 1–2 h is usually sufficient. Foods and beverages containing about 15 g carbohydrate include

1/2 cup regular gelatin	3/4 cup regular ginger ale
1/2 cup vanilla ice cream	1/2 cup regular soft drink
1/2 cup custard	1/2 cup orange or apple juice
1 regular double Popsicle	1 cup Gatorade
1/2 cup applesauce	1 cup clear soup

Fluid intake is essential during illness. If vomiting, diarrhea, or fever is present, take small quantities of liquids every 15–30 min. Clear broth, tea, and other fluids can supplement liquids containing carbohydrate.

Seek medical attention when you have

- Fever >100°F
- Persistent diarrhea
- Vomiting and are unable to take fluids for >4 h
- Blood glucose levels that are difficult to control with or without ketones (see information above on monitoring)

- Severe abdominal pain
- Other unexplained symptoms
- Illness that persists over 24 h

Physician's #   Pharmacy #

groups, including online diabetes networks, can help with denial and isolation.

■ **Developing personal strategies to promote health and behavior change:** Most aspects of diabetes management require changes in behavior. Behavior change is not simply willpower. Strategies such as goal setting, contracting, and developing problem-solving techniques based on patient experience are helpful in changing habits to reduce health risks and improve diabetes control. Risk factors for diabetic complications, including cardiovascular disease, should be addressed. Achieving optimal glucose control may deter the complications of diabetes, including those occurring during pregnancy. Women with type 1 diabetes need to achieve excellent blood glucose control before becoming pregnant (optimally for 3 months before conception) and maintain tight glucose control throughout pregnancy; however, tight control brings an increased risk of hypoglycemia. Individuals with diabetes need to be responsible for their diabetes management, which includes working with their diabetes management team to select the treatment plan that meets their personal goals for health. Because changing behavior underlies most aspects of diabetes self-management, presenting the content areas in action oriented, behavioral terms will help to underscore the importance of active patient participation in diabetes care and management.

ADDITIONAL TOPICS OF IMPORTANCE FOR TYPE 1 DIABETES

■ **Using the health care system and community resources:** People with diabetes need to be good consumers of the health care system and of community resources. Ongoing versus episodic care is important. Contact information, including phone numbers and Internet addresses of diabetes management team members and emergency services, should be readily available for use by family and friends as well as the individual with diabetes. Identifying accessible resources in the community and on the Internet for supplies, services, information, and support groups makes day-to-day diabetes management easier and helps the patient to maintain positive outcomes over time.

■ **Wearing an identification bracelet or necklace:** This is strongly encouraged and recommended at all times so that having diabetes can be quickly ascertained in the event of acute crises such as unconsciousness or motor vehicle accident.

■ **Driving a motor vehicle:** Special care should be taken to prevent hypoglycemia while driving a car, truck, motorboat, or any other powered vehicle. Blood glucose levels should be checked before driving, especially if the last meal was more than 3 h earlier or if the trip will be long, and low blood glucose values should be treated appropriately (Table 2.6). Supplies for SMBG and treating hypoglycemia should be carried in the vehicle at all times. If symptoms of hypoglycemia occur, driving should stop immediately and not be resumed until blood glucose levels are in the normal range for at least 10 min.

- **Traveling:** Insulin and diabetes supplies sufficient for the entire trip need to be carried with the traveler and not put into checked baggage. Food to treat hypoglycemia and for a meal that may be delayed by late arrival should be left in place or carried for security reasons. Additional prescriptions should be carried as well, in case the need to purchase supplies does occur.
- **Working:** Jobs that have erratic schedules, have long periods between meals, lack the flexibility to stop work and test blood glucose levels, or have other conditions make diabetes management more challenging. The Americans with Disabilities Act requires employers to make reasonable accommodations for employees with disabilities, including diabetes. The person with diabetes along with his or her supervisor and diabetes management team can identify ways to modify a job to accommodate the demands of work and diabetes management.
- **Orientation and continuing education for school personnel:** Children with diabetes in school are protected by Section 504 of the Rehabilitation Act of 1973, the Americans with Disabilities Act (ADA), and Individuals with Disabilities Education Act (IDEA) so that there is a medically safe environment and equal access to educational opportunities and school-related activities. The Diabetes Medical Management Plan, devised by the health care team and the student/parents, outlines what must be done in school with regard to administration of medication, monitoring, nutrition, activity, and diabetes-related emergencies. Parents, students, school personnel, and the diabetes management team work together to create a safe and supportive environment for school-age children.

INCORPORATING PATIENT EDUCATION IN CLINICAL PRACTICE

Patient education is essential for management of type 1 diabetes. However, all medical practice settings are not equipped to provide diabetes self-management training. Moreover, the complexity of type 1 diabetes, particularly when treated with intensive therapy, requires health care providers to have special expertise in diabetes. Physicians who specialize in the treatment of diabetes and who see many patients with type 1 diabetes can develop a team relationship with diabetes educators in the community, if hiring educators on a full- or part-time basis is not feasible. Systems such as health maintenance organizations, preferred provider organizations, telemedicine, and affiliations with hospitals offer potential resources for diabetes educators that can work with a number of physicians to maximize the economy of this specialized type of care. Physicians practicing in an area where there are education programs that have achieved American Diabetes Association Recognition may refer patients to programs that meet the National Standards. The local American Diabetes Association office maintains a list of recognized programs in their area, and this list is also available on the Association's website (*www.diabetes.org/findaprogram*).

To establish a team approach to diabetes self-management education, health professionals should *1)* share a common philosophy toward diabetes management and *2)* develop efficient methods for communicating about patient care and education to ensure that a consistent message is given to the patient. Forms, hand-written or electronic, can be helpful in documenting the educational process in a concise format that allows team members to keep abreast of each others' activities and to reinforce all areas of education. Communication by fax and computers offers the opportunity for expedient transfer of information among health professionals not working in the same location. Forms, if placed in the front of a chart or a similar place routinely used in providing patient care, or in the electronic medical record, can serve as a prompt to educate while providing routine medical care.

Diabetes education materials can be obtained from the American Diabetes Association, from companies manufacturing pharmaceuticals and diabetes equipment and supplies, and through a number of additional resources available through the National Diabetes Information Clearinghouse website at *www.niddk.nih.gov.*

CONCLUSION

Patients with type 1 diabetes need self-management education to be able to implement their treatment regimen. Education should be individualized to reflect the diabetes treatment regimen and learning characteristics of each patient. Self-management training is a systematic patient care process that requires educators with expertise in diabetes and resources of time and materials. Physicians should use a team approach to manage individuals with type 1 diabetes with self-management education integrated into the clinical care of the patient.

BIBLIOGRAPHY

American Association of Diabetes Educators: *A CORE Curriculum for Diabetes Educators.* 5th ed. Chicago, IL, American Association of Diabetes Educators, 2003

American Diabetes Association: *Diabetes Education Goals.* Alexandria, VA, American Diabetes Association, 2002

American Diabetes Association: *Life with Diabetes: A Series of Teaching Outlines by the Michigan Diabetes Research and Training Center.* 3rd ed. Alexandria, VA, American Diabetes Association, 2004

American Diabetes Association: Standards of medical care in diabetes—2012. *Diabetes Care* (Suppl. 1):S11–S63, 2012

American Diabetes Association: National Standards for Diabetes Self-Management Education. *Diabetes Care* (Suppl. 1):S101–S108, 2012

Anderson BJ, Rubin RR (Eds.): *Practical Psychology for Diabetes Clinicians.* 2nd ed. Alexandria, VA, American Diabetes Association, 2002

Anderson RM, Funnell MM, Burkhart N, Gillard ML, Nwankwo R: *101 Tips for Behavior Change in Diabetes Education.* Alexandria, VA, American Diabetes Association, 2002

Anderson RM: Taking diabetes self-management education to the next level. *Diabetes Spectrum* 20:202–203, 2007

Cheng YJ, Gregg EW, Geiss LS, Imperatore G, Williams DE, Zhang X, Albright AL, Cowie CC, Klein R, Saaddine JB: Association of A1C and fasting plasma glucose levels with diabetic retinopathy prevalence in the U.S. population: implications for diabetes diagnostic thresholds. Diabetes Care 32:2027–2032, 2009

Funnell MM, Brown TL, Childs BP, Haas LB, Hosey GM, Jensen B, Maryniuk M, Peyrot M, Piette JD, Reader D, Siminerio LM, Weinger K, Weiss MA: National standards for diabetes self-management education. *Diabetes Care* 34 (Suppl. 1):S89–S96, 2011

Funnell M, Peyrot M, Rubin RR, Siminerio L: Steering toward a new DAWN in diabetes management. *Diabetes Educ* 31 (Suppl.):1–18, 2005

Kanzer-Lewis G: *Patient Education: You Can Do It!* Alexandria, VA, American Diabetes Association, 2003

Michigan Diabetes Research and Training Center: *Teenagers with Type 1 Diabetes: A Curriculum for Adolescents and Families.* Alexandria, VA, American Diabetes Association, 2001

NDEP: *Helping the Student with Diabetes Succeed: A Guide for School Personnel.* Available from *www.ndep.nih.gov/media/youth_ndepschoolguide.pdf.*

Tools of Therapy

Highlights
Tools of Therapy

INSULIN TREATMENT

■ Patients with type 1 diabetes are dependent on insulin to survive.

■ The insulins primarily in use today are: recombinant human insulin, with the same amino acid sequence as native human insulin (with or without protamine to delay its absorption, onset, and duration) and recombinant human insulin analogs, in which the amino acid sequence of human insulin is altered to affect its absorption, onset, and duration of action.

■ Insulin preparations are classified by duration of action (rapid, short, intermediate, and long acting).

■ The insulin regimen should be tailored to the needs of the individual patient. Adjustments in the insulin regimen or specific insulin doses should be based on actual glycemic values obtained from patient self-monitoring of blood glucose (SMBG) or continuous glucose monitoring (CGM) rather than on "textbook" predictions of insulin action.

■ More physiological multiple-component "flexible" regimens emphasize the difference between basal and prandial (bolus) insulin. These insulin regimens consist of

- three or more daily injections (prandial/bolus and basal insulins)
- insulin pump therapy

■ Insulin needs may fluctuate during the first weeks or months of treatment. If a honeymoon or remission phase occurs, insulin dose must be appropriately reduced, occasionally to as little as 0.1–0.3 units/kg/day, but it should not be discontinued or replaced with an oral hypoglycemic agent.

■ Continuous subcutaneous insulin infusion is an alternative that offers advantages in lifestyle flexibility and glycemic variability.

■ Regimens using insulin algorithms place more demands on both patient and physician than does a fixed course of treatment, but they provide greater flexibility in lifestyle. All forms of intensive therapy require high degrees of long-term commitment and flexibility on the part of the patient, the family, and the diabetes management team.

■ Common problems associated with insulin therapy are detailed in Common Problems in Long-Term Therapy.

TREATMENT WITH THE AMYLIN ANALOG PRAMLINTIDE

■ Pramlintide is a soluble nonaggregating amylin analog that is an adjunct to patients receiving prandial insulin therapy. The clinical benefits of pramlintide are achieved by replacing the action of amylin, a naturally occurring β-cell hormone that is deficient in type 1 diabetes. Results from clinical studies showed that when pramlintide was added to insulin regimens, patients with type 1 diabetes had improved glycemic control with no increased body weight or severe hypoglycemia.

MONITORING

■ Patients can only manage type 1 diabetes effectively and safely if they self-monitor. This includes self-monitoring of blood glucose (SMBG) from the finger or an alternate site, alone or with the additional use of a continuous subcutaneous glucose (CGM) sensor, as well as urine or blood ketone monitoring as needed and careful record-keeping.

■ Monitoring allows objective goals for therapy and a means to measure the efficacy of changes in therapy.

■ SMBG is the established monitoring method that allows

- detection and prevention of hypoglycemia and hyperglycemia

- adjustment of insulin, diet, and physical activity to achieve target blood glucose levels

- analysis of data (from both SMBG and CGM) to look at patterns and trends, daily means (and standard deviations), means (and standard deviations) by time of day, and percentages of values in the hypoglycemic and hyperglycemic ranges. This can be done by keeping a log book, or with programs that analyze and display the information.

■ Four or more SMBG measurements every day—before breakfast, lunch, supper, and bedtime—usually provide the necessary information sufficient to adjust insulin, activity, and diet. Tests are done before meals and at bedtime at a minimum; additional testing may be warranted after meals (2 h after the start of the meal); in the middle of the night; before, during, and after exercising; on sick days; after an intervention to correct a high or low glucose value; or when a schedule change has occurred.

■ Continuous or intermittent glucose monitoring of interstitial fluid is available to provide additional information to adjust insulin, exercise, and diet to optimize glycemic control and prevent hypoglycemia.

■ A properly performed A1C provides the best available index of chronic glucose levels and is highly reliable.

NUTRITION

■ The overall goal of medical nutrition therapy (MNT) for type 1 diabetes is to enable patients to attain blood glucose levels as near normal as possible by integrating exogenous insulin into their usual eating and activity patterns. The MNT prescription should be individualized based on nutrition assessment and treatment goals. In general, recommendations follow nutrition guidelines for the general population:

- Calorie levels should be prescribed to achieve and maintain healthy body weight.
- Protein intakes of 10–20% of calories are adequate to support health; intakes of 0.8–1.0 g/kg/day (~10% of daily calories) are recommended for individuals showing evidence of diabetic nephropathy.
- Fat consumption should be moderate, with saturated fat limited to <7% of calories, and minimal to no trans fats.
- Carbohydrate foods, such as grains, dried beans, legumes, vegetables, fruits, and nonfat dairy products are rich sources of vitamins, minerals, and/or dietary fiber and are preferred choices for carbohydrate-containing foods. For type 1 diabetes, the total amount of carbohydrates in a meal, rather than the source (sugar or starch), should guide the estimation of insulin dosage. The glycemic effect of foods may provide an additional benefit to using total carbohydrate.
- Vitamin and mineral requirements of individuals with diabetes are the same as the general population.

Supplementation is advised if conditions create a deficiency.

■ Insulin therapy regimens using multiple daily doses of insulin allow greater flexibility in eating patterns than do conventional regimens. Blood glucose levels obtained by self-monitoring can be used to make adjustments in diet, activity, and insulin regimen to maximize blood glucose control.

■ The complexity of integrating nutrition and insulin therapies and the importance of diabetes self-management education require a coordinated team approach to care for individuals with type 1 diabetes.

■ MNT for diabetes is based on an assessment of the individual's metabolic and lifestyle parameters, implemented through a nutrition self-management plan and evaluated through nutrition-related outcomes such as blood glucose and lipid levels and achievement of a healthy weight and normal growth in children. Patients and their families should be actively involved in setting nutrition goals, developing the self-management plan, and evaluating treatment effectiveness through SMBG levels.

■ Registered dietitians have the expertise to design the nutrition intervention and to counsel patients on nutrition self-management. Nutritional counseling for newly diagnosed patients with type 1 diabetes should be provided in stages to allow the patient time to adjust to the treatment regimen. Nutritional care cannot be limited to diagnosis but must continue throughout the patient's life span. Follow-up may be appropriate every 3–6 months for children and every 6–12 months for adults.

EXERCISE

■ Exercise should be an integral part of the treatment plan for patients with type 1 diabetes.

■ Physiological responses to exercise in people without diabetes and in patients with type 1 diabetes are described in Table 3.13. For the type 1 diabetes patient, plasma insulin levels during and after exercise are critical determinants of response.

■ Potential benefits of exercise are explained on page 123. Some people do not consider that they exercise, but may be physically active because they use stairs, walk their dog, do house cleaning, or gardening. In this manner, physical activity, like regular exercise, can improve cardiovascular risk factors and may

- aid in achieving and maintaining a healthy weight
- heighten sense of well-being
- improve glucose control

■ Potential risks of exercise include destabilization of metabolic control, e.g.,

- hypoglycemia during or after exercise (most likely with sporadic or inconsistent exercise)
- hyperglycemia and ketosis (if diabetes is uncontrolled or ketones are present before beginning activity)

■ A pre-exercise medical evaluation should be performed regardless of the patient's age.

■ Exercise should be prescribed with caution in patients with

- unstable blood glucose values
- cardiovascular disease, neuropathy that results in loss of sensation, or proliferative retinopathy
- hypoglycemia unawareness

■ Guidelines for safe exercise are addressed in Table 3.17. They include

- monitoring blood glucose and taking appropriate action
- altering food or insulin if needed
- carrying short-acting carbohydrate and identification
- monitoring intensity of exercise
- avoiding trauma to joints, muscle, or ligaments as well as to the skin of the feet

Tools of Therapy

INSULIN TREATMENT

Type 1 diabetes is characterized by a near-absolute deficiency in endogenous insulin secretion within days or months after initial diagnosis. Affected patients are dependent on exogenous insulin to survive for the duration of their lives, and the insulin regimen must be individualized for each patient.

INSULIN PREPARATIONS

For the most part, insulin is no longer obtained from animal pancreas but rather it is made chemically identical to human insulin by recombinant DNA technology, then either provided in solution (human regular insulin) or complexed with protamine to delay its absorption and duration (human NPH insulin). In addition, there are a number of human insulin analogs, in which the amino acid sequence of the human insulin molecule has been modified to change its pharmacokinetics. Insulin preparations are generally classified by duration of action (rapid-, short-, intermediate-, and long-acting). Three rapid-onset, short-duration analogs (insulin lispro, insulin aspart, and insulin glulisine) are available. Human regular insulin and human NPH are characterized as short- and intermediate-acting, respectively, and two long-acting or basal analogs (insulin glargine and insulin detemir) are available. Lente (intermediate-acting) and ultralente (long-acting) insulin are no longer available. Other insulin preparations that may be either more rapid or longer acting are under development. Because there are many insulin preparations now available, and many more likely to be available soon, health professionals should familiarize themselves with several preparations and learn to use them rationally (Tables 3.1 and 3.2).

Species and Purity

In the US today, insulin is prepared by recombinant DNA technology and no longer derived from animal sources. All insulin preparations sold in the US are of the highest purity and contain less than one part per million of impurities. Such purification is associated with a reduced incidence of insulin antibodies, less insulin allergy, and less lipoatrophy at the injection site than previous less purified or more immunogenic animal preparations.

Duration of Action

Although insulins are classified into rapid-, short-, intermediate-, and long-acting preparations, actual insulin effects do not always coincide with such simple descriptions. For example, local subcutaneous tissue conditions not clearly understood may cause rates of absorption to vary by 20–40% from day to day

Table 3.1 Insulins Available in the United States (2012)

Product	Manufacturer
Rapid acting	
Humalog (insulin lispro)*	Lilly
NovoLog (insulin aspart)*	Novo Nordisk
Apidra (insulin glulisine)†	sanofi-aventis
Short acting	
Humulin R (regular)	Lilly
Novolin R (regular)	Novo Nordisk
Intermediate acting	
Humulin N (NPH)†	Lilly
Novolin N (NPH)	Novo Nordisk
Long acting	
Lantus (insulin glargine)*	sanofi-aventis
Levemir (insulin detemir)†	Novo Nordisk
Combinations	
Humulin 70/30 (70% NPH, 30% regular)†	Lilly
Humalog 75/25 (75% insulin lispro protamine suspension [NPL], 25% insulin lispro)†	Lilly
Humalog 50/50 (50% NPL, 50% lispro)†	Lilly
Novolin 70/30 (70% NPH, 30% regular)	Novo Nordisk
Novolog 70/30 (70% insulin aspart protamine, 30% insulin aspart)	Novo Nordisk

*Available in prefilled disposable pen injectors and cartridges for pen injectors in addition to vials.
†Available in cartridges for pen injectors in addition to vials.

in any one patient. In light of the many other variables influencing insulin pharmacokinetics, the clinician is cautioned against relying too heavily on textbook descriptions of insulin action. Health professionals should base therapy adjustments on actual glycemic values obtained from the patient's self-monitoring of blood glucose (SMBG) or CGM.

Rapid- and short-acting insulins are relatively predictable on a day-to-day basis in onset and duration of action. Therefore, they can be adjusted after a 2- to 3-day observation period to attempt to normalize postprandial glucose values. This adjustment can be made by changing a fixed dose or the insulin-to-carbohydrate ratio or the timing of insulin in relation to the meal or the amount of insulin used to correct a glucose value above the target range (correction algorithm). Any change in the dose of intermediate-acting (NPH) or long-acting (glargine or detemir) insulin requires a 2- to 5-day observation period before further dose adjustment because of the relatively slow absorption and long duration of action of these insulins and because of day-to-day variability in food, activity, and stress.

The use of SMBG to map out a profile of blood glucose values is invaluable in assisting the physician, patient, and diabetes management team with therapy. Blood glucose levels should be measured before and after meals and during the

Table 3.2 Insulins by Comparative Action

	Onset (h)	Peak (h)	Effective duration (h)
Rapid acting			
Insulin lispro (analog)	<0.25–0.5	0.5–2.5	3–6.5
Insulin aspart (analog)	<0.25	0.5–1.0	3–5
Insulin glulisine (analog)	<0.25	1–1.5	3–5
Short acting			
Regular (soluble)	0.5–1	2–3	3–6
Intermediate acting			
NPH (isophane)	2–4	4–10	10–16
Long acting			
Insulin glargine (analog)	2–4	Relatively flat	20–24
Insulin detemir (analog)	0.8–2 (dose dependent)	Relatively flat	Dose dependent 12 h for 0.2 U/kg; 20 h for 0.4 U/kg; up to 24 h. binds to albumin.
Combinations			
70% NPH, 30% regular	0.5–1	Dual	10–16
75% NPL, 25% lispro	<0.25	Dual	10–16
50% NPL, 50% lispro	<0.25	Dual	10–16
70% aspart protamine, 30%aspart	<0.25	Dual	15–18

night, particularly when initiating or intensifying insulin therapy or when seeking the cause of hypoglycemia or hyperglycemia. CGM may be a helpful tool because of the increase in number of glucose values obtained each day. Routine frequency of monitoring or use of CGM should be based on mutually defined goals described in Philosophy and Goals.

Insulin Pens and Apps

Most of the current human insulins and insulin analogs are available in insulin cartridges and/or disposable pens (Table 3.1). Such devices aid the patient in insulin measurement and simplify insulin administration with minimal added cost to therapy. Several manufacturers of insulin pens and pen needles exist; pens are either durable or disposable, and some devices deliver insulin by half units or have a memory device that records the prior doses. Use of pen devices, will not only facilitate the adaptation to basal-bolus therapy, and enhance the compliance to intensive insulin therapy but also improve outcomes when using flexible regimens. A cover to the pen has just been developed and released that keeps track of the last dose of insulin given. Applications on glucose meters and via the Internet on phones or computers can be used to record insulin doses as well.

Mixing Insulins

Mixing insulin is declining in the US because fixed regimens are being replaced by flexible basal-bolus regimens and pen usage is increasing. Insulin glargine and insulin detemir should not be mixed with other insulins. Mixing short- or rapid-acting insulin with NPH in the same syringe is an accepted and convenient way to produce differently timed pharmacologic actions with a single injection. Stable premixtures of intermediate- and short- or rapid-acting insulins in fixed proportion (e.g., 70% NPH/30% regular, 75% NPL/25% insulin lispro, 50% NPL/50% insulin lispro, and 70% NPA/30% insulin aspart) are also available commercially. Premixed insulins are not suitable when daily variation in the dose of short-acting insulin is required, which is the case for most patients with type 1 diabetes.

TREATING NEWLY DIAGNOSED PATIENTS

Diagnosis and Stabilization

At diagnosis, initial objectives of therapy are dependent on the degree of illness (e.g., resolving DKA if it exists, eliminating symptomatic hyperglycemia, or initiating insulin therapy in the asymptomatic patient). The goal is to resolve hyperglycemia, fluid deficit, and electrolyte disturbance while avoiding hypoglycemia. Therefore, glycemic targets should be approached gradually. Treatment should begin with ~0.6–0.75 units of insulin per kg body weight per day. However, during the first week of therapy, this amount can be expected to increase to an average of 1.0–1.5 unit/kg/day, because most patients are relatively insulin resistant at this time. This is particularly true for adolescents and those who present in DKA.

Immediately after diagnosis or after ketoacidosis has been resolved, therapy should begin with the insulin program that is negotiated and agreed upon between the patient/family and health care team, e.g., two or three daily insulin injections or a "flexible" intensive insulin program consisting of preprandial or bolus insulin at each meal and basal insulin once or twice per day. It is preferable to start with the flexible basal-bolus insulin program at the outset instead of learning twice-daily insulin injections, a therapy that eventually fails. Although twice- or once-daily insulin may suffice for a short time in patients who retain some of their β-cell function, psychological acceptance of flexible intensive injection programs is easier for both patient and family if introduced as soon as possible after diagnosis, even if glycemic control could be adequate on a different program with fewer injections. Moreover, there is evidence from the Diabetes Control and Complications Trial (DCCT) and EDIC that intensive exogenous insulin helps preserve β-cell function and should be given in adequate doses so that the patient does not need to utilize endogenous insulin for routine glycemic control.

Although not recommended, some clinicians start with two or three insulin injections per day, to acquaint the patient with basic diabetes management principles, before initiating a flexible intensive program. With the two-dose regimen, about two-thirds of the insulin dose is given in the morning before breakfast, and one-third is given before supper. The two doses may consist of premixed insulins (sometimes the case for infants and very young children) or two doses of a mixture of rapid- or short- and intermediate-acting or long-acting insulins. The prebreakfast dose consists of about two-thirds NPH and one-third regular or insulin aspart or lispro. The presupper dose is usually divided into equal amounts of NPH or insulin glargine or detemir, and regular insulin or insulin aspart, lispro, or glulisine. For the three shot regimen, the same is followed, however, the evening doses are split with the regular insulin or rapid-acting insulin before dinner and the NPH or insulin glargine or detemir before bed.

Patients and families should be taught the technique of blood glucose monitoring at diagnosis. They should determine blood glucose levels repeatedly under professional supervision to ensure the reliability of the readings. If premixed formulations (e.g., 70% NPH/30% regular; 75% NPL/25% insulin lispro) are used initially, patients should have supplies of short- or rapid-acting insulins for use when needed, such as supplementation for sick days.

Remission or Honeymoon Phase

Within weeks after diagnosis, with resolution of ketosis and hyperglycemia, there may be some recovery of β-cell function, and consequently, exogenous insulin requirements often decrease for weeks to months. This honeymoon phase of type 1 diabetes may be marked by the appearance of recurrent hypoglycemic reactions. A honeymoon phase occurs less frequently in younger children; it is more common in the late teenage years and in adults. During this period, insulin dosage must be appropriately reduced, occasionally to as little as 0.1–0.3 units/kg/day. Not all patients exhibit a profound honeymoon phase, but some period of stability in blood glucose levels is common, with insulin requirements at 0.2–0.5 units/kg/day. Evidence suggests that the honeymoon phase could be prolonged if blood glucose levels are kept in the near-normal range with basal/bolus therapy. There should not be an attempt to reduce insulin to the lowest dose possible nor to discontinue insulin, because of the apparent benefits of even modest preservation of β-cell function. Instead, the patient should receive the highest dose that does not induce hypoglycemia.

The TrialNet Study, a large multinational trial in the US, Canada, Australia, and Europe, has one of its goals to preserve β-cells, as assessed by C-peptide secretion, at the onset of type 1 diabetes. This study is investigating the use of immune-suppressive and immune-modulating agents, as well as intensive metabolic control. Patients should be informed of this study at the time of diagnosis. Patients and families can be referred to the TrialNet website *www2.diabetestrialnet.org*, to determine whether they are interested and eligible for any studies.

Chronic Phase: Developing a Long-Term Treatment Plan

As the honeymoon period comes to an end with the progressive decrease of β-cell function, insulin requirements increase gradually over several months. Prepubertal children and adults usually require between 0.6 and 0.9 units/kg/day, and pubertal children may require up to 1.5 units/kg/day because of relative insulin resistance, increased caloric intake during rapid growth spurts, and changes in hormone secretory patterns. After puberty, insulin doses should decrease to <1.0 units/kg/day to prevent excessive weight gain. Dose requirements for pregnant patients vary with gestational duration and are discussed in Pregnancy (page 161).

Careful balance of caloric and carbohydrate intake, activity, and insulin dose is required for an insulin regimen to be successful. It is most desirable to vary insulin doses to coincide with variations of food intake, activity, and prevailing blood glucose. On the other hand, if insulin dose is kept constant from day to day, food intake and activity should also be kept constant. The choice of insulin regimen should be based on individual characteristics, preferences, and habits, including age, stage of development, meal plans, and potential adherence to diabetes treatment. The diabetes management team should develop an acceptable and realistic treatment plan together with the patient/family. For example, an adolescent patient who is experiencing difficulties in following the treatment and has frequent episodes of hyperglycemia or ketoacidosis may have to be treated with two injections per day administered by a family member or visiting nurse until his or her problems are resolved. School can be used to administer one of the injections. On the other hand, the choice of insulin regimen should not be dictated by forces outside of the patient/family and health care team. For school-age children, the school must accommodate the delivery of a lunchtime injection of insulin if the child/family and health care team decide to use an intensive insulin regimen. Employed adults should similarly have flexibility for testing and injecting in the workplace.

After the initial dose adjustments, ongoing long-term adjustments are made on the basis of daily repeated blood glucose measurements or the use of CGM. Glucose levels should be assessed before meals, after meals, and at bedtime every day and periodically between 3:00 and 4:00 a.m. (perhaps once per week). With time and practice, patients and families are able to make the adjustments with relative ease and become progressively independent of the diabetes management team. This includes determining how to adjust the carbohydrate-to-insulin ratio and the insulin sensitivity factor used to calculate the amount of insulin needed to correct a glucose level above the target range. In addition to the long-term adjustments, insulin doses and waiting times between injections and food intake could be adjusted in response to high or low blood glucose levels, changes in food intake, activity level, or intercurrent illness. These adjustments can be made by patients who have been thoroughly trained and who can measure their blood glucose levels or use CGM and calculate dose changes precisely.

Patient education is time-consuming but essential and should be conducted by a skilled diabetes management team working together with the patient and his or her family. Many newly diagnosed patients will require an initial period of instruction of up to 10–12 h, with periodic review and follow-up sessions every few months until both patient and family feel comfortable with their knowledge and skills. Insulin regimens and blood glucose targets also should vary depending on the individual patient and should take into consideration the frequency and adherence to SMBG or CGM, the patient's ability to recognize and respond to hypoglycemic reactions, and the limitations imposed by what the patient and/or family are willing or ready to do. However, individualization should not prevent continued efforts toward the goal of achieving near-normoglycemia while avoiding severe hypoglycemia.

A frequent problem in the management of diabetes is the disappointment that sets in at the end of the honeymoon period when patients with or parents of children with type 1 diabetes realize that the efforts invested in the treatment are not rewarded by the achievement of normoglycemia. Often, minor deviations from treatment or even no deviations at all result in unexplained fluctuations of glucose levels. Because these fluctuations are part of the nature of type 1 diabetes, even under the strictest and most flexible treatment conditions, such as with the use of multiple injections and insulin pumps, it is helpful at diagnosis to warn patients and families that the treatment of diabetes is imperfect and that glucose fluctuations are to be expected. Adequate explanations about the unpredictability of blood glucose levels and their relationship to daily variations of insulin absorption, food composition and absorption, and changes in the level of physical activity often help to prevent the development of feelings of guilt and incompetence that can plague patients and families. A useful attitude on the part of the diabetes management team is to stress the importance of overall blood glucose control, such as assessing the mean glucose from meter or CGM readings, rather than individual values. However, if individual values are used, relatively wide fluctuations (70–160 mg/dL [3.9–8.9 mmol/L] preprandial, up to 200 mg/dL [11.1 mmol/L] postprandial, and between 90 and 200 mg/dL at bedtime and overnight [5.0–11.1 mmol/L]) can be suggested, even when narrower glycemic targets might be preferred.

INSULIN REGIMENS

General Principles

Normal insulin secretion is characterized by continuous basal release, with superimposed bursts of additional insulin integrated precisely to the rise in glucose after food intake. Additionally, insulin is secreted into the portal vein and approximately half is cleared by the liver before entering the general circulation. Ideally, exogenous insulin treatment regimens should mimic all aspects of this pattern. Unfortunately, with the available means of treatment, this is not entirely possible. Therefore, insulin treatment regimens represent varying degrees of compromise to achieve near-normalization of blood glucose levels, one of the most important goals of diabetes management. Ideally, insulin regimens should have both basal and bolus components to mimic normal insulin secretion.

The normal prandial burst of insulin is best mimicked by administering rapid-acting (insulin lispro, aspart, or glulisine) or short-acting (regular) insulin before meals at the appropriate time, depending on the blood glucose level. Prandial insulin typically comprises ~50–60% of the total daily dose. Advantages of rapid-acting insulin analogs over human regular insulin are convenience (injection before, at the time of or immediately after a meal instead of 30 min premeal), better postprandial control, and reduced risk of postprandial hypoglycemia occurring 3–6 h postinjection. Disadvantages of rapid-acting analogs are cost and inability to cover snacks without another bolus dose of insulin.

Basal insulin secretion comprises ~40–50% of the total daily insulin secretion. It can be mimicked best by giving long-acting insulin glargine or detemir once or twice a day or by delivering short- or rapid-acting insulin continuously by an insulin pump (continuous subcutaneous insulin infusion [CSII]). The basal insulin in CSII has the advantage of being variable and adjustable to cover the early morning rise in glucose levels (the dawn phenomenon) as well as periods of increased insulin sensitivity such as nighttime or during or after exercise. Compared to NPH, insulin glargine and detemir have the advantage of being relatively peakless. Insulin glargine has an onset of action of 1.5 h postinjection and mean duration of action being 23.5 h after several days of injections. As a result, clinical studies in type 1 diabetes have shown better fasting blood glucose with less nocturnal hypoglycemia than NPH once, twice, or four times daily. In ~20% of individuals, glargine lasts <20 h and may have to be given twice daily, usually in a 50:50 format. Insulin detemir achieves its longer duration by binding insulin with albumin and is injected once or twice daily. It has an onset of action between 0.8–2 h and a duration that is dose dependent lasting ~12 h at 0.2 units/kg and ~20–24 h at 0.4 units/kg. Disadvantages of glargine and detemir over NPH are that they are only basal insulins and do not cover snacks without a bolus injection, they cannot be mixed with other insulins in the same syringe, and they are more costly.

NPH can be used as a basal insulin and should be given twice daily at breakfast and bedtime. NPH has an onset of action ~2 h after the injection and produces peak levels ~6–10 h after injection. Morning NPH provides hyperinsulinemia, especially in mid- or late afternoon, when snacks may be needed to prevent hypoglycemia. Bedtime NPH provides progressive overnight basal hyperinsulinemia with peak serum insulins around breakfast time; giving the injection at bedtime rather than pre-supper reduces the risk of nocturnal hypoglycemia and may provide coverage for the dawn phenomenon. Long-acting insulin is given once daily before breakfast or at bedtime or twice daily at breakfast and bedtime or at breakfast and supper.

Starting Insulin Requirement

The starting insulin dose is usually based on body weight. On average, a patient will eventually require anywhere between 0.4 to 1.0 units/kg/day with higher amounts during puberty. It is best to start conservatively at 0.5 units/kg/day and increase insulin doses according to SMBG readings.

Two or Three Injections Daily

The twice-daily "split-mixed" insulin regimen (Fig. 3.1) was the most commonly used treatment regimen before results of the DCCT. Morning short- or rapid-acting insulin (regular or insulin aspart/lispro/glulisine) has major action between breakfast and lunch, and its effect is reflected in the prelunch blood glucose levels. Morning intermediate-acting (NPH) insulin has major action between breakfast and supper, and its effect is reflected in the presupper blood glucose levels. Evening short-acting insulin has major action between supper and bedtime, and its effect is reflected in the bedtime tests. The evening intermediate-acting insulin has its major action overnight, and its effect is reflected in the blood glucose level on arising the next morning. The evening intermediate-acting insulin can be replaced with long-acting insulin. The initial dose can be divided (based on % of total daily insulin) into a morning injection containing ~40% NPH and ~15% insulin aspart/lispro/glulisine or regular at breakfast, plus an evening injection containing ~30% NPH (or long-acting insulin) and ~15% insulin aspart/lispro/glulisine or regular at supper. In younger children, the proportions are closer to 80%/20% for both components.

The only advantages to this regimen are simplicity and a limited number of injections. The most frequent and serious disadvantage of this regimen is that, in many patients, attempts to achieve fasting normoglycemia result in nocturnal hypoglycemia (from midnight to 4:00 a.m.) and early morning hyperglycemia (from 4:00 to 8:00 a.m., due to the dawn phenomenon). In these cases, it is better to move the intermediate-acting insulin to bedtime and thus reduce the peak effect of insulin from 2:00 to 4:00 a.m. and increase it at dawn (Fig. 3.1B). In addition, post lunch hyperglycemia is often not controlled without the risk of daytime hypoglycemia from ratcheting up the morning NPH dose, and thus, an insulin injection at lunch or with an afternoon snack is often needed. Generally, it is not possible to achieve near-normal glycemic levels with two or three injections per day.

Multiple-Component Flexible Regimens

Basal insulin requirements typically account for ~50% (less in children and teens, closer to 35–45%) of the patient's total daily dose. Basal insulin may be provided as glargine, detemir, or NPH insulin or as a rapid-acting insulin with multiple-dose insulin programs or as a basal infusion of insulin analog with CSII (regular insulin is infrequently used in insulin pump therapy) (Fig. 3.2). The remaining ~50% (more in children and teens, closer to 55–65%) is given as prandial insulin, using a rapid-acting insulin analog delivered before meals and/or snacks either by syringe, pen, or an insulin pump bolus. Short-acting regular insulin is less frequently used in multiple-component flexible regimens. The amount of prandial insulin can be determined by calculating the insulin-to-carbohydrate ratio (discussed below) or by using a typical starting distribution of ~25% of the total daily dose as a rapid-acting insulin pulse before breakfast, ~10% before lunch, and ~20% before supper. These prandial boluses are varied based on the carbohydrate content of the meal as well as the actual blood glucose determined by SMBG at that time.

Glargine and detemir cannot be mixed in the same syringe with other insulin preparations. Another alternative is the combination of premeal injections (regular insulin or rapid-acting insulin analogs at breakfast, lunch, and supper, with NPH at bedtime; or with a small amount of NPH before breakfast (Fig. 3.3) or at every meal.

The combination of premeal rapid-acting insulin analogs with long-acting basal insulin (glargine or detemir) every 12 or 24 h is quite popular because, *1*) it offers flexibility in meal size and timing, *2*) it is very easily understood by most patients because each period of the day has a well-defined insulin component, *3*) the pharmacokinetics of analogs more closely mimics normal basal and prandial insulin secretion, and *4*) the introduction of insulin pens has made it very convenient. Bedtime administration of glargine or detemir allows the easy titration of the fasting glucose to normal with minimal risk of nocturnal hypoglycemia. If bedtime or presupper glucose levels are high with normal postlunch values and no afternoon snack, then consider the use of glargine twice a day. Another basal option is basal insulin only in the morning with titration to obtain the fasting morning glucose levels to be in the normal range. If this is not successful due either to daytime hypoglycemia or fasting hyperglycemia, then basal insulin should be given twice a day.

Continuous Subcutaneous Insulin Infusion (CSII)

The most precise way to mimic normal insulin secretion clinically is to use an insulin pump in a program of CSII. Pump devices provide continuous insulin administration to control blood glucose levels throughout the 24-h period. Because insulin delivery is continuous, it can more or less mimic normal insulin secretion. The pump delivers microliter amounts (as low as 0.025 units) of rapid-acting insulin on a continual basis, thus replicating basal insulin secretion (short acting insulin is rarely used in CSII). The basal rate may be programmed to vary at times of diurnal variation in insulin sensitivity. For example, the basal infusion rate may be programmed to decrease at night to avert nocturnal hypoglycemia and/or to increase in the early morning to counteract the dawn phenomenon. More than one basal pattern can be set if there are marked variations in insulin needs on different days (such as differences in activity levels between the weekdays and weekends, or for teenaged girls and women who experience a change in insulin requirements at different times in their menstrual cycle). Unique patterns of basal infusions may be needed by some patients, but most patients' circadian insulin requirements are met with two to four basal rates per day.

The pump is activated before meals to provide increments of insulin as meal "boluses" whenever a meal or snack is consumed. This allows total flexibility in meal timing. Meal boluses with rapid-acting insulin analogs are given 10–20 min before eating a meal. For small children with erratic eating patterns, the meal bolus may be delivered immediately after the meal when the amount of food consumed is known. A similar strategy can be used for the patient who is anorexic or nauseated (e.g., in early pregnancy or during illness). If a meal is skipped, the insulin bolus is omitted. If a meal is larger or smaller than usual, a larger or smaller insulin bolus is selected based on the carbohydrate content of the meal. Some pumps also offer variable bolus options including immediate delivery, square-wave delivery over a set amount of time (~2 h), or dual-wave delivery with both immediate and square-wave delivery together. Dual-wave delivery is useful for high-fat meals such as pizza and Mexican food, as well as for patients suspected of having gastroparesis. Frequent SMBG or the use of a continuous glucose monitor will help to determine the proper setting of the immediate and square-wave bolus. Thus, CSII patients have the potential of easily varying meal size, content, and timing, as well as omitting meals.

The ability to program insulin pumps also allows "suspension" of insulin delivery with increased physical activity, which serves to reduce the risk of exercise-related hypoglycemia. Caution should be taken regarding the duration of suspension of the basal insulin delivery because hyperglycemia and ketosis may rapidly supervene if insulin delivery is interrupted for >2 h. Switching to a reduced temporary basal for a set amount of time may be preferable.

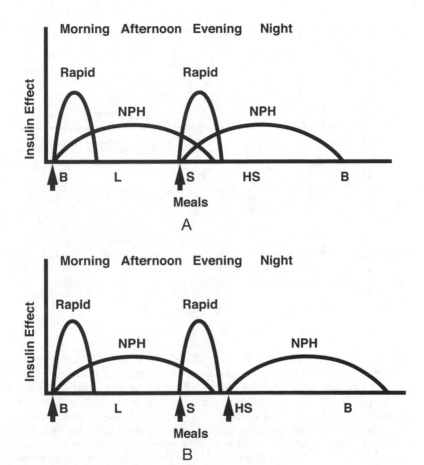

Figure 3.1 Schematic representation of idealized insulin effect provided by (A) "split-mixed" insulin regimen consisting of two daily injections of rapid- and intermediate-acting insulin given before breakfast and supper and (B) three daily injections with rapid- and intermediate-acting insulin before breakfast, rapid-acting insulin at supper, and intermediate-acting insulin at bedtime. B, breakfast; L, lunch; S, supper; HS, bedtime; *Arrow*, time of insulin injection, before meals.

Infusion pumps are relatively small, lightweight, portable, battery-driven devices; they are either attached directly to the body (patch pump) or worn on clothing or in a pouch (traditional pump). The patch pump is placed on the skin with adhesive and the small needle catheter is automatically inserted under the skin; after insertion they cannot be removed temporarily. The patch pump is controlled by a handheld personal digital assistant (PDA). The traditional pump is attached via plastic tubing to a small subcutaneous catheter that is taped to the

Figure 3.2 Schematic representation of idealized insulin effect provided by three daily injections with rapid-acting insulin at meals and once-daily insulin glargine or detemir at bedtime. Detemir sometimes is given twice daily (dashed arrow). B, breakfast; L, lunch; S, supper; HS, bedtime; *Arrow,* time of insulin injection.

skin; most of these catheters offer a quick-release device to remove the pump for such activities as swimming, contact sports, showering, sexual activity, or dressing. The devices on the market have such features as alarms for low battery, blocked delivery, and empty reservoir. Other options found in pumps include calculating meal or correction boluses based on insulin-to-carbohydrate ratio algorithms and insulin sensitivity factors, setting glucose targets, determining the amount of active insulin so as to avert hypoglycemia when giving multiple correction doses, alerting to recommend SMBG tests and changing the infusion sets at specified times, and wireless connections to blood glucose meters. Insulin pumps can be integrated with continuous glucose monitors. The information from the pump or PDA memory can be extracted for review of total daily insulin doses, number and timing of insulin boluses, carbohydrate intake used in bolus calculations, pump settings, and glucose levels from SMBG or CGM by the patient, family, and the health care team.

Treatment with insulin pumps is extremely effective in improving glucose control in patients with type 1 diabetes, particularly those motivated patients most interested in meticulous glycemic control. As long- and rapid-acting insulin analogs have been developed, however, multiple-dose insulin regimens have become increasingly comparable to pump therapy in terms of the ability to mimic normal physiology. However, the results of a meta-analysis of 12 randomized controlled trials comparing pumps to optimized MDI showed less insulin is used and glycemic control is better during pump therapy. Although the difference is small, it should be sufficient to reduce risk of microvascular disease. Disadvantages of pump therapy include cost and the need to overcome the psychological aversion some patients

Figure 3.3 Schematic representation of idealized insulin effect provided by three daily injections with rapid-acting insulin at meals and two daily injections of intermediate-acting insulin at breakfast and at bedtime. B, breakfast; L, lunch; S, supper; HS, bedtime; *Arrow,* time of insulin injection.

have to "always being hooked to something." In addition, due to the short duration of rapid-acting analogs and the lack of a subcutaneous depot of basal insulin, patients on pump therapy can develop severe hyperglycemia or ketosis rapidly with interruption of insulin delivery (such as kinking or disconnection of the subcutaneous cannula, empty insulin reservoir, or pump malfunction). Such episodes can be prevented or averted quickly with proper attention and education. Indications for CSII are listed in Table 3.3.

On initiating CSII therapy, the patient must receive instruction from the diabetes management team, including

- accurate monitoring of capillary blood glucose before each meal, after each meal, at bedtime, and at mid-sleep
- knowing safe blood glucose targets during the day and night and the duration of active insulin to avoid hypoglycemia, the most frequent complication of intensive therapy
- learning strategies to reduce the risk of nocturnal hypoglycemia, if it ensues, including increasing the target fasting blood glucose to 100–140 mg/dL (5.6–7.8 mmol/L), decreasing the basal rate if 3:00 a.m. blood glucose levels are <80 mg/dL (<4.4 mmol/L), and daily measurements of blood glucose levels at bedtime followed by ingestion of carbohydrate (or carbohydrate in combination with protein and/or fat) or use of temporary basal rates if the values are ≤100 mg/dL (≤5.5 mmol/L)
- understanding how to avoid hypoglycemia during and after exercise by suspending or decreasing basal insulin infusion and/or ingesting additional carbohydrate

Figure 3.4 Schematic representation of idealized insulin effect provided by continuous subcutaneous insulin infusion (insulin pump) with rapid analog. B, breakfast; L, lunch; S, supper; HS, bedtime. *Arrow,* time of insulin bolus, at meals.

- caring for infusion site with changes of the catheter every 2–3 days to avoid infection and inflammation
- understanding the urgency of preventing or reversing hyperglycemic crises from insulin underdelivery by taking the following steps with detection of moderate unexplained hyperglycemia: monitoring urine or blood ketones, changing the infusion set or taking an insulin injection immediately, contacting the medical team for persistent problems, and troubleshooting the reasons for insulin underdelivery (crimped cannula, leaking, obstruction, pump failure) after correcting the hyperglycemia
- knowing how to contact experienced medical personnel by phone 24 hours per day, 7 days per week
- having the constant presence of a relative or friend until the patient becomes familiar with the pump

The initial programming of the pump is based on the total daily insulin dose of the previous regimen. Approximately 35–50% of the total dose is given as the basal rate, and the rest is divided between breakfast, lunch, supper, and snacks. For insulin-to-carbohydrate ratio, divide 450 by the average total daily insulin dosage, and for insulin sensitivity factor, divide 1700 (or 1500 if more insulin resistant) by the average total daily insulin dosage. The patient is generally started with a single basal rate over a 24-h period. Bedtime snacks are not given until the basal rate is correct overnight. The basal rate is adjusted every second or third day on the basis of the blood glucose levels at bedtime, mid-sleep, and on rising until the desired blood glucose target is obtained. Increments should be in the order of 10–15% or 0.1 units/h (or 0.025–0.05 units/h for young children). In the case of nocturnal hypoglycemia, basal rate should be lowered starting 2–3 h before the

Table 3.3 Indications for Insulin Pump Therapy (CSII)

■Inadequate glycemic control, defined as:
  ◆ A1C above target (>7.0% nonpregnant, >6.5% if planning pregnancy, >6.0% if pregnant)
  ◆ Dawn phenomenon with fasting glucose >140 mg/dL (>8 mmol/L)
  ◆ Marked variability in glucose levels on a day-to-day basis

■History of severe hypoglycemia or hypoglycemia unawareness

■Desire for flexibility in lifestyle (e.g., shift worker, traveler, or worker in safety-sensitive job, student, erratic schedule day to day)

■Commitment to frequent SMBG or CGM and skilled in intensive diabetes management

time of the hypoglycemic event. Patients exhibiting the dawn phenomenon may require increased basal rates in the early morning hours starting 2–3 h before waking and lasting 4–6 h. Children may have a reverse dawn phenomenon requiring higher basal rates between 10:00 p.m. and 2:00 a.m. Basal rates are adjusted during the day by delaying meals to determine if the blood glucose levels rise or fall >30 mg/dL (>1.7 mmol/L) during that time. Daytime basal rates for those on rapid-acting analogs can often be determined by observing late postprandial glucose patterns (for example, pre-lunch and pre-supper glucose levels, when the effects of the prior meal bolus are no longer in effect) or by skipping a meal and seeing the effect of basal rates alone.

Even when a patient's initial commitment persists, the use of pumps may be associated with various problems. These include local inflammation at catheter sites from infection or tape irritation, pump breakdown and/or malfunction, forgetting to refill reservoirs on time, or forgetting to give meal boluses. Appropriate education in troubleshooting hyperglycemia, hypoglycemia, as well as other problems must be provided. Many of the problems with CSII of the past have been solved; there is less local irritation at insertion sites and less insulin precipitation, there are more programmable features to calculate bolus doses and duration of active insulin, and more alerts, and pump therapy can be combined with CGM. As a result, pump therapy continues to increase in patients of all ages. Once initiated, most patients remain on CSII, and although there are no large-scale randomized trials, except for sensor augmented pump studies, clinical reports and experience suggest that patients (including toddlers and young children) have improved glycemic control, less hypoglycemia, and improved quality of life.

Insulin pumps coupled with CGM and control algorithms are now able to have automation of some aspects of insulin delivery. For example, insulin delivery can be suspended automatically after a pre-set glycemic threshold has been reached, referred to as the "low glucose suspend" feature. This feature appears to be able to reduce time spent in hypoglycemia without increasing hyperglycemia. Predictive algorithms are being evaluated that will suspend insulin prior to reaching the threshold to prevent, not just reduce, hypoglycemia. These automated steps are part of the "artificial pancreas" that someday may allow for the full automation of insulin delivery.

ALTERNATIVE INSULIN DELIVERY SYSTEMS

Multiple alternative methods for delivering insulin into the bloodstream have either been developed or are under development and investigation. These include pulmonary insulin delivered through inhalation, peritoneal insulin delivered via implantable pumps, and transdermal and buccal insulin delivery.

Pulmonary delivery of insulin in humans was initially reported in 1925, with further studies in the 1970s and 1980s confirming the feasibility of administering insulin by the aerosol route. In these studies, ~10–30% of the insulin inhaled was absorbed into the circulation and the aerosols appeared to be well tolerated. The first pulmonary insulin preparation was approved by the FDA in January 2006, but was subsequently removed from the market by the manufacturer in late 2007 for financial/business reasons. However, many other preparations remain under development.

Studies in patients with type 1 or type 2 diabetes have shown that inhaled insulin is absorbed more rapidly than subcutaneous regular insulin and as quickly or quicker than rapid-acting insulin (aspart/lispro). The bioavailability of inhaled insulin relative to subcutaneous regular insulin is ~10% with all the current inhaled systems in development except for technosphere insulin, which has ~30% bioavailability. The intrasubject variability of inhaled insulin is comparable to subcutaneous regular insulin. Studies in smokers and chronic obstructive pulmonary disease patients have shown enhanced absorption of inhaled insulin, with studies in asthma patients showing some decreased absorption.

Results of studies in patients with rhinovirus infection have been mixed, with most showing no substantial change in the pharmacokinetics of inhaled insulin. Results from studies of the use of inhaled pulmonary insulin have shown that they are as effective as subcutaneous insulin regimens in type 1 and type 2 diabetes patients. Quality of life and treatment satisfaction assessments have shown inhaled insulin therapy is preferred over subcutaneous insulin therapy by many patients. The most frequently reported adverse event is hypoglycemia. Mild changes in pulmonary function have been reported but have been felt to be reversible and of little clinical significance.

Continuous peritoneal insulin infusions via programmable implantable insulin pumps have been used for over 20 years, although only in research settings in the US. Intraperitoneal insulin is rapidly and predictably absorbed into the portal circulation, simulating physiologic insulin delivery and absorption. Such rapid and predictable absorption may avoid the peripheral hyperinsulinemia seen with subcutaneous insulin regimens and the theoretical risk of accelerated atherosclerosis. Clinical studies have proven implantable pump therapy to be safe and effective for achieving glycemic control (significant reductions in A1C, average glucose level, and glucose variability), decreasing the rate of severe hypoglycemia, and improving glucagon responses to hypoglycemia.

OPTIMIZING BLOOD GLUCOSE CONTROL

Physiologic insulin secretion in nondiabetic individuals involves *1*) meal-related increased insulin secretion initiated by neural and gut factors before the hyperglycemic stimulus that is responsible for tissue uptake and storage of nutrients, followed by a rapid return of insulin secretion to the baseline level, and 2) basal insulin secretion between meals and during the night to regulate amino acids and fatty acids in the fasting state and to prevent excessive fasting gluconeogenesis. It is presumed that only an artificial or bioengineered β-cell with continuous glucose monitoring and the administration of short-acting insulin into the portal circulation can replicate the function of the normal pancreas.

Proper diabetes management has the goal of approaching normal blood glucose levels without severe hypoglycemia. The preprandial plasma blood glucose levels will most likely be outside the desired premeal values of 90–130 mg/dL (5.0–7.2 mmol/L) and peak postprandial values of <180 mg/dL (<10.0 mmol/L). Safe middle-of-the-night values are in the range of 70–120 mg/dL (3.9–6.7 mmol/L). These targets are difficult to maintain safely except under very intensive programs with selected patients, although use of CGM has been shown to reduce hyperglycemia by 30%.

The implications of the DCCT findings are that optimal treatment should be offered to all patients. Such treatment has the goal of approaching normal blood glucose levels without severe hypoglycemia. This generally means a progression from two or three daily injections, to multiple injections or the insulin pump depending on the response to treatment. Critical in determining success are the patient's and family's priorities, abilities, and willingness to adhere.

To achieve near-normal glycemic levels, it is advisable to use algorithms for adjusting the dose and timing of insulin and meals based on regularly monitored blood glucose levels or continuous glucose monitoring. They also allow patients to adjust insulin dose in relation to amount and composition of food and exercise. Although flexible, such regimens tend to place a great demand on both patient and physician. The efficacy of insulin algorithms is predicated on

- reasonable and consistent adherence to carbohydrate counting
- adjustment of insulin based on SMBG
- appropriate dosing of insulin before the meal (in young children, the dose may be given immediately after the meal or split with some pre-bolus and the rest delivered once the total amount consumed is known)
- a regular pattern of activity and willingness to make adjustments for unscheduled activities

Algorithms are used to correct for a given glucose value based on the sensitivity factor or to adjust insulin dosing in anticipation of any blood glucose–altering factors, e.g., increased carbohydrate intake, most intercurrent stress, or changing physical activity.

Timing of Prandial Insulin

If using regular insulin, it is preferable to give the insulin injection 30–45 min before meals so that the peak corresponds to the postmeal glycemic peak, allowing for more optimal glucose disposal. If using a rapid-acting analog, the injections are given at least 15 minutes before eating. In very young children or persons with nausea, for whom it is not possible to estimate meal intake before eating, rapid-acting insulin may be given immediately after the meal or split with some pre-bolus and the rest delivered once the total amount consumed is known.

Insulin-to-Carbohydrate Ratios

Patients with type 1 diabetes should be encouraged to learn carbohydrate counting and to calculate their insulin-to-carbohydrate ratio (I:C) to enhance flexibility in their diet and improve postprandial glucose control. The I:C can vary, for example, between 1 unit insulin/5 g carbohydrate to 1 unit insulin/25 g carbohydrate. For young children, the I:C may be 0.25–0.5 units insulin for every 20–30 g carbohydrate. To determine the I:C ratio, the patient can either *1*) eat a fixed amount of carbohydrates with a meal, adjust the premeal insulin to obtain adequate postmeal glucose control, and then determine the ratio, or *2*) start with an estimated ratio and adjust it based on the resulting patterns of postprandial glucose concentrations to obtain adequate postmeal control. The I:C can be determined by a statistically established formula initially: I:C is estimated at 450 divided by the total daily dose (TDD) of insulin. For example, the initial estimate of I:C for a patient taking 25 units of insulin per day would be 18 (1 unit of insulin per 18 grams of carbohydrate). Subsequently, the I:C can be adjusted by 2–5 g carbohydrates at a time based on analysis of postprandial glucose records. The I:C is usually the same at all meals but may be higher (1 unit of insulin to more carbohydrate) in the morning because of insulin resistance at that time or lower at bedtime. I:C can also change when there are changes in body weight or the total daily insulin dose.

Correction Bolus Algorithms

All patients on insulin should be provided with correction bolus algorithms to correct out-of-range glucose values. To do this, the insulin sensitivity, or correction factor (CF), must be determined for each patient. The insulin CF is defined as the estimated number of mg/dL (mmol/L) the blood glucose will drop over a 2- to 4-h period following administration of 1 unit rapid-acting insulin. Once this factor is determined, a corrective bolus or supplemental dose can be estimated and added to the normal premeal dose or can be given at other times to correct hyperglycemia.

The CF can be determined by using the "1700 rule," in which CF = 1700/TDD. For example, if a patient's TDD is 50 units insulin, the CF = 1700/50 = 35. In this case, 1 unit insulin should lower the patient's blood glucose level by 35 mg/dL (2 mmol/L). The CF can be used to calculate an individual's supplemental or correction bolus dose, where

correction dose = (actual blood glucose [BG] – midtarget BG)/CF.

For most people, midtarget blood glucose is 100 mg/dL (5.5 mmol/L). However, patients prone to hypoglycemia may have a higher target (120 mg/dL [6.7 mmol/L]), and pregnant patients may have a lower target (80 mg/dL [4.4 mmol/L]). The correction dose is added to the premeal dose to optimize postmeal glucose levels. When this is done, it is best to give the dose at least 15–30 minutes before the meal to start correcting hyperglycemia before eating. A patient's CF and correction dose are adjusted upon review of the SMBG records. The correction dose is also used in sick-day management for correcting hyperglycemia. Because of overlapping dosing effect when insulin is given again in less than 4 h, the target glucose should be increased to 140 when dosing at 2 h, i.e.,

correction dose = (BG – 140)/CF.

With CSII, active insulin or insulin on board will help prevent insulin stacking.

Glycemic Targets and Insulin Adjustments

Adjustments of the insulin doses are made on the basis of SMBG measurements and are aimed at achieving target blood glucose values. Target glucose values are individualized based on the patient's ability to detect hypoglycemia and his or her current state of health. In most cases, targets are the normal values of a person without diabetes. If a child or a person has a proven problem coping with hypoglycemia, the target may be set higher. If the patient is pregnant, the target is set toward normal values for a pregnant woman without diabetes.

Adjustments of insulin should be made with care to avoid hypoglycemia and overinsulinization. Dose adjustments should generally not surpass 1–2 units (decreases or increases) and should be made only when patterns of out-of-range glucose levels occur at the same time of day and are not attributed to transient changes in activity, food intake, or erroneous insulin injection. Ideally, adjustments upward should be made every 2–3 days for short- or rapid-acting insulin and every 3–5 days for long-acting insulin until the desired blood glucose targets are achieved. Adjustments downward should be made the next day for unexplained hypoglycemia, especially if severe.

There are different ways to achieve treatment targets. One method is to change the basal insulin to normalize the morning blood glucose level while avoiding hypoglycemia at 1:00–3:00 a.m. Basal insulin during the day can best be adjusted when the patient delays or skips a meal and no food intake has occurred for a minimum of 4 h. Glucose levels should not fluctuate more or less than 30 mg/dL. Bolus insulin is adjusted based on the postmeal glucose values if using rapid-acting analogs or the glucose values prior to the next meal if using regular. Once blood glucose levels are normalized postmeal after a known amount of carbohydrates for that meal, an I:C can be calculated for that mealtime. Correction bolus algorithms are also adjusted if the glycemic response does not bring the glucose into the desired range. If the glycemic response consistently remains above target range, the insulin CF is lowered. If the glycemic response is too great and the glucose falls below target range, the insulin CF is increased.

Treatment options should be individualized according to meal plan, exercise, patient preferences, and lifestyle requirements. SMBG or CGM should be used frequently to profile glycemic values and to adjust therapy. Optimal type 1 therapy requires a high degree of knowledge, time, and commitment on the part of the patient, the family, and the diabetes management team. Insulin pump therapy requires even more rigorous adherence to SMBG or CGM and other aspects of management and careful coordination by a team of experienced professionals.

Barriers to Adherence

Even with initial commitment to intensified insulin therapy from the patient and diabetes management team, problems can arise. When the goals of the patient and the diabetes management team are not congruent, attempts at intensive insulin therapy are problematic. Patients may become frustrated by the normal variability of glucose levels in type 1 diabetes, despite their best efforts. Clinicians should be alert for signs of "diabetes burnout," eating disorders, or depression.

COMMON PROBLEMS IN LONG-TERM THERAPY

Problems with insulin therapy arise regardless of the insulin regimen, and they must be addressed. Detecting and eliminating patterns of hypoglycemia and hyperglycemia are the cornerstone of caring for patients with diabetes. This is as true for the individual with diabetes of several years' duration as for the newly diagnosed patient.

Recurrent moderate or severe hypoglycemic reactions signal the need for evaluation of the insulin regimen, eating and exercise patterns, other diseases or autoimmune disorders (celiac, Addison's, thyroiditis) and other lifestyle factors (e.g., alcohol consumption). Exceptionally low A1C levels may identify patients at risk for moderate and/or severe hypoglycemia. Some patients have diminished symptoms of impending hypoglycemia (hypoglycemia unawareness) and, thus, suffer from recurrent hypoglycemic reactions and/or hypoglycemic seizures. Hypoglycemia unawareness is more common with longer duration of diabetes. It also can be exacerbated by antecedent hypoglycemia and conversely partially reversed by stringent avoidance of hypoglycemia. In patients with hypoglycemia unawareness, blood glucose targets must be increased, and insulin pump therapy and use of continuous glucose monitoring should be considered.

Fasting hyperglycemia may occur due to either over- or under-insulinization overnight. If glucose levels between 2:00 and 4:00 a.m. reveal nocturnal hypo-glycemia, rebound hyperglycemia (Somogyi effect) may be operative, although blood glucose levels >200 mg/dL (>11.1 mmol/L) usually do not occur unless carbohydrates are given to treat hypoglycemia. In this case, a decrease in eve-ning intermediate- or long-acting insulin or overnight basal rates on the pump is needed. However, if no nocturnal hypoglycemia can be documented, inadequate insulin in the early morning hours, due to the dawn phenomenon and/or too little basal insulin at night may be causative. This should be addressed with either an increase in presupper or bedtime insulin or a change from a presupper injection to a bedtime injection schedule. If this fails, insulin pump therapy needs to be considered with appropriate titration of overnight basal rates.

Disordered eating and inconsistencies in food intake and/or activity, often associated with psychosocial factors, can be causes of unacceptable day-to-day glucose control and elevated A1C levels. Additional problems of insulin therapy, including changes in insulin absorption or sensitivity, surgery, hypoglycemia, and insulin allergy are discussed in subsequent parts of this chapter or in other chapters.

INSULIN ALLERGY

Allergic reactions to insulin are increasingly rare with the widespread use of human insulin. However, patients, particularly those with known atopic diseases, may exhibit local or systemic allergy to human insulin itself, protamine in NPH, or the low pH of glargine insulin.

Some allergic-type reactions may be transient or artifactual. Burning, itching, and hives at injection sites may result from improper injection technique (intra-dermal rather than subcutaneous injection or injection of cold insulin) or from localized allergic phenomena.

If symptoms do not resolve and the patient's injection technique is sound, a change from one brand or type to another may be in order. True anaphylaxis or severe asthma, although rare, occurs occasionally and should be treated according to well-established protocols (e.g., antihistamines, epinephrine). If changing insulin type does not result in improvement, antihistamines can be prescribed. If atopic phenomena continue or if systemic symptoms occur, consultation with an allergist or endocrinologist is recommended for alternative approaches, including insulin desensitization.

Local Reactions

Lipohypertrophy at the injection site is the most common local complication of insulin therapy. It is thought to occur as a result of insulin stimulation of fat cell growth; the exact incidence is unknown. Lipoatrophy is rare with human insulin. If it does occur, changing brands of insulin may help. If either lipohypertrophy or lipoatrophy occur, rotation of injection sites with avoidance of the affected sites is recommended.

Insulin Resistance

Immunological insulin resistance due to antibodies to insulin is exceedingly rare, particularly since the introduction of purified insulins and human insulin. If it is suspected in a patient with unexplained severe insulin resistance, i.e., >2 units/kg/day after correction of ketosis with intravenous insulin, insulin antibody titers should be obtained in a reliable research laboratory. If high, change in insulin brands and type of insulin should be considered. If problems persist, such patients should be seen by a consultant diabetologist experienced in the assessment and management of complex problems. Patients with insulin resistance due to high insulin antibodies sometimes improve with corticosteroid treatment or other immune suppression therapy. Apparent insulin resistance is much more likely to occur as the result of the patient's not taking insulin as prescribed or using insulin that has precipitated or aggregated from excessive shaking or heating.

SPECIAL CONSIDERATIONS

Exercise

Because physical activity offers numerous health benefits, it should be encouraged in every patient with diabetes. In anticipation of the glucose-lowering effects of exercise, e.g., 30–45 min of moderate to vigorous physical activity, it may be necessary to increase carbohydrate intake or decrease the insulin dose to avoid hypoglycemia during or after exercise. Exercise-related hypoglycemia results from increased glucose uptake and utilization by the exercising muscle. In the case of prolonged exercise (lasting >1–2 h), it is necessary to reduce the insulin dose because hypoglycemia can occur many hours after exercise. General guidelines for avoiding exercise-related hypoglycemia are given in Table 3.4.

■ A decrease in prebreakfast rapid- or short-acting insulin is recommended if exercise is done within 3 h of breakfast.

■ Decrease prelunch rapid- or short-acting insulin and/or morning NPH or exercise occurring in the late morning or early afternoon.

■ Decrease presupper rapid- or short-acting insulin in anticipation of exercise occurring after supper.

■ Suspend or decrease basal insulin delivery with the pump during and after strenuous exercise.

Management During Acute Illnesses

The increased secretion of counterregulatory hormones and decreased activity even in the face of reduced caloric intake or vomiting may increase insulin requirements. Blood glucose and urine or blood ketone levels should be tested frequently (e.g., every 1–4 h or each time the patient urinates). The physician should be contacted immediately for advice if prior written guidelines are not known by the patient or family member. The following guidelines, based on whether the patient is able to take food or liquids by mouth, are useful for managing a patient during an illness.

An illness not accompanied by nausea or vomiting (e.g., minor infection or trauma requiring bed rest). If activity is normal, give the usual dose of basal insulin plus a correction bolus every 2–4 h as needed according to the blood glucose and ketone tests. If able to drink or eat, give, in addition to the correction bolus, the meal bolus insulin to cover the carbohydrate consumed. If an I:C is not known, give ~1–1.5 units insulin for every 15 g carbohydrate consumed.

Table 3.4 General Guidelines for Avoiding Exercise-Induced Hypoglycemia in Insulin-Treated Patients

■ Measure blood glucose before, during, and after exercise.

■ Unplanned exercise should be preceded by extra carbohydrate, e.g., 15–30 g per 30 min exercise; insulin may need to be decreased after exercise.

■ If exercise is planned, insulin dosages can be decreased before and after exercise according to the exercise intensity and duration as well as the personal experience of the individual with diabetes.

■ Patients on pumps may suspend or decrease their basal rate during and after exercise.

■ During exercise, easily absorbable carbohydrate may need to be consumed.

■ After exercise, extra carbohydrate may be necessary and may be added to meals and snacks.

■ Athletes and those who exercise for fitness need specific instructions and training on self-management skills for exercise.

■ Exercise can cause hypoglycemia during the night and bedtime snacks or reduction in basal insulin needs to be considered.

Adapted from Berger M: Adjustment of insulin and oral agent therapy. In *Handbook of Exercise and Diabetes*. Ruderman N, Devlin JT, Schneider SH, Kriska A, Eds. Alexandria, VA, American Diabetes Association, 2002, p. 374.

If activity is reduced and the patient is confined to bed, caloric intake should be reduced by approximately one-third. The reduction in caloric intake compensates for the inactivity. The insulin adjustment is the same as for an illness without bed rest.

An illness accompanied by nausea, vomiting, or marked anorexia. Blood glucose and urine or blood ketones should be measured as soon as possible and every 2–4 h until the illness or situation has resolved. If there are initial aberrations of glycemia, repeat glucose measurements may need to be done hourly, The insulin dose must never be omitted, because this could lead to ketoacidosis. If glucose is >240 mg/dL (>13.3 mmol/L) and ketones are large, the patient should give a correction bolus by syringe, call the health care team, and consider emergency department care for probable diabetic ketoacidosis. If glucose is >240 mg/dL (>13.3 mmol/L) and ketones are not large, the patient can take a correction bolus every 2–4 h and drink noncaloric fluids until the situation has resolved. If on CSII, the infusion set and tubing must be changed and the correction bolus given by injection. If the glucose is <240 mg/dL (<13.3 mmol/L) and ketones are large, the patient can take a correction bolus or an insulin injection every 2–4 h and consume caloric fluids as tolerated until the situation is resolved. When in doubt or the situation is not resolving, the patient should contact the health care provider.

Vomiting that occurs after administration of the usual morning dose of insulin. Sips of sugar-containing fluids should be given every 20–30 min to maintain blood glucose levels between 100 and 180 mg/dL (5.67 and 10.0 mmol/L). If vomiting persists and blood glucose level falls to <100 mg/dL (<5.6 mmol/L), consider giving "low-dose" glucagon at 1 unit of mixed glucagon on the insulin syringe for every year, up to 15–20 units. This might be sufficient to resolve hypoglycemia and associated nausea/vomiting and allow for the ingestion of small amounts of sugar-containing fluids as above. If hypoglycemia persists, the patient may require intravenous glucose therapy. A subcutaneous injection of remaining dosage of glucagon, or if not previously given "low-dose" glucagon, a full dose of glucagon depending on age should be given at home before departing if the patient lives some distance from the hospital.

Whenever the patient is sick and has blood glucose levels >240 mg/dL (>13.3 mmol/L) and moderate or large ketonuria, the diabetes team should be advised immediately or the patient should be brought to the emergency room, because this could reflect impending ketoacidosis. Repeated vomiting lasting more than 4–6 h or accompanied by high fever, abdominal pain, severe headache, or drowsiness may require that the patient be evaluated by a health care provider to ascertain whether he or she has a serious infection, appendicitis, meningitis, or other condition requiring antibiotics, surgery, or intensive medical care in a hospital setting.

Treatment of Diabetes in Newborns and Infants

Transient or permanent neonatal diabetes (NDM) occurs before 6 months of age, including in newborn infants. Neonatal diabetes is a rare monogenic form of diabetes occurring in 1 in 100,000–500,000 live births. Affected infants are insulin deficient leading to hyperglycemia, dehydration, and ketoacidosis; neonatal diabetes can be mistaken for the much more common type 1 diabetes, but type 1 diabetes usually does not occur before 6 months of age. In about half of the cases of neonatal diabetes, the condition is lifelong and is called permanent neonatal diabetes, and in half, it is transient and disappears during infancy, although it can reappear later in life. Specific genes that can cause NDM have been identified.

Due to insulin deficiency, these babies usually suffer from severe intrauterine malnutrition and, therefore, are small for their gestational age. As a result of hypoinsulinema, and intrauterine growth failure, these infants must be treated with exogenous insulin and may require high doses of 1–2 units/kg/day. Insulin requirements are best established by starting a continuous intravenous insulin infusion at rates that provide at least 0.5 units/kg/day. Insulin treatment is simplified by using diluted insulins (e.g., a solution containing 10 units/ml) so that inadvertent overdoses do not occur. It is very important to dilute the insulin with diluents received directly from the manufacturer. After birth, some infants fail to gain weight and grow as rapidly as expected; however, appropriate diabetes management improves and may normalize growth and development.

Type 1 diabetes can start in infancy, usually after 6 months of age. To differentiate type 1 from a monogenic form of neonatal diabetes, antibodies should be obtained as well as specific gene analyses. The treatment of type 1 diabetes in infancy is similar to that described for the infant with neonatal diabetes. Insulin requirements vary, and care of these patients should be supervised by an experienced specialist. The type of regimen used must be individualized depending on the ability to control hyperglycemia without an excess of hypoglycemia, since both may be particularly detrimental to the developing brain. Many infants are placed on CSII with dilute insulin, since this treatment might best facilitate decreasing extremes of glycemic variability.

CONCLUSION

Type 1 diabetes is characterized by a progressive decline of insulin secretion until its disappearance 1–5 years after diagnosis. Thus, people with type 1 diabetes are dependent on insulin to survive. Insulin therapy should always be coupled with SMBG, monitoring of carbohydrate intake, and proper precautions for illness and physical activity. CGM should be considered as a method to improve glucose control. In this way, insulin therapy can be adjusted safely and effectively and individualized to age, lifestyle, eating habits, state of health, and physical activity. Effective insulin therapy helps the patient avoid extreme metabolic crises, such as hypoglycemia and ketoacidosis, achieve and maintain good glycemic control, and reduce the risk of diabetes complications.

BIBLIOGRAPHY

Ahern JAH, Boland EA, Doane R, Ahern JJ, Rose P, Vincent M, Tamborlane WV: Insulin pump therapy in pediatrics: a therapeutic alternative to safely lower HbA1c levels across all age groups. *Pediatr Diabetes* 3:10–15, 2002

Agrawal P, Welsh JB, Kannard B, Askari S, Yan Q, Kaufman FR: Usage and effectiveness of the low glucose suspend feature of the Medtronic Paradigm Veo insulin pump. *J Diabetes Sci Technol* 5:1137–1141, 2011

American Diabetes Association: *Intensive Diabetes Management*. 5th ed. Wolfsdorf J, Ed. Alexandria, VA, American Diabetes Association, 2012

American Diabetes Association: *Practical Insulin: A Handbook for Prescribers*. 3rd ed. Alexandria, VA, American Diabetes Association, 2011

Armstrong DU, King AB: Basal insulin: continuous glucose monitoring reveals less overnight hypoglycemia with continuous subcutaneous insulin infusion than with glargine (Abstract). *Diabetes* 51 (Suppl. 2):A92, 2002

Bode BW, Tamborlane WV, Davidson PC: Insulin pump therapy in the 21st century. *Postgrad Med* 111:69–77, 2002

Bolderman K: *Putting Your Patients on the Pump*. Alexandria, VA, American Diabetes Association, 2002

Bruttomesso D, Pianta A, Crazzola D, Scaldaferri E, Lora L, Guarneri G, Mongillo A, Gennaro R, Miola M, Moretti M, Confortin L, Beltramello GP, Pais M, Baritusso A, Casiglia E, Tienga A: Continuous subcutaneous insulin infusion (CSII) in the Veneto region: efficacy, acceptability, and quality of life. *Diabet Med* 19:628–634, 2002

Cersosimo E, Jornsay D, Arce C, Rieff M, Feldman E, DeFronzo R: Improved clinical outcomes with intensive insulin pump therapy in type 1 diabetes (Abstract). *Diabetes* 51 (Suppl. 2):A128, 2002

Davidson PC, Hebblewhite HR, Bode BW, Richardson PL, Steed RD, Welch NS, Johnson J: Statistical estimates for CSII parameters: carbohydrate-to-insulin ratio (CIR); correction factor (CF); and basal insulin. *Diabetes Technol Ther* 5:A28, 2003

DeVries JH, Snoek FJ, Kostense PJ, Masurel N, Heine RJ: A randomized trial of continuous subcutaneous insulin infusion and intensive injection therapy in type 1 diabetes for patients with long-standing poor glycemic control. *Diabetes Care* 25:2074–2080, 2002

Dunn FL, Nathan DM, Scavini M, Selam JL, Wingrove TG: The Implantable Insulin Pump Trial Study Group: Long-term therapy of IDDM with an implantable insulin pump. *Diabetes Care* 20:59–63, 1997

Hanaire-Broutin H, Broussolie C, Jeandidier N, Renard E, Guerci B, Haardt M-J, Lassmann-Vague V: The EVADIAC Study Group (Evaluation dans le Diabète du Traitement par Implants Actifs): Feasibility of intraperitoneal insulin therapy with programmable implantable pumps in IDDM: a multicenter study. *Diabetes Care* 18:388–392, 1995

Hattersley A, Bruining J, Shield J, Njølstad P, Donaghue K: International Society for Pediatric and Adolescent Diabetes (ISPAD) Clinical Practice Consensus Guidelines 2006–2007: The diagnosis and management of monogenic diabetes in children. *Pediatric Diabetes* 7:352–360, 2006

Henry RR, Mudaliar SRD, Howland WC III, Chu N, Kim D, An B, Reinhardt RR: Inhaled insulin using the AERx insulin Diabetes Management System in healthy and asthmatic subjects. *Diabetes Care* 26:764-769, 2003

Lepore G, Dodesini AR, Nosari I, Trevisan R: Both continuous subcutaneous insulin infusion and a multiple daily insulin injection regimen with glargine as basal insulin are equally better than traditional multiple daily insulin injection treatment. *Diabetes Care* 26:1321–1322, 2003

Linkeschova R, Raoul M, Bott U, Berger M, Spraul M: Less severe hypoglycaemia, better metabolic control, and improved quality of life in type 1 diabetes mellitus with continuous subcutaneous insulin infusion (CSII) therapy: an observational study of 100 consecutive patients followed for a mean of 2 years. *Diabetic Med* 19:746–751, 2002

Litton J, Rice A, Friedman N, Oden J, Lee MM, Freemark M: Insulin pump therapy in toddlers and preschool children with type 1 diabetes mellitus. *J Pediatr* 141:490–495, 2002

National Center for Biotechnology Information, National Library of Medicine, National Institutes of Health, National Institute of Diabetes and Digestive and Kidney Diseases. The genetic landscape of diabetes. Available at: *http://www.ncbi.nlm.nih.gov/books/NBK1667*. Accessed 29 March 2012

Phillip M, Battelino T, Rodriques H, Danne T, Kaufman F: Use of insulin pump therapy in the pediatric age group. Consensus statement from the European Society for Pediatric Endocrinology, the Lawson Wilkins Pediatric Endocrine Society, and the International Society for Pediatric and Adolescent Diabetes. Endorsed by the American Diabetes Association and the European Association for the Study of Diabetes. *Diabetes Care* 30:1653–1662, 2007

Pickup J, Matack M, Kerry S: Glycaemic control with continuous subcutaneous insulin infusion compared with intensive insulin injections in patients with type 1 diabetes: meta-analysis of randomized control trials. *BMJ* 324 (7339):705, 2002.

Rudolph JW, Hirsch IB: Assessment of therapy with continuous subcutaneous insulin infusion in an academic diabetes clinic. *Endocrine Pract* 8:401–405, 2002

Santiago JV, White N: Diabetes in childhood and adolescence. In *International Textbook of Diabetes Mellitus*. 2nd ed. Alberti KGMM, Zimmet P, DeFronzo RA, Eds. Chichester, U.K., Wiley, 1997, p. 1095–1122

Skyler JS: Insulin therapy in type 1 diabetes mellitus. In *Current Therapy of Diabetes Mellitus*. DeFronzo RA, Ed. St. Louis, MO, Mosby, 1998, p. 36–49

Skyler JS, Cefalu WT, Kourides IA, Landschulz WH, Balagtas CC, Cheng SL, Gelfard RA: Efficacy of inhaled human insulin in type 1 diabetes mellitus: a randomized proof-of-concept study. *Lancet* 357:331–335, 2001

Wolpert H (Ed.): *Smart Pumping for People with Diabetes: A Practical Approach to Mastering the Insulin Pump*. Alexandria, VA, American Diabetes Association, 2002

TREATMENT WITH AMYLIN ANALOG PRAMLINTIDE

Type 1 diabetes manifests with absolute insulin deficiency, and for the past 80 years, insulin replacement therapy has been the only pharmacological treatment available for this disease. Despite considerable advances in insulin therapy, such as the development of insulin pumps and, more recently, rapid- and long-acting insulin analogs, many patients with type 1 diabetes are still unable to achieve and maintain optimal glycemic control.

Among the clinical barriers that hinder the attainment of glycemic goals with insulin therapy alone are the increased risk of hypoglycemia, postprandial hyperglycemia, excessive glucose fluctuations throughout the day, and undesired weight gain. More recently, it has been recognized that pancreatic β-cells secrete another glucoregulatory hormone, amylin, which is normally cosecreted with insulin in response to meals. Consequently, the autoimmune-mediated destruction of pancreatic β-cells in type 1 diabetes results in an absolute deficiency not only of insulin, but also of amylin.

Amylin is a 37-amino acid neuroendocrine hormone that binds with high affinity to certain areas of the brain and complements the effects of insulin in postprandial glucose control. Specifically, while insulin is the major hormone in the regulation of glucose disposal (efflux) out of the circulation, amylin regulates the inflow of glucose into the circulation after meals. This is achieved by suppression of glucagon secretion and regulation of gastric emptying. In addition, amylin has been shown to reduce food intake and body weight in laboratory animals, suggesting that it may also act as a physiological satiety signal.

The findings that amylin is normally cosecreted with insulin, that it complements the effect of insulin, and that it is completely deficient in type 1 diabetes led to the hypothesis that amylin replacement may convey additional benefits to patients with type 1 diabetes when added to existing insulin regimens. Human amylin itself is not optimal for clinical use because of its insolubility and tendency to self-aggregate; thus, a soluble nonaggregating equipotent amylin analog, pramlintide, was developed.

Pramlintide is an adjunct to insulin therapy in people with type 1 or type 2 diabetes. Like insulin, pramlintide is given via subcutaneous injection. In short-term studies (days or weeks) of patients with type 1 diabetes, addition of pramlintide to insulin injections before meals reduced postprandial glucose excursions by at least 75%, regardless of whether pramlintide was used with regular insulin or a rapid-acting insulin analog. Adjunctive treatment with pramlintide reduced excessive glucose fluctuations over the course of the day, as demonstrated in a 4-week study with a continuous glucose-monitoring device in an intensively treated type 1 diabetes patient. Note that these effects were achieved with pramlintide doses (30 and 60 μg) that yield a plasma pramlintide profile similar to the normal postprandial amylin response in healthy subjects, indicating that the improvement in postprandial glucose control is achieved via physiological replacement of the absent amylin action. Additional studies in patients with type 1 diabetes have shown that the improvement in postprandial glucose control with pramlintide is attributable to both a correction of postprandial glucagon hypersecretion, thereby controlling excessive glucose output from the liver, and a slowing of gastric emptying, thereby controlling glucose inflow from the gut.

These pramlintide effects are entirely consistent with the known physiological functions of amylin.

In studies of 6–12 months duration in patients with type 1 diabetes, addition of pramlintide to preexisting insulin regimens led to a significant A1C reduction of ~0.3–0.5% compared to placebo and a doubling of the proportion of patients achieving recommended glycemic targets (A1C <7%). In a longer term study (29 weeks), the safety, efficacy, and dose escalation of pramlintide showed with mealtime insulin reduction, followed by insulin optimization. Pramilintide was shown to drecrease postprandial glucose excursions and weight, and with a decreased prandial insulin dose and without severe hypoglycemia.

This makes pramlintide the first pharmacological agent and hormone replacement other than insulin shown to improve long-term glycemic control in patients with type 1 diabetes. It is important to note that the glycemic improvement with pramlintide was not accompanied by the long-term increases in body weight and severe hypoglycemia typically seen when glycemic control is improved by increasing the dose of insulin. On the contrary, compared to placebo, pramlintide treatment was associated with a relative decrease in insulin use and reduction in body weight that was most pronounced (~1.5–3 kg) in overweight and obese patients (lean patients did not have unwarranted weight loss). Pramlintide treatment was generally well tolerated; the most common adverse event was mild nausea, which typically occurred during the first few weeks of therapy and dissipated over time.

In summary, amylin replacement with pramlintide elicits a combination of clinical benefits that addresses some of the unresolved challenges with insulin therapy in type 1 diabetes. Adjunctive therapy with pramlintide is useful for those patients with type 1 diabetes in whom there are excessive unpredictable glucose fluctuations, postprandial hyperglycemia, undesired weight gain, or repeated episodes of insulin-induced hypoglycemia that hinder the achievement of glycemic targets. The clinical benefits of pramlintide are achieved by replacing the action of a second, naturally occurring β-cell hormone that is deficient in type 1 diabetes. By better matching the rate of glucose inflow to the rate of insulin-mediated glucose disposal, pramlintide improves glucose control via a unique mechanism of action that is distinct from, and complementary to, the action of insulin and its analogs.

BIBLIOGRAPHY

Baron AD, Kim D, Weyer C: Novel peptides under development for the treatment of type 1 and type 2 diabetes. *Curr Drug Targets Immune Endocr Metabol Disord* 2:63–82, 2002

Buse JB, Weyer C, Maggs DG: Amylin replacement with pramlintide in type 1 and type 2 diabetes: a physiological approach to overcome barriers with insulin therapy. *Clinical Diabetes* 20:137–144, 2002

Edelman SV, Weyer C: Unresolved challenges with insulin therapy in type 1 and type 2 diabetes: potential benefit of replacing amylin, a second β-cell hormone. *Diabetes Technol Ther* 4:175–189, 2002

Edelman S, Garg S, Frias J, Maggs D, Wang Y, Zhang B, Strobel S, Lutz K, Kolterman O: A double-blind, placebo-controlled trial assessing pramlintide treatment in the setting of intensive insulin therapy in type 1 diabetes. *Diabetes Care* 29:2189–2195, 2006

Gottlieb A, Velte M, Fineman M, Kolterman O: Pramlintide as an adjunct to insulin therapy improved glycemic and weight control in people with type 1 diabetes during treatment for 52 weeks (Abstract). *Diabetes* 49 (Suppl. 1):A109, 2000

Levetan C, Want LL, Weyer C, Strobel SA, Crean J, Wang Y, Maggs DG, Kolterman OG, Chandran M, Mudaliar SR, Henry RR: Impact of pramlintide on glucose fluctuations and postprandial glucose, glucagon, and triglyceride excursions among patients with type 1 diabetes intensively treated with insulin pumps. *Diabetes Care* 26:1–8, 2003

Nyholm B, Brock B, Ørskov L, Schmitz O: Amylin receptor agonists: a novel pharmacological approach in the management of insulin-treated diabetes mellitus. *Expert Opin Investig Drugs* 10:1–12, 2001

Weyer C, Maggs DG, Kim D, Crean J, Wang Y, Burrell T, Fineman M, Kornstein J, Schwartz S, Guiterrez M, Kolterman OG: Mealtime amylin replacement with pramlintide markedly improves postprandial glucose excursions when added to regular insulin or insulin lispro in patients with type 1 diabetes: a dose-timing study. *Diabetologia* 45 (Suppl. 2):A240, 2002

Weyer C, Maggs DG, Young AA, Kolterman OG: Amylin replacement with pramlintide as an adjunct to insulin therapy in type 1 and type 2 diabetes mellitus: a physiological approach toward improved metabolic control. *Curr Pharm Des* 7:1353–1373, 2001

Whitehouse F, Kruger DF, Fineman M, Shen L, Ruggles JA, Maggs DG, Weyer C, Kolterman OG: A randomized study and open-label extension evaluating the long-term efficacy of pramlintide as an adjunct to insulin therapy in type 1 diabetes. *Diabetes Care* 25:724–730, 2002

MONITORING

Monitoring, performed by patients, families, and their diabetes management teams, is an integral feature of diabetes care. Specifically, results of blood or interstitial glucose monitoring are useful in preventing hyperglycemia and hypoglycemia, reducing glycemic excursions, and adjusting insulin and other medications such as pramlintide, diet, and exercise so that target blood glucose levels are achieved. Additionally, testing for urine or blood ketones provides an early warning sign of impending ketoacidosis.

PATIENT-PERFORMED MONITORING

Patients can manage their diabetes effectively and safely only if they are able to perform SMBG. In certain circumstances (infants, young children, hospitalized or incapacitated patients), monitoring may be performed by family members, school personnel, child care providers, and health care providers.

SMBG is a direct method of testing glucose that allows patients to determine their glucose levels anywhere (at home, school, or work) and to adjust therapy on the basis of accurate and timely results. To perform SMBG, a drop of blood is obtained from a fingertip or alternative site by use of a sharp lancet, usually with the aid of an automatic spring-loaded puncturing device. The blood is then applied to a chemically impregnated or electrochemical strip, and after a specified time, the result is quantitated and displayed on the meter. In most meters, the results, as well as additional data (date, time, and, in some cases, additional data entered by the patient, such as whether the reading is pre or postprandial), are stored in memory for later analysis.

Alternative site testing is available with some meters that need only a small amount of blood (<1 mL). Such testing, usually performed on the forearm but also possible at other sites (heel of hand, thigh), is reliable and correlates well with fingerstick testing in the premeal or fasting state but can have up to a 15- to 30-min lag if testing is done when glucose levels are changing rapidly (postmeal or with hypoglycemia). Therefore, it is recommended that patients be aware of this lag and not make decisions based on alternative testing at these times, but rather test the fingertip.

Many commercially available strips and meters have been evaluated and are relatively reliable and reasonably accurate. Lists of SMBG products are found in the *Resource Guide*, published annually in the January issue of *Diabetes Forecast*, the American Diabetes Association's magazine. With appropriate education, most patients can perform the technique successfully. However, office return demonstrations of the patient's skills and the use of quality control techniques at home are essential. Patients should be encouraged to bring their meters to every office visit to assess their accuracy and, if possible, to download the memory. Downloads have log book displays calling out values above and below target, mean values, pie charts, graphs, etc. Inaccurate measurements can be obtained with faulty meters, wrong coding of strips, unclean or wet hands, or use of control solutions instead of blood for testing. Using inaccurate measurements to make treatment adjustments can be more dangerous than having no measurements at all.

Frequency of SMBG

The frequency and timing of glucose monitoring should be dictated by the particular needs and goals of the patient. If the goal is to obtain near-normal glucose levels and prevent hyperglycemia and hypoglycemia and extremes of glycemic excursions, then most patients with type 1 diabetes should do a minimum of 4–6 tests per day (before meals to calculate prandial insulin doses and before bedtime to protect against hypoglycemia at night.) Additional testing after meals may be needed periodically or regularly to adjust prandial insulin doses. Testing before, during, and/or after exercise can help the patient avoid serious hypoglycemia (see Exercise, page 122). Adding a test periodically in the middle of the night is particularly important for patients who aim for near-normal blood glucose levels, those with unexplained fasting hyperglycemia, and for any patient during illness or after intense physical activity. Patients should vary testing times to learn about their blood glucose patterns over the entire day. Patients who are ill (Table 2.7), pregnant, or whose usual schedule has changed require more frequent monitoring.

Adjusting Insulin Dose

SMBG results are crucial in making appropriate insulin adjustments to optimize glycemic control and prevent hypoglycemia and avoid hyperglycemic crisis. Insulin dose adjustments are covered earlier in this chapter under the section Glycemic Targets and Insulin Adjustments. SMBG results are also used at mealtimes to calculate a correction bolus in addition to the meal bolus needed to cover that meal. Thus, most patients should be encouraged to monitor a minimum of 4–6 times a day (before and after meals and at bedtime and during the night), with additional monitoring at other times (during hypoglycemia, exercise, illness) to ensure safe and effective therapy. Since there is evidence that more monitoring improves glucose levels, it is not uncommon to see patients monitoring 8–10 or more times per 24 hours, either routinely or occasionally.

Pregnant women need to perform SMBG more frequently (8–10, or more, times daily) to adjust insulin doses to obtain stringent glycemic targets and to avoid hypoglycemia. As with other elements of diabetes management, the prescription for glucose monitoring must be individualized.

The value of SMBG is not limited to adjustments in insulin dose. Patients with suspected nocturnal hypoglycemia can check their blood glucose levels at 3:00 a.m. SMBG is a valuable educational tool to help the patient differentiate between symptoms truly arising from hypoglycemia or hyperglycemia and those from other causes.

Common Causes of Errors

Despite the relative simplicity of SMBG, the information is not free of errors. Many of the previous problems with SMBG have been resolved with test strips that do not require wiping, meters with built-in timers, meters with memory, and strips that do not require coding. The most common problems now with SMBG, independent of specific methodologies, include the use of an inadequate drop of blood on the strip, wet or dirty hands, use of the control solution instead of blood, or a poorly calibrated meter. These problems stress the need to provide proper patient education and training in SMBG. Finally, some patients report their results inaccurately, perhaps to please their spouses, parents, or diabetes management team with the right results. The use of meters that automatically store glucose results in an electronic memory may simplify the recording, reporting, and analysis of SMBG; these results should be downloaded before or during office visits. Faxing data or transmitting through emails, with proper precautions to protect patient privacy, saves considerable amounts of time and enhances compliance to SMBG and intensive diabetes management.

Successful SMBG

If the goal of SMBG is to improve glycemic control, the diabetes management team should ensure that the patient

- reviews results of glycemic patterns with the diabetes management team
- responds to the results by making appropriate changes in the insulin regimen
- receives the necessary psychosocial support and technical guidance
- monitors as frequently as recommended
- reads and reports tests accurately
- uses additional SMBG during intercurrent illnesses, exercise, traveling, and when routine not followed

To support successful glycemic control, there should be mutual efforts to maintain education, motivation, and adherence. Furthermore, it is essential for the diabetes management team to provide feedback by monitoring progress with A1C (eAG) tests every 3 months.

GLUCOSE SENSORS

Continuous interstitial glucose sensing is an adjunct to SMBG that provides additional data to optimize glycemic control and alarms to help prevent hypoglycemic and hyperglycemic crises. Several different systems have been approved in the US by the FDA, and others are in development. The devices that are available are calibrated by fingerstick SMBG measurements and then sense glucose in the interstitial fluid using glucose oxidase enzymatic methodology. Interstitial fluid has been shown to correlate well with blood glucose, and the glucose concentration in the interstitial fluid has been shown to reflect glucose concentrations and glucose dynamics in the brain. However, there is a physiological lag between the interstitial fluid and the blood. This lag is usually <5 min in the fasting or premeal state but can be up to 13 min in the postprandial state. As a result of the lag time and other factors, these devices are currently recommended for use as an adjunct to, not a replacement for, SMBG. The glucose trends and alarms/alerts, rather than the absolute glucose values, obtained from these devices are used to make therapy changes to optimize glucose control. For immediate therapy decisions, such as deciding on premeal insulin doses or treatment of hypoglycemia, patients should use the SMBG results. Most continuous glucose sensors can be worn for 3–7 days.

The original continuous glucose monitoring system (CGM) was used like a Holter-style monitor system and measured glucose continuously in interstitial fluid for up to 72 h. The data was not displayed to the patient in real-time, but was used by a physician or member of the diabetes team for retrospective monitoring and interpretation of the readings. To use this system, an electrochemical sensor was inserted by an insertion device into the subcutaneous tissue (usually the abdomen, buttocks, or back) and worn for up to 72 h. The sensor used in the original systems measured glucose every 10 s and provided an average glucose every 5 min for up to 288 readings per day. These readings were collected and stored in a monitor connected by a cable to the sensor. Calibration by fingerstick blood glucose measurements was done at least three times per day with entry of the value into the monitor. Patients were also instructed to keep a food diary and enter event markers for specific behaviors such as eating, insulin administration, exercise, and hypoglycemia symptoms. After wearing the device, the sensor was removed and the monitor was downloaded into a computer for further analysis and evaluation by the health care provider and the patient.

Retrospective (also called professional or blinded) CGM devices used now employ the same sensor that is used with real-time CGM, and instead of transmitting the interstitial glucose values to a monitor, the information is stored and downloaded to a computer program at the end of the sensor wear (3–7 days depending on sensor life). During the use of retrospective CGM, the patient must calibrate the sensor with SMBG and use SMBG to manage their diabetes. Patients are also instructed to keep a food diary and enter event markers for specific behaviors such as eating, insulin administration, exercise, and hypoglycemia symptoms. These systems are used one time or at repeated intervals to obtain continuous glucose monitoring information when the patient is not ready to wear a real-time device. The 288 glucose values per day can be used to determine the presence of hypoglycemia, particularly at night, the dawn phenomenon, and postprandial hyperglycemia. It is of particular value in those suspected of having hypoglycemia unawareness and can be used at the time of a change in the diabetes regimen, such as when switching from MDI to CSII. Retrospective CGM can also be used to help patients understand the effect of certain lifestyle choices, such as glycemic patterns associated with exercise or after the ingestion of specific foods. The uploaded data is displayed on a number of pages including a log book that calls out values above and below glycemic targets, individual tracings by day, mean glucose by day and time of day, pie charts, and area and percent above and below targets. Retrospective CGM is also used in research protocols to compare the glycemic outcomes between the groups being evaluated in the research study.

Real-time Continuous Glucose Monitoring System (CGM)

Continuous glucose monitoring systems are meant to be worn chronically or intermittently by the same patient and provide real-time as well as stored glucose data (which can be uploaded through a computer program for retrospective analysis). The system consists of a sensor, a monitor, and a transmitting device (which sends in real-time the signal from the sensor to the monitor). When CGM is integrated with an insulin pump, referred to as sensor-augmented pump therapy, the pump itself is used as the monitor and the stored glucose and pump data can be uploaded together. Real-time CGM systems have alarms for present high and low glucose levels, alarms for a rapid change in glucose value, and predictive alarms to warn of impending hypoglycemia and hyperglycemia.

The first linkage between sensor glucose and insulin delivery (an automated step in the path to the "closed loop" pump or artificial pancreas) is low glucose suspend. Low glucose suspend allows for suspension of insulin delivery when a low glucose threshold, determined by the patient and health care team, has been reached. Insulin is suspended for a maximum of 2 h; however, the patient may interrupt the suspension and resume insulin delivery at any time. Early data on the use of this system suggests that it decreases the time spent in hypoglycemia without increasing hyperglycemia. The predictive low glucose suspend feature uses a prediction algorithm to prevent, not just mitigate, hypoglycemia. In addition, investigators across the globe are working on closed-loop algorithms for nighttime, as well as fully closed-loop systems that would automate insulin delivery day and night.

Although originally there were only short-term and not rigorously controlled studies on CGM, there have been an increasing number of longer-term studies (6–12 month study phase with up to 12-18 month continuation phase) in adults and children showing that CGM is associated with reduced glycemic variability (less time spent in the hyperglycemic and hypoglycemic ranges) and improved glycemic control. In subjects with A1C < 7%, CGM usage has been shown to assist in maintaining target A1C levels while limiting the risk of hypoglycemia. These studies have also shown that the greater the sensor usage, the more the reduction in A1C levels. A recent meta-analysis of 6 randomized controlled trials involving 449 patients showed that CGM was associated with significant reduction in A1C. Those with the highest A1C and those who used sensors the most had the greatest reduction in A1C. The devices and sensors are expensive and may not be covered by third-party payors. However, the devices are increasingly being prescribed, especially for children and adults with severe hypoglycemia. In 2008, the ADA recommendation (level E, based on expert opinion) was that such systems may be a useful supplemental tool to SMBG for selected patients with type 1 diabetes, who have demonstrated they can use these devices.

Advances continue to be made with next generation glucose oxidase sensors being more accurate, smaller, more comfortable, and of longer duration. Research continues not only with this methodology, but with other methods to measure glucose in the interstitial fluid as well as in other parts of the body. The ultimate goal is to develop CGM methodologies that will replace SMBG and be reliable enough for the artificial pancreas.

KETONE TESTING

The ketone bodies acetoacetate (AcAc), acetone, and β-hydroxybutyric acid (β-HBA) are catabolic products of free fatty acids. Determinations of ketones in the urine and blood are widely used as adjuncts for both the diagnosis and ongoing monitoring of DKA. Measurements of ketone bodies can be routinely performed both in the office/hospital setting and by patients at home.

Urine ketone testing remains the most commonly used method to detect impending ketosis at home. Most urine methods use reagent strips containing nitroprusside that form a colorimetric reaction on contact with AcAc (and in some strips acetone), resulting in a purple color. Care should be taken not to use out-of-date strips. The strips are manually read as measuring negative, small, moderate, or large ketones. Urine methodologies do not measure β-HBA and are thus not useful in monitoring the response to DKA treatment, because AcAc and acetone may increase as β-HBA falls during successful treatment of DKA.

Testing for ketonuria should be a regular feature of sick-day instructions and should be done every time blood glucose levels are consistently >240 mg/dL (>13.3 mmol/L). The presence of persistent moderate or large amounts of ketones in the urine suggests the possibility of impending or established DKA and should prompt patients to adjust insulin as recommended or seek assistance by calling their health care provider. Note that positive urine ketone readings are found in up to 30% of first morning urine specimens from pregnant woman (with and without diabetes), during starvation, and after hypoglycemia.

Blood ketone testing is also available for home and office/hospital use. Most blood methods measure β-HBA, which is the predominant ketone in DKA. Reference intervals for β-HBA differ among the assay methods, but concentrations <0.5 mmol/L are considered normal, 0.6–1.5 mmol/L indicate the potential for DKA, and >1.5 mmol/L indicate high risk for DKA or that DKA is already present.

Specific measurements of β-HBA in blood can be used by both the patient and health care provider for the diagnosis and monitoring of DKA. Testing for blood ketones is not mandatory for either the patient or the health care provider because the patient can use urine testing to troubleshoot hyperglycemia and the health care provider can use measurements of serum CO_2, anion gap, and pH to diagnose and monitor DKA treatment. However, blood ketone testing is much more specific than urine testing and much quicker and easier than these hospital laboratory methods, and thus has a role in the prevention, diagnosis, and management of DKA.

PHYSICIAN-PERFORMED GLUCOSE MONITORING

Because blood glucose levels can fluctuate widely in type 1 diabetes, sporadic testing in the physician's office is not sufficient as the sole means of monitoring. Intermittent testing does not reliably predict glucose levels at other times or the level of chronic glycemic control. Laboratory glucose determinations by a calibrated meter or approved instrument can be performed, if needed, to validate the accuracy of patient-performed monitoring and meter accuracy.

Glycated Hemoglobin (A1C Test)

The introduction of the A1C assay has revolutionized the ability to follow glucose control over time. When hemoglobin and other proteins are exposed to glucose, the glucose becomes attached to the protein in a slow, nonenzymatic, and concentration-dependent fashion. The concentration of glycated hemoglobin best reflects the mean blood glucose concentration over the preceding 6–10 weeks.

This measurement is performed on a single tube of blood or with a fingerstick capillary sample, and when correctly performed by a reliable laboratory or certified kit, the test is unaffected by acute changes in blood glucose; therefore, the test can be performed at any time during the day.

The Diabetes Control and Complications Trial (DCCT) established the major role of glycemic control in the development and progression of microvascular complications in type 1 diabetes. Although glycemic control can be assessed directly by analyzing multiple blood glucose levels over time, the A1C is strongly associated with the mean of the blood glucose values and easier to obtain. However, factors other than just mean blood glucose have been shown to affect A1C; these include biological variation for glycation and glucose variability or instability. The contribution of glycemic variability or instability to A1C in studies derived from DCCT data appears to be minor. This suggests that glucose variability, particularly the instability of postprandial values, may influence outcome through other pathways, such as oxidative stress.

Assay methods. Many different types of glycohemoglobin assay methods were available in the past, differing considerably with respect to the glycated components measured, interferences, and nondiabetic range. Glycated hemoglobin A1C (A1C) has become the preferred standard for assessing glycemic control and, in 1996, the National Glycohemoglobin Standardization Program (NGSP) was formed to standardize the A1C test to DCCT values. Since then, A1C measurements in North America have been almost universally standardized to the DCCT assay range.

In recent years, the International Federation of Clinical Chemistry (IFCC) developed a new standard for A1C that results in a measurement of concentration (mmol A1C/mol HbA) rather than percent and a reference range that is different than the DCCT standard. Although small studies had suggested this to be the case for type 1 populations, a recent multicenter study in subjects with type 1, type 2, and no diabetes; of multiple ethnic groups; and on multiple types of diabetes therapies confirmed that there is a close association of A1C with the mean blood glucose over the prior 2–3 months across the entire study population.

Hemoglobin variants have the potential to cause falsely low or high A1C readings, especially with older assays. In 2008, only ~5% of assays done in labs in the US give spurious results with Hb AS or A1C. A list of assays and whether or not they are accurate in patients with hemoglobin variants can be found on the NGSP website (*http://www.ngsp.org/prog/index.html*). Additionally, patient comorbidities affecting red blood cell turnover (hemolytic anemias, chronic kidney disease) will make interpretation of the test difficult.

Utility. A properly performed A1C test provides the best available index of chronic glucose levels. Other glycated protein molecules can be measured for this purpose (e.g., glycated albumin or fructosamine), especially in patients with abnormalities of red blood cell turnover, but their role in clinical practice is less well established.

A1C testing is invaluable in identifying patients who have relatively high, average, or near-normal levels of chronic glucose control. Discrepancies between the A1C level and the results of SMBG may indicate that the latter is either inaccurately performed or fabricated, or that the patient has an interfering hemoglobinopathy or disorder of red blood cell turnover.

The measurement of A1C allows physician and patient to set objective goals for therapy and to measure the efficacy of changes in therapy. The usual frequency for performing this assay in type 1 diabetes should be four times per year.

A1C testing at the time of the patient's visit with immediate results at that time is available by several NGSP-certified instruments. Such testing allows the patient and physician to discuss the results at that visit and make immediate changes in treatment if needed to optimize glycemic control. Such point-of-care testing has resulted in a 0.5– to 1–percentage point drop in the A1C value. A1C testing by home NGSP-certified kits is also commercially available, but the value of such testing remains to be determined.

A1C can also be used to make the diagnosis of diabetes in adults, and likely children although this has not been confirmed. A value ≥6.5% is sufficient to suggest diabetes, while a value of ≥5.7–6.4% suggests prediabetes.

The GlycoMark blood glucose test measures monosaccharide 1,5-anhydroglycitol in the blood, which is a specific index of elevated postmeal glucose levels and short-term glycemic control. This test has proven useful in pharmaceutical research, as well as in patient care, when methods are being employed that specifically target glucose instability after meals.

OTHER MONITORING

In addition to monitoring for glycemia and A1C, patients need ongoing monitoring of fasting lipid profiles, urine albumin excretion, and kidney function, as further described in the Complications section and in the American Diabetes Association's Standards of Medical Care. TSH testing is recommended periodically for all patients with type 1 diabetes. Screening for celiac disease or other auto-immune diseases may be indicated in patients with signs or symptoms.

CONCLUSION

The appropriate application of SMBG techniques provides the patient with type 1 diabetes the opportunity to adjust therapy safely and effectively. The type and frequency of monitoring must be individualized and will be dictated primarily by the patient's lifestyle and the intensity of insulin therapy. A1C testing provides an objective index of long-term glucose levels and can be used to determine efficacy of treatment.

BIBLIOGRAPHY

American Diabetes Association: Tests of glycemia in diabetes (Position Statement). *Diabetes Care* 27 (Suppl. 1):S91–S93, 2004

Bergenstal RM, Tamborlane WV, Ahmann A, Buse JB, Dailey G, Davis SN, Joyce C, Perkins BA, Welsh JB, Willi SM, Wood MA and the STAR 3 Study Group: Effectiveness of sensor-augmented insulin-pump therapy in type 1 diabetes. *N Engl J Med* 363:311–320, 2010

Bergenstal RM, Tamborlane WV, Ahmann A, Buse JB, Dailey G, Davis SN, Joyce C, Perkins BA, Welsh JB, Willi SM, Wood MA and the STAR 3 Study Group: Sensor-augmented pump therapy for A1C reduction (STAR 3) study. *Diabetes Care* 34:2403–2405, 2011

Bode BW, Sabbah H, Davidson PC: What's ahead in glucose monitoring? *Postgrad Med* 109:41–44, 2001

Boland EA, Delucia M, Brandt CA, Grey MJ, Tamborlane WV: Limitations of conventional methods of self blood glucose monitoring: lessons learned from three days of continuous glucose monitoring (CGM) in pediatric patients with type 1 diabetes. *Diabetes* 49 (Suppl. 1):397, 2000

Chase HP, Kim LM, Owen SL, MacKenzie TA, Klingensmith GJ, Murtfeldt R, Garg SK: Continuous subcutaneous glucose monitoring in children with type 1 diabetes. *Pediatrics* 107:222–226, 2001

Cheyne EH, Cavan DA, Kerr D: Performance of a continuous glucose monitoring system during controlled hypoglycaemia in healthy volunteers. *Diabetes Technol Ther* 4:607–613, 2002

Diabetes Research in Children Network (DirecNet) Study Group; Continuous glucose monitoring in children with type 1. *J Pediatr* 151:388–393, 2007

Garb S, Zisser H, Schwartz S, Bailey T, Kaplan R, Ellis S, Jovanovic L: Improvement in glycemic excursions with a transcutaneous, real-time continuous glucose sensor: a randomized controlled trial. *Diabetes Care* 29:44–50, 2006

Garg SK, Schwartz S, Edelman SV: Improved glucose excursions using an implantable real-rime continuous glucose sensor in adults with type 1 diabetes. *Diabetes Care* 27:734–738, 2004

Jungheim K, Koschinsky T: Risky delay of hypoglycemia detection by glucose monitoring at the arm. *Diabetes Care* 24:1303–1304, 2001

Juvenile Diabetes Research Foundation Continuous Glucose Monitoring Study Group: Continuous glucose monitoring and intensive treatment of type 1 diabetes. *N Engl J Med* 359:1464–1476, 2008

Kerr D, Cheyne EH, Weiss M, Ryder J, Cavan DA: Accuracy of MiniMed continuous glucose monitoring system during hypoglycaemia. *Diabetology* 44 (Suppl. 1):A239, 2001

Klonoff DC, Buckingham B, Christiansen JS, Montori VM, Tamborlane WV, Vigerskky RA, Wolpert H: Continuous glucose monitoring: An Endocrine Society Practice Guideline. *J Clin Endocrinol Metab* 96:2968–2979, 2011

McCarter RJ, Hempe JM, Chalew SA: Mean blood glucose and biological variation have greater influence on HbA1C levels than glucose instability: an analysis of data from the Diabetes Control and Complications Trial. *Diabetes Care* 29:352–355, 2006

Nielsen JK, Djurhuus CB, Gravholt CH, Carus AC, Granild-Jensen J, Orskov H, Christiansen JS: Continuous glucose monitoring in interstitial subcutaneous adipose tissue and skeletal muscle reflects excursions in cerebral cortex. *Diabetes* 54:1635–1639, 2005.

Pickup JC, Freeman SC, Sutton AJ: Glycaemic control in type 1 diabetes during real-time continuous glucose monitoring compared with self monitoring of blood glucose: meta-analysis of randomized controlled trials using individual patient data. *BMJ* 343:d3805 doi: 10.1136/bmj.d3805, 2011

Sacks DB, Bruns DE, Goldstein DE, Maclaren NK, McDonald JM, Parrott M: Guidelines and recommendations for laboratory analysis in the diagnosis and management of diabetes mellitus. *Clin Chem* 48:436–472, 2002

Schiaffini R, Ciampalini P, Fierabracci A, Spera S, Borrelli P, Bottazzo G, Crinò A: The continuous glucose monitoring system (CGM) in type 1 diabetic children is the way to reduce hypoglycemic risk. *Diabetes Metab Res Rev* 18:324–329, 2002

NUTRITION

The effectiveness of medical nutrition therapy (MNT) in the medical management of type 1 diabetes is well established. MNT includes a comprehensive assessment of the patient's nutritional status, diabetes and health status, weight for height or BMI, lifestyle, support systems, and willingness and ability to make changes or initiate new behaviors. MNT is implemented in a nutrition care plan based on individual goals negotiated with the patient and monitoring and evaluation of goal-directed activities. Success and satisfaction are measured by goal achievement and improved metabolic and other health outcomes.

Managing eating is one of the most challenging aspects of diabetes self-management and requires knowledge, time, effort, and commitment from those involved. Although there are many other variables beside food that affect blood glucose levels, physicians and other diabetes management care team members often attribute poor glycemic control to a lack of dietary adherence. In the best-case scenario, all team members are knowledgeable about nutrition therapy and supportive of the person with diabetes who is struggling to make lifestyle changes. Because of the complexity of nutrition issues, it is recommended that a registered dietitian, knowledgeable and skilled in implementing diabetes MNT, be the team member providing MNT. Patients with type 1 diabetes should be referred when diagnosed, then routinely consult with a registered dietitian as part of the continuing medical care of their diabetes. Follow-up may be appropriate every 3–6 months for children and every 6–12 months for adults.

NUTRITION RECOMMENDATIONS

The American Diabetes Association has published evidence-based nutrition recommendations and interventions for diabetes. These recommendations attempt to translate research data and clinically applicable evidence into nutrition care. The Institute of Medicine's Food and Nutrition Board of the National Institutes of Health (NIH) has published dietary reference values for the intake of macronutrients. This report covers dietary reference intakes (DRIs) for energy, carbohydrates, fiber, fat, fatty acids, cholesterol, protein, and amino acids. Competing with the science-based recommendations are media and commercially generated nutrition recommendations based on misinformation, opinion, and a desire to sell a product or program. The target audience for these questionable products and practices is often individuals with chronic disease lured by the promise of a quick or easy solution.

The diabetes management team members must not only be knowledgeable about science- or evidence-based recommendations, but must also be aware of the latest health or nutrition fad or product in the marketplace. When applying scientific principles and recommendations, team members will continue to focus on the patient's individual circumstances and preferences. The patient is the central team member and the one who most actively manages his or her diabetes.

The Nutrition Prescription

The "ADA Diet" as a formulated prescription of calorie and macronutrient composition has been replaced by an individualized nutrition prescription based on nutrition assessment and treatment goals. Specific goals of diabetes MNT are to

- achieve and maintain
  - blood glucose levels in the normal range or as close to normal as is safely possible
  - a lipid and lipoprotein profile that reduces the risk for vascular disease
  - blood pressure levels in the normal range or as close to normal as is safely possible
- prevent, or at least slow, the rate of development of the chronic complications of diabetes by modifying nutrient intake and lifestyle
- address individual nutritional needs, taking into account personal and cultural preferences and willingness to change

Additional MNT goals for specific situations include

- for youth with type 1 diabetes, pregnant and lactating women, and older adults, to meet the nutritional needs of these unique times in the life cycle
- for all type 1 patients, to provide self-management training for safe conduct of exercise, including the prevention and treatment of hypoglycemia, and diabetes treatment during acute illness

Nutrition recommendations advise that macronutrient composition and distribution be individualized to achieve desired metabolic outcomes (Table 3.5).

Table 3.5 Nutrition Recommendations: Historical Perspective

Year	Distribution of Calories		
	Carbohydrate (%)	Protein (%)	Fat (%)
Before 1921	Starvation diets		
1921	20	10	70
1950	40	20	40
1971	45	20	35
1986	50–60	12–20	30
1994	A	10–20	A, B
2002	A, C	15–20*	A, B, C, D
2008	A	15–20 E = saturated fat < 7%	

A, based on nutrition assessment; B, <10% saturated fat; C, carbohydrate and monounsaturated fatty acids together = 60–70% energy intake; D, minimize intake of trans fatty acids.
*If renal function is normal.

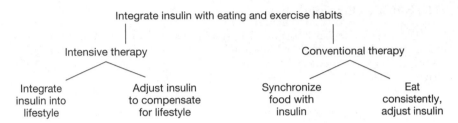

Figure 3.5 Medical nutrition therapy for type 1 diabetes.

NUTRITION THERAPY FOR TYPE 1 DIABETES

Nutritional management of type 1 diabetes requires careful attention to the glycemic effect of foods to contain postprandial blood glucose excursions, maximize the effectiveness of exogenous insulin, and minimize hypoglycemia. MNT also must provide for optimal growth and development of the individual and reduce nutrition-related health risks. Although individuals with diabetes have the same nutritional needs as individuals without diabetes, the amount and type of food and coordination with insulin delivery directly affect blood glucose levels.

Insulin Regimens

Individuals on multiple daily injections (MDIs) of insulin or CSII therapy, i.e., insulin pumps, should adjust their premeal short- or rapid-acting insulin based on the total amount of carbohydrate in their meals. Those receiving fixed daily insulin doses should emphasize consistency of daily carbohydrate content at meals and snacks. Along with the type of insulin regimen, the nutrition care plan addresses caloric requirements, macro- and micronutrient intake, the glycemic effect of foods and meal patterns, lifestyle, exercise, overall health status, and patient goals.

Caloric Requirements

Calories should be prescribed to achieve and maintain reasonable body weight in all patients and normal linear growth for children. Note that reasonable weight is defined as the weight an individual and health care provider acknowledge as achievable and maintainable, both short and long term. This may not be the same as traditionally defined desirable or ideal body weight. In addition to weight, body mass index (BMI, weight in kg/height in meters squared) may also be measured with the goal of having a healthy BMI, out of the obese and overweight range. Daily caloric requirements vary depending on age, gender, body size, and activity patterns. Additional calories are needed to promote growth during childhood, adolescence, pregnancy, and lactation and for catabolic illnesses.

The Estimated Energy Requirement (EER) is defined by the Food and Nutrition Board of the Institute of Medicine as "the dietary energy intake that is predicted to maintain energy balance in a healthy individual of a defined age,

Table 3.6 Estimating Adult Daily Energy Needs

Adults

Basal calories	20–25 kcal/kg desirable body wt 25–35 kcal/kg for catabolic illness	
Add calories for activity	If sedentary	30% more calories
	If moderately active	50% more calories
	If strenuously active	100% more calories
Adjustments	Add 500 kcal/day to gain 1 lb/week Subtract 500 kcal/day to lose 1 lb/week Pregnancy: add 340 kcal/day during 2nd trimester, 452 kcal/day during 3rd trimester* Lactation: add 330 kcal/day during 1st 6 months, 400 kcal/day during 2nd 6 months*	

Adapted from Joyce M: Issues in prescribing calories. In *Handbook of Diabetes Medical Nutrition Therapy*, p. 368.
*Food and Nutrition Board Institute of Medicine: *Dietary Reference Intakes for Energy, Carbohydrate, Fiber, Fat, Fatty Acids, Cholesterol, Protein, and Amino Acids (Macronutrients)*. See Bibliography.

gender, weight, height, and level of physical activity consistent with good health." The Food and Nutrition Board has published several tables of EER for adults based on BMI and four physical activity levels: sedentary, low active, active, and very active. The board also published gender- and age-based EER tables for infants, children, and adolescents. These tables are available on the Internet from the National Academies Press website (see Resources for Professionals). Several other methods for estimating caloric requirements are available, including the Harris-Benedict or World Health Organization equations, which compute calories for basal or resting energy expenditure (REE) and then add activity calories to the basal requirement. Simple methods for routine use are outlined in Table 3.6. Accurate records of food intake offer another means for estimating energy requirements and provide useful information on food preferences and eating patterns. Adjustments in caloric intake will need to be made to promote growth, weight gain, weight loss, or weight maintenance. In addition to meeting energy requirements, the caloric prescription promotes a consistency in daily food intake that is helpful in managing type 1 diabetes.

Macronutrients

In general, recommendations for the macronutrient composition of the meal plan for diabetes correspond to guidelines for healthy eating for all Americans. The composition and distribution will be guided by the individual's needs and preferences.

Carbohydrate

The primary role of carbohydrates (sugars and starches) is to provide energy to cells in the body. The RDA for carbohydrate is set at 130 g/day for adults and

Table 3.7 Classification of Carbohydrates

Class	Subgroup	Components
Sugars	Monosaccharides	Glucose, galactose, fructose
	Disaccharides	Sucrose, lactose
	Polyols	Sorbitol, mannitol, xylitol
Polysaccharides	Starch	Amylose, amylopectin, modified starches
	Nonstarch polysaccharides (fiber)	Cellulose, hemicellulose, pectins, hydrocolloids

children and is based on the average minimum amount of glucose utilized by the brain.

Carbohydrate Classification

Carbohydrates are divided into categories based on the number of sugar units. The categories of greatest interest in diabetes care and education are sugars (monosaccharides, disaccharides, and polyols) and polysaccharides (starches and nonstarch polysaccharides [fiber]) (Table 3.7). The terms "complex carbohydrates" and "simple sugars" are no longer used. Intrinsic sugars are sugars that are present within the cell walls of plants (naturally occurring), whereas extrinsic sugars are those that are typically added to foods. Added sugars are defined as sugars and syrups that are added to foods during production and do not include naturally occurring sugars such as lactose in milk or fructose in fruits. Foods and beverages with a high added sugar content include soft drinks, cookies, cakes, pastries, and candy. These foods and beverages have lower micronutrient densities compared to those that are major sources of naturally occurring sugars. Current US food labels do not distinguish between sugars naturally present in foods and added sugars. Traditionally, sugars, particularly sucrose, have been restricted in diets for individuals with diabetes. However, studies show that this restriction is not warranted metabolically. The USDA Food Guide Pyramid guidelines allow for added sugars as part of discretionary calories once food is consumed from nutrient-dense food groups. Generally speaking, this would be <10% of calories for most calorie levels. Carbohydrates providing essential nutrients should receive first priority in food choices over selecting foods and beverages high in added sugars and low in nutrient density.

Healthy carbohydrates. Foods containing carbohydrate from whole grains, fruits, vegetables, legumes and dry beans, and fat-free or low-fat milk are important sources of vitamins, minerals, phytochemicals, and fiber and are preferred choices for carbohydrate-containing foods. Healthy eating programs such as MyPlate from the USDA, Fruits and Veggies, More Matters (previously Five a Day) program, and the Dietary Approaches to Stop Hypertension (DASH) diet encourage increased intake of fruits and vegetables, whole grains, and low-fat milk.

Glycemic effect of carbohydrate. The American Diabetes Association's position states that the total amount of carbohydrate in meals and snacks is usually the primary determinant of postprandial response, but the type of carbohydrate may also affect this response. A key strategy in achieving glycemic control is by monitoring carbohydrate, whether by carbohydrate counting, exchanges, or experienced-based estimation. The use of the glycemic index and load may provide a modest additional benefit over that observed when total carbohydrate is considered alone.

Individuals using MDI or CSII therapy should adjust premeal insulin doses based on the total carbohydrate content of the meal. Those on fixed doses of insulin should be consistent with their carbohydrate intake. There is widespread interest and controversy surrounding the concepts of glycemic index and glycemic load. See Fig. 3.6 and Fig. 3.7 for definitions.

Glycemic index. Glycemic index (GI) is a concept and meal-planning approach based on published tables ranking carbohydrate foods according to glycemic response (Fig. 3.6). The tables propose that, per gram of carbohydrate, foods with a high GI produce a higher peak in postprandial blood glucose and a greater overall glucose response during the first 2–3 h after consumption than do foods with a low GI. The International Table of Glycemic Index and Glycemic Load Values: 2002 contains 1,300 data entries representing 750 different types of foods tested. Study subjects included "healthy" volunteers and those with type 1 or type 2 diabetes. Type 1 diabetes subjects participated in the study of 17% of the foods included in the table.

"The glycemic index is a classification proposed to quantify the relative blood glucose response to carbohydrate-containing foods. It is defined as the area under the curve for the increase in blood glucose after the ingestion of a set amount of carbohydrate in an individual food (e.g., 50 g) in the 2-h postingestion period as compared with ingestion of the same amount of carbohydrate from a reference food (white bread or glucose) tested in the same individual under the same conditions using the initial blood glucose concentration as a baseline."

Figure 3.6 Glycemic Index: Institute of Medicine's Food and Nutrition Board definition.

"Thus, the GL of a typical serving of food is the product of the amount of available carbohydrate in that serving and the GI of the food." The GL values in the tables were calculated "by multiplying the amount of carbohydrate contained in a specified serving size of the food by the GI value of that food (with the use of glucose as the reference food), which was then divided by 100." Because portion sizes vary from country to country, researchers and health professionals are advised to calculate their own GL data by using appropriate serving sizes and carbohydrate composition data.

Figure 3.7 Glycemic load (GL): International Table of Glycemic Index and Glycemic Load Values: 2002 definition.

Table 3.8 Factors Affecting the Rate of Digestibility and Glycemic Response

Factors inherent in a food	Grain, particle size
	Amylose-amylopectin (starch) ratio
	Fiber content
	Enzyme inhibitors
	Physical interaction with fat or protein within a food
	Degree of ripeness in fruit
Factors related to preparation	State of hydration
	Raw vs. cooked
	Amount of food processing
Factors related to consumption	Addition of protein, fat, other foods
	Acidity of a meal
	Preceding meal
	Time of day
	Palatability
	Duration of the meal
	Rate of gastric emptying

The concept of GI seemed straightforward when it was first introduced as a research tool in the 1980s, but the use of GI in preventing and treating disease has created much controversy. Proponents of GI support its role in treating and preventing chronic disease, including diabetes, obesity, coronary heart disease, and cancer. Critics of GI point out flaws in epidemiologic studies cited in support of GI as a public health tool. Additional concerns are related to the utility of the tables as a tool for nutritional management. Within each food category, there is wide variability; values can vary as much as fivefold, depending on the food form, study setting, and other factors. In earlier studies, cooked carrots received a GI rating of 92 ± 20, whereas in more recent studies, they are rated at 32 ± 5. Many factors affect the glycemic response, including variation in the food and its preparation and the circumstances under which it is ingested (Table 3.8). Additionally, variability within and between subjects is large.

Glycemic load. The portion sizes for many of the foods studied for GI were not realistic or usual. To obtain 50 g carbohydrate from carrots, almost five cups of cooked carrots would need to be ingested. The concept of glycemic load (GL) was introduced to take into account the amount of carbohydrate in a usual serving of a particular food. The GL is calculated using the average GI of the particular food, multiplied by the grams of carbohydrate available in a typical serving of that food (Fig. 3.4). GL has been calculated for the foods listed in the International

Table. Concerns about GL are based on the use of imprecise values multiplied to give yet another imprecise number. To use GI, or GL, as a meal-planning tool, one would select foods with low or medium GI versus those with a high GI or, if consuming high-GI foods, also select low-GI foods for balance. The assumption is that the higher the GI or GL, the greater the expected elevation in blood glucose and insulin requirements.

Using GI for meal planning. The American Diabetes Association position is that GI adds another level of complexity to meal planning without scientific evidence to recommend its use as a primary strategy. However, a recent meta-analysis of low glycemic index or low glycemic load diets in diabetes involving 11 randomized controlled trials and 402 participants with poorly controlled diabetes showed that compared to higher glycemic diets there was a significant decrease in A1C by -0.5% (with either parallel or crossover studies). In addition, the proportion of participants with more than 15 episodes of hyperglycemia per month was less and there was no increase in hypoglycemia, morbidity, or costs. This suggests that people with type 1 diabetes may find value in identifying foods and circumstances to determine their own personal GI of preferred and frequently used foods and meals. Based on their unique response, they can develop strategies to adjust meal-related insulin accordingly. The starting point is to match premeal insulin doses to the total carbohydrate content of the meal.

Resistant starch. There are no published long-term studies proving benefit from use of resistant starch in subjects with diabetes.

Nutritive Sweeteners

Sucrose. Sucrose restriction in the diet for diabetes cannot be justified on the basis of its glycemic effect. Sucrose can be included in diets of people with diabetes by making appropriate substitutions for other carbohydrate sources to maintain consistent carbohydrate intake. If the sucrose-containing food is added as an extra, it can be covered with additional short- or rapid-acting insulin. However, patients should consider the potential for a decrease in nutrient value and an increase in fat intake and calories that often accompanies sucrose-containing foods.

Fructose. Fructose has a low glycemic effect, which suggests that it could be a useful sweetener for individuals with diabetes. Large amounts of fructose, however, can have an adverse effect on blood lipids. Like other sugars, fructose provides 4 cal/g and in general does not offer strong advantages over other sweeteners.

Natural sweetener. Fruit juice, honey, molasses, corn syrup, and other natural sweeteners require the same considerations as sucrose. They contribute 4 cal/g and need to be counted as carbohydrate in meal planning.

Sugar alcohols. Sugar alcohols (e.g., sorbitol) and hydrogenated starch hydrolysates have less of a glycemic effect than sucrose and yield about 2 cal/g on average. Some individuals report gastric discomfort after eating foods sweetened with these products, and consumption of large quantities can cause diarrhea.

Nonnutritive Sweeteners

Nonnutritive sweeteners available in the US include acesulfame potassium, aspartame, neotame, saccharin, stevia, and sucralose. The FDA determines an acceptable daily intake (ADI) for products it approves that is defined as a safe amount for daily consumption over a lifetime. The ADI includes a 100-fold safety factor and greatly exceeds average consumption levels. All FDA-approved sweeteners can be used by individuals with diabetes, including pregnant women. However, moderation is often recommended.

Fiber

Dietary fiber appears to benefit overall bowel health, including prevention and treatment of constipation and possible prevention of colon cancer. Soluble fiber in large amounts has been shown to be effective in reducing total and LDL cholesterol levels in diabetic and nondiabetic subjects. The beneficial effect of soluble dietary fiber on glycemic control, although intuitively attractive, is difficult to substantiate. An overall benefit to blood glucose control from dietary fiber has not been established and may require large amounts (>50 g fiber) to achieve a significant effect. The Food and Nutrition Board of the NIH, for the first time, has indicated an adequate intake (AI) for fiber (Table 3.9). The *Choose Your Foods: Exchange Lists for Meal Planning*'s starch, vegetable, fruit, and plant-based protein lists identify foods that provide more than 3 g of dietary fiber per serving.

Protein

Daily requirements. The RDA for protein is 0.8 g/kg/day of high-quality protein for adults, which corresponds to ~10% of calories. This is lower than the usual protein intake of 15–20% of calories consumed by adults in the general US population. The long-term effects of diets with 20% of energy as protein on renal function have not been determined. Protein requirements for children range from 1.5 g/kg/day for infants to 0.85 g/kg/day for adolescent males through 18 years of age. Some patients who are interested in strength training and muscle development are advised by trainers, coaches, and others to take large amounts of protein or amino acids, often in powdered form, to build muscle. When patients indicate an interest in strength training activities, diabetes clinicians must be prepared

Table 3.9 Adequate Intake for Total Fiber

	Men	Women
Adults aged <50 years	38 g	25 g
Adults aged ≥50 years	30 g	21 g

Adapted from Food and Nutrition Board Institute of Medicine: *Dietary, Reference Intakes for Energy, Carbohydrate, Fiber, Fat, Fatty Acids, Cholesterol, Protein, and Amino Acids (Macronutrients).* See Bibliography.

to discuss with them safe amounts of protein intake for their individual kidney function status.

Protein and nephropathy. There is no evidence to suggest that the usual intake of protein needs modification if renal function is normal. In patients with diabetic nephropathy, reduction of dietary protein to 0.8–1.0 g/kg/day for people with earlier stages of chronic kidney disease and to 0.8 g/kg/day in the later stages of CKD may improve measures of renal function.

Protein and insulin requirements. Meal doses of insulin are calculated based on the carbohydrate content of the meal, with the assumption that the basal insulin will cover the attenuated glycemic effects of the protein in the meal. The addition of larger than usual amounts of protein to meals may require a small amount of additional insulin 3–5 h following the meal. Individuals using CSII may use extended delivery of meal bolus insulin for this type of meal. A dual-wave bolus can deliver part of the meal bolus before the meal and the remainder over 2–4 h following the meal.

Fat

The 80–85% of daily calories not allocated to dietary protein are distributed between carbohydrate and fat sources. Saturated fat and *trans* unsaturated fatty acids (*trans* fats) are highly atherogenic and have a greater impact on serum cholesterol than dietary cholesterol. Because diabetes is an independent risk factor for cardiovascular disease, the ADA recommends restricting saturated fat intake to <7% of calories and that *trans* fats be minimized. Dietary cholesterol intake should be <200 mg/day. Content of the diet from monounsaturated and polyunsaturated fats should be individualized to reach goals.

Foods that contain omega-3 fatty acids have cardioprotective effects; the ADA recommends that people with diabetes (as is true of the general population) eat 2–3 servings per week of foods providing omega-3 polyunsaturated fat, such as fish.

Alcohol

Most adults with type 1 diabetes may drink alcohol in moderation if they so choose. Exceptions include individuals whose blood glucose is out of control, those with elevated blood triglycerides, and pregnant women. Daily intake should be limited to one drink for women and two drinks for men. One drink is 12 oz beer, 5 oz wine, or 1.5 oz 80-proof distilled spirits. Each drink contains 15 g alcohol.

In addition to the precautions regarding alcohol use that apply to the general public, people with type 1 diabetes risk alcohol-induced hypoglycemia for up to 24 h after ingestion, especially if meals are skipped or delayed or during fasting. Therefore, alcoholic beverages should be ingested with food. If the patient is overweight and consumes alcohol on a regular basis, adjustments to the meal plan to account for calories from alcohol (7 cal/g) without increasing risk for hypoglycemia should be considered. A reduction in fat (9 cal/g) intake is preferable to a reduction in carbohydrate intake, because of the hypoglycemia implications, to offset calories consumed in an alcoholic beverage.

Micronutrients

Sodium and hypertension. People differ greatly in their sensitivity to sodium and its effect on blood pressure. The recommendation for people with normotension is a reduced sodium intake of ≤2,300 mg/day sodium 1500 mg/day and a diet high in fruits, vegetables, and low-fat dairy products. For individuals with symptomatic heart failure, reducing sodium to ≤2,000 mg/day may help reduce symptoms. Sodium intake can be minimized by reducing the use of table salt, processed and convenience foods, and fast foods. *Choose Your Foods: Exchange Lists for Meal Planning* highlights foods with a sodium content >480 mg/serving. The Nutrition Facts panel on food labels provides useful information by indicating, for a single serving, the amount of sodium in milligrams and the percent of the daily value (the % of 2,400 mg). A consumer may wish to reconsider use of a food containing >25% of the daily value.

Potassium. Individuals taking diuretics may experience a loss of potassium sufficient to warrant supplementation. Potassium restriction may be required if hyperkalemia occurs in patients with renal insufficiency or in those taking angiotensin-converting enzyme inhibitors or angiotensin receptor blockers.

Magnesium. Magnesium deficiency can be easily detected and treated. The deficiency may occur as a result of poorly controlled diabetes and the accompanying urinary loss.

Calcium. The Food and Nutrition Board of the Institute of Medicine has established AIs for calcium based on age (Table 3.10). The values are the same for males and females. Because of enhanced absorption of calcium during pregnancy and lactation, calcium requirements are similar to the nonpregnant and nonlactating state and are based on age.

Vitamin and mineral supplementation. At this time, there is no clear evidence that vitamin and mineral requirements of individuals with type 1 diabetes are different from those of other healthy people. If a nutrition assessment reveals a deficiency, individuals should be counseled on how to adjust food intake to meet these needs. If they are unable to do so, supplements should be recommended. When caloric intake is ≤1,200 cal/day, use of a multivitamin and mineral supplement should be advised. Several conditions may create a deficiency in one or more micronutrients that would warrant supplementation. These include poor diabetes control, celiac (fat soluble vitamins), use of diuretics, critical care environments, medications that alter micronutrient metabolism, strict vegetarian diets, nutritional intakes that do not meet established RDAs or AIs, pregnancy, and lactation. Pregnancy increases requirements for folate and iron.

Herbal and botanical supplements. Many people who balk at taking prescription or over-the-counter medications view herbal and botanical products as a safe and natural alternative or adjunct to their diabetes management plan. Very few randomized, clinical trials have examined the safety and efficacy of these products, especially for people with diabetes. Herbal and botanical supplements, sports supplements, vitamins, minerals and other specialty products represent a

Table 3.10 Adequate Intake for Calcium

Age	Adequate Intake (mg/day)
0–6 months	210
7–12 months	270
1–3 years	700
4–8 years	1,000
9–18 years	1,300
19–50 years	1,000
≥51 years	1,200

Dietary Reference Intakes for Calcium and Vitamin D (2011, Food and Nutrition Board, Institute of Medicine, National Academies, www.nap.edu)

$22 billion industry in the US. The 1994 Dietary Supplement Health and Education Act (DSHEA) changed the regulation of dietary supplements and associated label claims. DSHEA places the burden of proof of unsafe or adulterated products or of false or misleading labeling on the FDA rather than on the manufacturer. However, DSHEA restricts the FDA in regulation of these products. The Federal Trade Commission regulates the advertising of dietary supplements and has taken action against sponsors of false and misleading information. Until proven otherwise, consumers have no assurance that a product contains what the label says it docs or that it is free from harmful contaminants. Some herbal preparations have been found to surreptitiously contain pharmaceutical agents that produce hypoglycemia. Health care providers should ask whether their patients are using these products, as many patients do not voluntarily share this information. While providing individualized, science-based information, it is also important to be sensitive to the patient's decisions to use products that might be considered questionable. The FDA Center for Food Safety & Applied Nutrition and the National Institute of Health Office of Dietary Supplements can provide reliable information about many of these products (see Resources for Patient Education, page 119).

ADDITIONAL NUTRITION CONSIDERATIONS

Sick-Day Management

Individuals with type 1 diabetes must be educated to manage brief periods when they cannot ingest solid foods. They must understand the need to continue insulin therapy and carbohydrate consumption. Fruit juices and sugar-containing soda, sports drinks, or gelatin can replace the usual carbohydrate in the meal plan. Frequent intermittent intake of small amounts of these foods and beverages helps to provide fluids and energy and helps to avoid hypoglycemia. Individuals should also be taught the value of ingesting fluids containing sodium and potassium (e.g., vegetable and fruit juices and broths) to help replace electrolytes lost from diarrhea and vomiting. The usual meal plan should be reintroduced gradually (see Table 2.7, page 47).

Growth Years

For infants, children, and adolescents, height and weight data can be plotted on standardized growth grids. The caloric prescription for children with diabetes should include adequate calories for growth and development. Poor diabetes control during the growth years can contribute to failure to attain height potential. During these years, it is helpful to schedule visits with the dietitian every 3–6 months to adjust calories and other nutrients and to account for changes in food preferences and habits. Parents of infants and young children with diabetes may need frequent nutrition counseling to deal with eating challenges common to children that present particular difficulty when coupled with type 1 diabetes.

Pregnancy

The 2005 RDA for pregnant women sets increased calorie requirements at 340 kcal during the 2nd trimester and 452 kcal during the 3rd trimester. The RDA for protein during pregnancy is 1.1 g/kg, or approximately an additional 25 g/day protein. The 1990 National Academy of Sciences recommendations for optimum weight gain for pregnant women are based on prepregnancy BMI (Table 3.11). These guidelines anticipate delivery of babies weighing 3–4 kg at term. The 1998 Food and Nutrition Board publication recommends that, to reduce the risk of neural tube defects for women capable of becoming pregnant, 400 µg folic acid should be taken daily from fortified foods, supplements, or both in addition to consuming folate from a varied diet. Therefore, prescribing a multivitamin plus up to 400 µg/day folate from preconception through the 1st trimester is recommended. The RDA for iron during pregnancy is 27 mg/day. Assessment of nutritional status and dietary intake should guide prescription of supplements. Because of the additional metabolic stress of diabetes on pregnancy, nutritional guidelines need to be individualized for each pregnant diabetes patient to promote optimal blood glucose levels and appropriate maternal and fetal weight gain.

A plan of three meals and three to four snacks will help patients minimize blood glucose excursions and facilitate tight glycemic control. If there is morning ketosis with normal blood glucose levels, the amount of food in the pre-bedtime snack can be increased or a snack at 3:00 a.m. considered. In the 1st trimester, hyperemesis may be a problem. A very liberal meal plan allowing the patient to eat whatever is tolerated can be helpful. Insulin dosage should be adjusted to allow for minimum food intake at critical points during the day.

Lactation

The protein RDA for lactation is an additional 25 g/day above pre-pregnancy requirements. Additional EER for lactation is based on a milk energy output of 330 kcal/day in the first 6 months and 400 kcal/day in the second 6 months. Many women with diabetes report wide swings in blood glucose levels while they are

Table 3.11 Recommendations for Total and Rate of Weight Gain during Pregnancy, by Prepregnancy BMI

| Prepregnancy BMI | Total weight gain | | Rates of weight gain* 2nd and 3rd trimester | |
	Range in kg	Range in lbs	Mean (range) in kg/ week	Mean (range) in lbs/week
Underweight (<18.5 kg/m²)	12.5–18	28–40	0.51 (0.44–0.58)	1 (1–1.3)
Normal weight (18.5–24.9 kg/m²)	11.5–16	25–35	0.42 (0.35–0.50)	1 (0.8–1)
Overweight (25.0–29.9 kg/m²)	7–11.5	15–25	0.28 (0.23–0.33)	0.6 (0.5–0.7)
Obese (≥30.0 kg/m²)	5–9	11–20	0.22 (0.17–0.27)	0.5 (0.4–0.6)

BMI: body mass index.
* Calculations assume a 0.5–2 kg (1.1–4.4 lbs) weight gain in the first trimester.
From Weight Gain During Pregnancy: Reexamining the Guidelines. Institute of Medicine (US) and National Research Council (US) Committee to Reexamine IOM Pregnancy Weight Guidelines, Rasmussen KM, Yaktine AL (Eds), National Academies Press (US), The National Academies Collection: Reports funded by National Institutes of Health, Washington (DC) 2009. Available at http://www.nap.edu/catalog/12584.html. Reprinted with permission from the National Academies Press, Copyright © 2009

breast-feeding, which may be related to the amount of milk produced and the frequency of feedings. Continuing the pregnancy meal pattern of three meals and three to four snacks may help prevent hypoglycemia and decrease the need for additional insulin to cover the extra calories.

Obesity Management

People with type 1 diabetes may gain excessive weight for several reasons:

- overinsulinization
- frequent and inappropriate treatment of insulin reactions
- efforts to avoid insulin reactions with the use of extra food
- failure to decrease caloric intake to compensate for decreased urinary caloric loss with improved glucose control
- general overemphasis on food intake

Individuals and parents of children with diabetes should be advised about the consequences of obesity on general health. Individuals with diabetes who are attempting to lose weight should avoid fad diets that promote inappropriate food combinations or omissions and rapid weight loss, because dehydration, fluid and electrolyte imbalances, and starvation ketosis may result. Weight loss programs for individuals with type 1 diabetes must include advice about insulin dose adjustment, careful monitoring of diabetes control, and realistic weight loss goals.

The American Diabetes Association advises that either low-carbohydrate low-fat or Mediterranean style calorie-restricted diets may be effective for short-term weight loss (up to 2 years, the duration of comparative studies). If patients are following a low-carbohydrate diet, clinicians should monitor lipid profiles, because these diets can raise LDL cholesterol. Because low-carbohydrate diets may be high in protein, those with nephropathy should be counseled about appropriate protein intake, and renal function should be monitored. Patients using I:C can adjust their prandial insulin downward to account for the lower carbohydrate intake. Patients who lose weight from either type of diet are likely to need changes in their I:C due to the effects of weight loss on insulin sensitivity.

To enable the overweight or obese patient with type 1 diabetes to alter his or her eating, motivational interviewing can be employed to initiate behavior change. Motivational interviewing is a patient-centered method for enhancing intrinsic motivation to change by exploring and resolving ambivalence; however, the basic tenet is that the patient must be ready to change, and that desire must emanate from within, and not be thrust upon the patient by a member of the health care team.

Long-term maintenance of weight loss is a challenge. Strategies for successful weight management are emerging from the National Weight Control Registry (NWCR), a prospective study of individuals age ≥ 18 years who have successfully maintained a 30-lb weight loss for a minimum of 1 year. The NWCR, a collaborative effort between the University of Colorado Health Sciences Center and the University of Pittsburgh School of Medicine, currently includes over 5,000 individuals and offers the opportunity to study the eating and exercise habits of successful weight loss maintainers (*www.nwcr.ws*). The average registrant was overweight as a child (66%), has a family history of obesity, and has a lifetime average gain and loss of 271 lb. Half followed a formal weight loss program. Additional characteristics of the average registrant include:

- has a resting metabolic rate equal to the rate of a nondieting counterpart in the same weight range
- has lost 66 lb and kept it off for 5.5 years
- takes in an average of 1,400 calories/day (macronutrient composition is 49% carbohydrate, 22% protein, and 29% fat)
- exercises, on average, about 1 h per day
- walks for exercise
- eats breakfast every day

NWCR registrants indicate that weight loss maintenance becomes easier over time. Additional strategies used by these registrants include keeping many healthy foods in the house (87%), keeping records of food intake or exercise (43%), and buying books or magazines related to nutrition or exercise (74%).

Disordered Eating

An increasing number of children, adolescents, and adults in the general population appear to be affected with anorexia nervosa, bulimia, or a combination of the two. Disordered eating in type 1 diabetes is more common than previously thought. A meta-analysis evaluating the prevalence of eating disorders in type 1 diabetes in 748 and 1,587 female subjects with and without diabetes, respectively, showed the prevalence of anorexia nervosa was not different between controls and subjects with type 1 diabetes. However, the prevalence of bulimia nervosa and bulimia plus anorexia combined was significantly higher in patients with diabetes. Type 1 diabetes complicated by an eating disorder is very difficult to manage because of erratic eating patterns and purging behaviors such as vomiting, laxative abuse, or excessive exercise. A purging behavior unique to type 1 diabetes is self-induced glycosuria, achieved by insulin omission. These destructive behaviors can lead to recurrent diabetic ketoacidosis and early development of long-term complications. Risk factors for disordered eating in girls and women with type 1 diabetes include higher BMI, increased body weight and shape dissatisfaction, low self-esteem and depression, and dietary restraint. Recognition and treatment are critical, along with referral to experienced medical, psychological, and nutrition counselors (see Resources for Patient Education, page 119).

THE PROCESS OF MEDICAL NUTRITION THERAPY

The process of MNT begins with a comprehensive assessment of the patient's diabetes status and nutritional status. Following the assessment, the intervention includes collaboration on setting metabolic and self-care goals determined by patient and dietitian as priorities and a plan for action. Achievement of goals will be monitored by ongoing communication between the patient and dietitian. Follow-up visits will provide opportunities to evaluate progress, identify barriers to success, solve problems, and make necessary changes in the plan of care. Although the dietitian is the primary provider of MNT, this component of diabetes management must be integrated into the care provided by all members of the core team. Coordination of this effort is supported by concise and accurate documentation, communication among team members, and consistency of diabetes and nutrition messages provided to the patient.

Assessment

A comprehensive nutrition assessment (Table 3.12) contains components of the medical evaluation and the education assessment for overall diabetes education needs. Recognizing that the other members of the patient's diabetes care team need similar information should encourage communication among clinicians, collaboration on treatment goals, and consistency of messages provided to the patient.

Goal-Setting

Specific goals for MNT are identified through the nutrition assessment. These goals must correspond with the overall treatment goals for the individual and must agree with the patient's personal goals for therapy. Goal-setting is often a negotiation process involving clinicians and the patient. Goals should be realistic and specific.

Table 3.12 Nutrition Assessment

Clinical Data

- Height, weight, BMI
- Body frame
- Reasonable weight
- Blood pressure
- Family history
- Blood glucose and lipids
- A1C
- Abnormal laboratory findings

Nutrition History

- Usual food intake
- Attitudes toward nutrition and health
- Previous nutrition education and outcomes
- Cultural food practices
- Physical activity
- Allergies and intolerances

Nutrient Intake

- Overall nutritional adequacy
- Caloric intake
- Nutrient distribution

- Type of carbohydrate, protein, and fat
- Use of vitamins, minerals, and herbal and botanical products

Social History

- Daily schedule
- Family relationships
- Friends—social support
- Finances and living environment
- Education—learning style
- Self-efficacy

Diabetes and Health Status

- Duration of diabetes
- Insulin regimen
- Hypoglycemia treatment and history
- Diabetes knowledge and skills
- Complications history and current status
- Other medications
- Smoking
- Alcohol

Nutrition Care Plan

The meal plan for type 1 diabetes is directed by the insulin deficiency that characterizes the condition. Food intake and insulin regimens must be coordinated to accommodate the patient's food preferences and lifestyle while achieving goal glucose levels as closely as is safely possible. Fortunately, SMBG, basal-bolus insulin regimens, and CSII support this coordination effort. Specific strategies for nutritional management of type 1 diabetes are to

- integrate insulin therapy with an individual's food and physical activity preferences
- base the food plan on assessment of appetite, preferred foods, and usual eating and exercise habits
- use information from SMBG, CGM, insulin, food, and physical activity records and uploads to make adjustments in food intake or insulin dose to achieve target glucose levels
- modify caloric and nutrient composition of the food plan as appropriate to achieve metabolic and weight goals and for different stages of the life cycle

The individualized self-management plan should also reflect the patient's lifestyle, exercise patterns, and resources. Important considerations include

- daily schedule (weekday and weekend), travel to and from work or school, during work/school, recreational and social activities
- individual's and family's eating patterns, including usual time and size of meals, where meals are eaten, food preferences, social habits, and cultural customs
- availability of food at home, school, or work; and food budget
- facilities and equipment for preparation and storage of food

Evaluation

The effectiveness of the nutrition treatment plan is evaluated by outcomes specifically related to the goals of therapy. Outcomes would include metabolic and behavior change measures.

Practice Guidelines for MNT of Type 1 Diabetes

Practice guidelines offer a systematic approach to disease management designed to increase assurance that desired outcomes will be achieved. Nutrition practice guidelines for type 1 and type 2 diabetes were developed using criteria set forth by the Institute of Medicine. In field tests of the nutrition practice guidelines for type 1 diabetes, practice guideline patients achieved greater reduction in A1C than usual care patients. These guidelines are available from the Academy of Nutrition and Dietetics (see Resources for Patient Education, page 119).

PRACTICAL APPROACHES TO NUTRITION COUNSELING

Pattern Management

SMBG, CGM, insulin, food, and physical activity records and uploads provide patients and clinicians an evaluation mechanism that can be used to closely examine the effectiveness of the treatment regimen and to make adjustments to improve glycemic control. Finding and interpreting blood glucose patterns leads to possible changes in either the amount or timing of insulin, food, or physical activity.

Carbohydrate Counting for Intensive Insulin Therapy

Carbohydrate counting is a meal planning approach that focuses on carbohydrate as the primary nutrient affecting postprandial glycemic response. Carbohydrate counting can be used at basic or advanced levels depending on the interest and skills of the individual.

Basic carbohydrate counting. Carbohydrate counting can be used at a basic level by patients whose goals include consistency of carbohydrate intake to support improved glycemic control. Patients first learn to estimate how much carbohydrate is in their meals and snacks by becoming familiar with reference amounts of foods similar to the exchange lists or other published carbohydrate food lists. Other skills include reading food labels accurately for carbohydrate values and estimating carbohydrate amounts in combination foods such as pizza and in restaurants or meals prepared by others. A person must be willing to spend time and effort learning and practicing measuring and weighing foods, reading food labels, and using reference books to develop the skills necessary to accurately estimate carbohydrate amounts in portions usually eaten. These skills require moderate levels of literacy and numeracy. Nutrient databases are available on the Internet and as software for loading into personal computers or personal digital assistants.

Advanced carbohydrate counting. Individuals on intensive insulin therapy, either basal-bolus regimens or CSII, can learn to match their premeal insulin to their carbohydrate foods using an individualized insulin-to-carbohydrate ratio. Patients striving for tight glucose control while maintaining flexibility in meals and snacks are candidates for using this counting method.

The insulin-to-carbohydrate ratio is determined for individuals based on records of SMBG, CGM, insulin doses, food intake, and physical activity. The ratio is based on the amount of short- or rapid-acting insulin needed to cover a specific amount of carbohydrate to achieve postprandial glucose targets. For example, a patient uses 1 unit rapid-acting insulin for every 10 g carbohydrate eaten to achieve a specific blood glucose target 2 h postprandially. Therefore, this person has an insulin-to-carbohydrate ratio of 1:10, i.e., 1 unit insulin covers 10 g carbohydrate. To adjust insulin for varying amounts of carbohydrate, divide the total grams of carbohydrate to be consumed by the insulin-to-carbohydrate ratio. A meal with 100 g carbohydrate would require 10 units of premeal insulin (100 g divided by 10 = 10 units insulin). Some formulas for initially calculating insulin-to-carbohydrate ratio include weight and total daily insulin dose as part of the equation (e.g., 450 divided by total daily dose; see Optimizing Blood Glucose Control, page 74).

An absolute prerequisite for insulin-to-carbohydrate ratio use is that the patient must already be extremely well versed in carbohydrate counting. The insulin-to-carbohydrate ratio's effectiveness depends on the patient's ability to accurately estimate carbohydrate amounts that can be covered by insulin. Miscalculation of consumed carbohydrate will result in taking too much or too little insulin. Time, effort, and practice are needed to become proficient enough in carbohydrate counting to use it safely and effectively in insulin dose calculation and adjustment.

Individuals using insulin-to-carbohydrate ratios also need to consider other factors that affect glycemic response and be aware that they may need to adjust timing of insulin delivery as well as amount of insulin for specific situations. For example, high-fat meals can delay stomach emptying and may require delivery of a divided dose of insulin, such as part of the dose before and part after the meal. CSII allows delivery of extended boluses that help to accommodate this type of insulin delivery.

Nutrition Self-Management Tools

Meal planning tools, such as the *Basic Carbohydrate Counting, Match Your Carb to Your Insulin, Choose Your Foods: Exchange Lists for Diabetes*, or its simplified version, *Healthy Food Choices*, can be used to guide patients in implementing their nutrition management plan. These tools are available from the American Diabetes Association and the Academy of Nutrition and Dietetics. These associations also offer nutrition education materials related to several ethnic and regional food practices. The American Diabetes Association has published a variety of cookbooks and meal planning books, and in addition has nutrition resources for patients on its website, *www.diabetes.org*. A meal planning resource should be selected that is appropriate for the patient's lifestyle, reading level, culture, and intensity of diabetes management.

Staged Nutrition Counseling

Eating habits are not easy to change. For the person with type 1 diabetes, the need to balance food intake and activity, the potential for hypoglycemia, and the psychological stress of managing a chronic disease make changing food habits even more difficult. Nutrition counseling should be provided in stages to allow the patient time to absorb information, try out self-management skills, and test the nutrition plan in daily living. Staged nutrition counseling also provides an opportunity to evaluate the effectiveness of the treatment plan and to make modifications to improve diabetes control. MNT is a lifetime treatment of diabetes. Therefore, nutrition counseling must be included in the ongoing care of the patient with type 1 diabetes.

CONCLUSION

Diabetes MNT is more than mere calculation of a caloric prescription with appropriate macronutrient composition and distribution of foods into meals and snacks. It is a complex process that requires commitment on the part of clinicians and the patient to design an individualized nutrition self-management plan. The effectiveness of MNT is evaluated by success in achieving nutrition-related goals. MNT cannot be limited to the time of diagnosis, but must continue through life with adjustments made for growth and development; changes in lifestyle, diabetes status, and health status; and advances in the field of diabetes nutritional care.

BIBLIOGRAPHY

American Diabetes Association: Nutrition recommendations and interventions for diabetes (Position Statement). *Diabetes Care* 31:S61–S78, 2008

Dietary Supplement Health and Education Act of 1994, Public Law 103–417 (S.784) (1994) (codified at 42 USC 287C–11)

Elliott TD: Low glycaemic index, or low glycaemic load, diets for diabetes mellitus (review): *The Cochrane Collaboration*, Published by John Wiley and Sons, Ltd. 3:1–31, 2009 or *Cochrane Database of Systematic Reviews* 2009, Issue 1, Art. No.: CD006296, DOI: 10.1002/14651858,CD006296.pub 2

Food and Nutrition Board Institute of Medicine: *Dietary Reference Intakes for Calcium, Phosphorus, Magnesium, Vitamin D and Fluoride.* Washington, DC, National Academy Press, 1999

Food and Nutrition Board Institute of Medicine: *Dietary Reference Intakes for Energy, Carbohydrate, Fiber, Fat, Fatty Acids, Cholesterol, Protein, and Amino Acids* (Macronutrients). Washington, DC, National Academy Press, 2005

Food and Nutrition Board Institute of Medicine: *Dietary Reference Intakes for Thiamin, Riboflavin, Niacin, Vitamin B6, Folate, Vitamin B12, Pantothenic Acid, Biotin, and Choline.* Washington, DC, National Academy Press, 1998

Food and Nutrition Board Institute of Medicine: *Dietary Reference Intakes for Vitamin A, Vitamin K, Arsenic, Boron, Chromium, Copper, Iodine, Iron, Manganese, Molybdenum, Nickel, Silicon, Vanadium, and Zinc.* Washington, DC, National Academy Press, 2002

Foster-Powell K, Holt S, Brand-Miller, JC: International table of glycemic index and glycemic load values. *Am J Clin Nutr* 76:5–56, 2002

Franz MJ, Bantle JP, Beebe CA, Brunzell JD, Chiasson JL, Garg A, Holzmeister LA, Hoogwerf B, Mayer-Davis E, Mooradian AD, Purnell JQ, Wheeler M: Evidence-based nutrition principles and recommendations for the treatment and prevention of diabetes and related complications (Technical Review). *Diabetes Care* 25:148–198, 2002

Goebel-Fabbri AE: Disturbed eating behaviors and eating disorders in type 1 diabetes: clinical significance and treatment recommendations. *Current Diabetes Reports* 9:133–139, 2009

Institute of Medicine: *Nutrition During Pregnancy Part I: Weight Gain.* Washington, DC, National Academy Press, 1990

Jenkins DJA, Kendall CWC, Augustin LSA, Franceschi S, Hamidi M, Marchie A, Jenkins AL, Axelsen M: Glycemic index: overview of implications in health and disease. *Am J Clin Nutr* 76 (Suppl.):266S–273S, 2002

Joint National Committee on the Prevention, Detection, Evaluation, and Treatment of High Blood Pressure: *Seventh Report of the Joint National Committee on the Prevention, Detection, Evaluation, and Treatment of High Blood Pressure.* Washington, DC, National Institutes of Health National Heart Lung and Blood Institute, 2004

Klem ML, Wing RR, Lang W, McGuire MT, Hill JO: Does weight loss maintenance become easier over time? *Obesity Res* 8:438–444, 2000

Mannucci E, Rotella F, Ricca V, Moretti S, Placidi GF, Rotella CM: Eating disorders in patients with type 1 diabetes: a meta-analysis. *J Endocrinol Invest* 28 (5):417–419, 2005

Marsh K, Barclay A, Colagiuri S, Brand-Miller J: Glycemic index and glycemic load of carbohydrates in the diabetes diet. *Curr Diab Rep* 11:120–127, 2011

Miller WR, Rollnick S, (Eds): *Motivational Interviewing: Preparing People for Change*, 2nd edition. New York, Guilford Press, 2002

National Institutes of Health: *National Cancer Institute: 5 a Day for Better Health Program Monograph.* Washington, DC, National Institutes of Health, 2002

Peters AL, Davidson MB: Protein and fat effects on glucose response and insulin requirements in subjects with insulin-dependent diabetes mellitus. *Am J Clin Nutr* 58:555–560, 1993

Pi-Sunyer FX: Glycemic index and disease. *Am J Clin Nutr* 76 (Suppl.):290S–298S, 2002

Polonsky WH: Identifying and treating eating disorders in persons with diabetes. In *Handbook of Diabetes Medical Nutrition Therapy.* Powers MA, Ed. Gaithersburg, MD, Aspen, 1996, p. 585–601

Pastors JG, Franz MJ, Warshaw H, Daly A, Arnold MS: How effective is medical nutrition therapy in diabetes care? *J Am Diet Assoc* 103:827–831, 2003

Pastors JG, Warshaw H, Daly A, Franz M, Kulkarni K: The evidence for the effectiveness of medical nutrition therapy in diabetes management. *Diabetes Care* 25:608–613, 2002

Report of a Joint FAO/WHO Expert Consultation: *Carbohydrates in Human Nutrition.* Rome, Italy, Food and Agriculture Organization of the United Nations and World Health Organization, 1998

Sacks FM, Appel LJ, Moore TJ, Obarzanek E, Vollmer WM, Svetkey LP, Bray GA: Dietary approaches to prevent hypertension: a review of the Dietary Approaches to Stop Hypertension (DASH) study. *Clin Cardiol* 22 (Suppl. 7):III6–III10, 1999

Toeller M, Buyken A, Heitkamp G, Bramswig S, Mann J, Milne R, Gries FA, Keen H, the EURODIAB IDDM Complications Study: Protein intake and urinary albumin excretion rates in the EURODIAB IDDM Complications Study. *Diabetologia* 40:1219–1226, 1997

USDA (US Department of Agriculture): *My Pyramid: Steps to a Healthier You.* 2005, accessed January 2008.

RESOURCES FOR PATIENT EDUCATION

Count Your Carbs: Getting Started. Alexandria, VA, American Diabetes Association, and Chicago, American Dietetic Association, 2010

Choose Your Foods: Exchange Lists for Meal Planning. Alexandria, VA, American Diabetes Association, and Chicago, American Dietetic Association, 2007

Choose Your Foods: Plan Your Meals. Alexandria, VA, American Diabetes Association, and Chicago, American Dietetic Association, 2009

Diabetes Care and Education Practice Group of the American Dietetic Association: Ethnic and Regional Food Practices: A Series. Alexandria, VA, American Diabetes Association, and Chicago, American Dietetic Association, various publication dates

Healthy Food Choices. Alexandria, VA, American Diabetes Association, and Chicago, American Dietetic Association, 2009

Match Your Insulin to Your Carbs. Alexandria, VA, American Diabetes Association, and Chicago, IL, Academy of Nutrition and Dietetics, 2011

McCarren M. *Carb Counting Made Easy for People with Diabetes.* Alexandria, VA, American Diabetes Association, 2002

Warshaw HS: *Diabetes Meal Planning Made Easy,* 4th ed. Alexandria, VA, American Diabetes Association, 2010

Warshaw HS, Kulkarni K: *Complete Guide to Carb Counting,* 3rd ed. Alexandria, VA, American Diabetes Association, 2011

Warshaw HS, Webb R: *Diabetes Food and Nutrition Bible.* Alexandria, VA, American Diabetes Association, 2001

RESOURCES FOR PROFESSIONALS

American Dietetic Association: *Nutrition Practice Guidelines for Type 1 and Type 2 Diabetes Mellitus.* Chicago, American Dietetic Association, 1998

Diabetes Care and Education Practice Group of the American Dietetic Association: *The American Dietetic Association Guide to Diabetes Medical Nutrition Therapy and Diabetes Education.* Chicago, American Dietetic Association, 2003

Franz MJ, Evert A (Eds.): *American Diabetes Association Guide to Medical Nutrition Therapy for Diabetes.* Alexandria, VA, American Diabetes Association, 2012

National Academies Press website for online review of publications on dietary reference intakes for macronutrients and micronutrients: www.nap.edu

NIH Office of Dietary Supplements website (with IBIDS-International Bibliographic Information on Dietary Supplements, which contains over 690,000 scientific citations and abstracts about dietary supplements): http://ods.od.nih.gov/

Pastors J (Ed.): *Diabetes Nutrition Q & A for Health Professionals: 101 Essential Questions Answered by Experts.* Alexandria, VA, American Diabetes Association, 2003

Powers M (Ed.): *Handbook of Diabetes Medical Nutrition Therapy.* Gaithersburg, MD, Aspen, 1996

Sarubin A: *The Health Professional's Guide to Popular Dietary Supplements.* Chicago, American Dietetic Association, 2000

Shane-McWhorter L: *Complementary and Alternative Medicine (CAM) Supplement Use in People with Diabetes: A Clinician's Guide.* Alexandria, VA, American Diabetes Association, 2007

U.S. Food and Drug Administration, Center for Food Safety and Applied Nutrition Dietary Supplements website. http://www.fda.gov/food/dietarysupplements/default.htm

Warshaw HS, Bolderman KM: *Practical Carbohydrate Counting: A How-to-Teach Guide for Health Professionals*, 2nd ed. Alexandria, VA, American Diabetes Association, 2008

EXERCISE

In addition to insulin and medical nutrition therapy, physical activity and exercise play a key role in diabetes management. Important health benefits of physical activity for individuals with diabetes include a reduction in cardiovascular risk factors, increased sensitivity to insulin, better ability to maintain a healthy weight and level of body fat, and a heightened sense of well-being. Given these health benefits, regular physical activity should be considered an integral part of the treatment plan for individuals with type 1 diabetes.

Because exercise can significantly affect blood glucose levels, it must be carefully integrated into the diabetes management regimen. When individuals with type 1 diabetes are given appropriate guidance and support and attain good self-management skills, they can achieve optimal glycemic control, exercise safely, and achieve desired levels of exercise performance. Children and adolescents can participate fully in gym classes, team sports, and other activities and have at least 60 min of moderate to vigorous physical activity a day. In the absence of contraindications, all adults should accumulate at least 30 min of moderate daily activity to improve health and reduce risk of chronic disease. Adults with type 1 diabetes should be encouraged to achieve at least this level of daily activity. Individuals with physical limitations should be encouraged to maintain an active lifestyle and offered guidance about safe and appropriate exercise options that will enable them to do so.

Success with any physical activity program is greatly enhanced when exercise goals are appropriately established. Goals must be individualized based on a person's interests, likes and dislikes, unique lifestyle and psychosocial variables, age, general health, level of physical fitness, and prior exercise experience.

GLYCEMIC RESPONSE TO EXERCISE

Exercise requires rapid mobilization and redistribution of metabolic fuels to ensure an adequate energy supply for working muscles. For individuals who do not have diabetes, this complex process is coordinated via neural and hormonal responses that increase production of glucose and free fatty acids (FFAs) and facilitate uptake and utilization of these fuels by working muscle (Table 3.13). Insulin levels fall while counterregulatory hormones rise, so that increased glucose utilization by exercising muscle is matched precisely by increased glucose production by the liver. For individuals with type 1 diabetes, the metabolic adjustments that maintain fuel homeostasis during and after exercise are lacking. The result can be a mismatch between hepatic glucose production and muscle glucose utilization and significant deviation from normal glycemia. The glycemic response to exercise can be variable and is influenced by multiple factors. These include

- overall metabolic control
- circulating insulin level
- plasma glucose at the start of exercise
- timing of exercise in relation to food intake
- glycogen stores
- level of training and fitness
- intensity, duration, time, and type of exercise

Table 3.13 Metabolic Response to Light and Moderate Exercise: Normal vs. Type 1 Diabetes

Normal Response	Response in Type 1 Diabetes
Insulin level decreases ■ ↑glucose release from liver ■ ↑FFA mobilization ■restricts use of glucose by nonexercising skeletal muscle	Insulin level fails to change at the onset of exercise ■insulin excess: muscle glucose uptake exceeds liver glucose production ■insulin deficiency: liver glucose production exceeds muscle uptake; FFA release and ketone body formation increase ■adequate insulin level: liver glucose output matches muscle glucose uptake
Counterregulatory hormones increase ■ ↑hepatic glucose production and release ■ ↑muscle glycogenolysis ■adipose tissue lipolysis	Counterregulatory hormones generally increase, although response may be blunted in some individuals
Glucose uptake and utilization by working muscle increases	Glucose uptake and utilization by working muscle may or may not increase depending on insulin availability
Precise integration of glucose production and utilization and stable blood glucose levels	Potential mismatch between glucose production and utilization and variable blood glucose levels

Plasma insulin level is a primary determinant of the glycemic response to exercise. In individuals who do not have diabetes, the circulating insulin level normally falls at the onset of light or moderate-intensity exercise. In those with type 1 diabetes, this response is absent, and insulin adjustments need to be made in anticipation of exercise. If circulating insulin levels are too high, a state of relative hyperinsulinemia results, which leads to enhanced muscle glucose uptake, inhibited hepatic glucose production, and potentiation of hypoglycemia. In contrast, if circulating insulin levels are too low, as evidenced by pre-exercise hyperglycemia and poor metabolic control, an inadequate level of insulin combined with a heightened counterregulatory hormone release associated with exercise can lead to a marked increase in glucose production and FFA mobilization from the liver. When availability of these substrates exceeds muscle uptake, a further worsening of hyperglycemia and ketosis may result.

POTENTIAL BENEFITS OF EXERCISE

Because individuals with type 1 diabetes are at high risk for the development of cardiovascular disease, exercise, through its ability to improve multiple cardiovascular risk factors, offers important health benefits. Regular exercise can improve the lipoprotein profile by lowering VLDL cholesterol and triglycerides and by increasing HDL cholesterol. It also can reduce blood pressure, decrease adiposity, improve cardiac work capacity, decrease platelet adhesiveness, and lower the adrenergic response to stress.

Beyond cardiovascular benefits, participation in regular exercise assists with weight loss and is essential for long-term success with maintaining a healthy weight. It enhances sense of well-being and reduces feelings of stress and anxiety. It improves muscle strength and agility, reduces bone loss, and prevents loss of functional capacity that can occur with aging.

Although exercise increases insulin sensitivity and can lower the requirement for insulin, it has not consistently been shown to lead to improvements in glycemic control in individuals with type 1 diabetes as measured by A1C. However, when exercising individuals learn to self-adjust their management to accommodate physical activity through careful meal planning, frequent SMBG and record keeping, and correct application of insulin-adjustment strategies, they can achieve excellent glycemic control and A1C levels.

POTENTIAL RISKS OF EXERCISE

Although exercise offers many health benefits, it also carries potential risks for those with type 1 diabetes. Both acute complications, hyper- and hypoglycemia, and long-term microvascular and macrovascular complications may be exacerbated by physical activity, especially if an exercise option is contraindicated given existing complications or physical limitations or is incorrectly performed.

Hyperglycemia and Hypoglycemia

Because exercise potentiates the effects of insulin, hypoglycemia may occur during, immediately after, or many hours after a period of physical activity. Hypoglycemia poses a risk to individuals who perform unusually long-duration or strenuous exercise or to those who exercise sporadically without adjusting their usual insulin dose or meal plan. In contrast, hyperglycemia can occur if pre-exercise metabolic control is poor or if exercise is performed at a very high intensity, anaerobic level (>80% of VO_{2max}).

Individual glycemic response patterns can differ markedly with exercise. SMBG, use of continuous glucose sensing, careful record keeping, and recognition of glucose patterns with activity are important skills that can enable individuals with type 1 diabetes to understand unique glycemic responses to exercise, enhance their ability to make self-management decisions that support optimal glycemic control, and exercise safety and enhance performance. Frequent SMBG helps with anticipation of the onset of hypo- or hyperglycemia and enables individuals to make decisions about taking corrective actions before either complication becomes severe. When data from monitoring are carefully recorded and analyzed, they can provide a valuable basis for making decisions about adjustments in management for subsequent exercise sessions. In the future, it may be possible to use computer-based algorithms and sensor-augmented pumps with threshold or predictive low glucose suspend features to help avoid aberrations of glycemia during and after exercise.

Macrovascular and Microvascular Complications

Although regular participation in physical activity tends to reduce cardio-vascular risk factors, the risk of arrhythmias, myocardial ischemia or infarction, and cardiac arrest is transiently elevated during exercise. Because individuals with type 1 diabetes are at high risk for cardiovascular disease, careful evaluation to assess risk for preexisting disease is advisable before an exercise program is initiated, especially in previously sedentary adults with long duration of diabetes. For those with known or suspected disease, a moderate, safe level of exercise that will minimize risk of negative cardiac events should be prescribed.

Screening for microvascular diabetes complications before initiation of exercise is also advisable. Worsening of complications is possible (Table 3.14) if exercise is not carefully prescribed. As for the general population, exercise can aggravate preexisting joint disease or lead to musculoskeletal injuries.

REDUCING EXERCISE RISKS

Potential exercise risks can be reduced if a thorough medical evaluation that includes screenings for microvascular, macrovascular, and neurologic complications of diabetes precedes initiation of exercise (Table 3.15). Based on findings of this exam, an individualized physical activity program should be carefully planned and supported by an appropriate level of supervision to minimize exercise risks and promote progressive gains in health and fitness. Exercise should be prescribed with caution in individuals with previous poor metabolic control, including severe hyperglycemia and ketonuria, frequent hypoglycemia or hypoglycemia unawareness, cardiovascular disease, neuropathy, proliferative retinopathy, or

Table 3.14 Potential Risks of Exercise with Microvascular Diabetes Complications

Microvascular Complication	Potential Exercise Risk
Proliferative retinopathy	Retinal detachment, vitreous or retinal hemorrhage, blood pressure elevation
Peripheral neuropathy	Loss of protective sensation, soft tissue injury, foot ulcers, injury to bones and joints, infection
Autonomic neuropathy	Reduced heart rate and blood pressure response to exercise, silent ischemia, orthostatic hypotension, impaired counterregulatory response to exercise, hypoglycemia unawareness, impaired body temperature regulation, dehydration, reduced exercise tolerance
Nephropathy	Marked blood pressure elevations with high intensity, which may lead to transient increases in proteinuria/albuminuria

Table 3.15 Pre-exercise Testing Indications for Exercise Program Greater Than Brisk Walking

- Age >40 years
- Age >35 years and
  - ✳ Type 1 or type 2 diabetes of >10 years duration
  - ✳ Hypertension
  - ✳ Cigarette smoking
  - ✳ Dyslipidemia
  - ✳ Proliferative or preproliferative retinopathy

- ✳ Nephropathy, including microalbuminuria
- Any of the following, regardless of age:
  - ✳ Known or suspected coronary artery disease, cerebrovascular disease, and/or peripheral vascular disease
  - ✳ Autonomic neuropathy
  - ✳ Renal failure

nephropathy. Individuals with these complications should be offered guidance about safe exercise options as well as activities that should be avoided (Table 3.16). Some individuals may benefit from initially participating in a supervised exercise program. Performance of frequent SMBG before, during, and after exercise should be encouraged.

Participation in a cardiac rehabilitation program may benefit individuals with known cardiovascular disease. For these individuals, the exercise prescription should be based on results of a graded exercise test. Special precautions and monitoring are warranted for those who have hypertension or thyroid disease

Table 3.16 Exercise Options with Diabetes Complications

Diabetes Complication	Best Exercise Options	Inadvisable Exercise Options
Proliferative retinopathy	Low-impact activities like walking, swimming, low-impact aerobics, stationary cycling	Pounding, jarring, or "head-low" activities, high impact sports, heavy lifting, breath-holding and Valsalva-like maneuvers
Insensitive feet/peripheral vascular insufficiency	Non-weight-bearing activities like cycling, swimming, arm chair exercises, light weight lifting, yoga, tai chi	Repetitive weight-bearing or high-impact activities like prolonged walking or jogging
Nephropathy	Light to moderate daily activities, low-intensity aerobic activity, light weight lifting	Heavy lifting or intensive exercise that results in blood pressure increase
Hypertension	Dynamic exercises that primarily use large, lower-extremity muscle groups	Heavy lifting and Valsalva-like maneuvers

and for anyone who is taking cardiac or blood pressure medications that can mask hypoglycemia, alter heart rate response to exercise, or influence cardiac work capacity (e.g., β-blockers).

EXERCISE PRESCRIPTION

Before initiating exercise, all individuals should be given specific guidance about appropriate exercise options, exercise goal-setting, methods for self-monitoring exercise performance, strategies for maintaining optimal glycemic control, and exercise safety precautions (Table 3.17).

The purpose of an exercise prescription is to offer specific exercise recommendations that will safely and successfully guide an individual toward achieving a level of physical activity that will improve health, fitness, functional capacity, and quality of life. Individualization is the key to success of any exercise program. Unique lifestyle variables, likes and dislikes regarding exercise options, stage of readiness to make necessary lifestyle changes, age, prior exercise experience, and level of fitness should all be considered.

Recommendations regarding frequency, intensity, duration, and type of exercise should similarly be individualized. The most precise exercise prescriptions are based on exercise testing that determines heart rate and blood pressure response to exercise and aerobic capacity ($VO_{2\,max}$).

An aerobic conditioning program is desirable for most individuals with diabetes. In addition, all people can benefit from informally increasing daily lifestyle activities (e.g., walking and climbing stairs). The very unfit person may benefit from beginning with a lifestyle activity program before progressing to structured, aerobic exercise.

Whenever possible, an exercise contract that guides an individual toward achieving exercise goals should be established. Goals should be established collaboratively with input from the exercising individual. The person's progress toward achieving goals should regularly be assessed and the exercise plan adjusted as needed. Specific recommendations that are established with active involvement and input from the individual with diabetes are most likely to lead to successful exercise outcomes.

AEROBIC TRAINING

Individuals who are interested and physically able should be encouraged to participate in aerobic activity. Aerobic training, which uses large muscle groups repetitively and continuously for an extended time, promotes optimal improvements in cardiorespiratory fitness, body composition, functional capacity, and overall health when it is consistently done at a level that accrues an energy expenditure of 1,000–2,000 calories per week. Generally, aerobic activity should be performed

- 20–60 min per session
- 150 min/week

Table 3.17 Exercise Safety Guidelines

General

■Carry a medical identification card and wear an identification bracelet, necklace, or tag that alerts others that individual has diabetes

■Exercise with an informed partner

■Measure pre-exercise blood glucose and take appropriate action:
  ◆ If <100 mg/dL: eat a carbohydrate-containing snack before exercising
  ◆ If >250 mg/dL: test for ketones and troubleshoot reason for hyperglycemia; if ketones present, delay exercising until ketones are negative

■Frequently consume fluids before, during, and after exercise to prevent dehydration

■Do visual and tactile inspections of feet before and after exercise

■Wear footwear and clothing that is appropriate for the activity you plan to do and for the exercise climate

■Avoid exercising in extreme heat, humidity, or cold

To Prevent Hypoglycemia

■Perform SMBG periodically during prolonged exercise; monitor more frequently postexercise

■Be alert for signs of hypoglycemia during and several hours after an exercise session

■Avoid exercising during peak insulin action

■Administer insulin away from working limbs if exercise is to be initiated within 30 min of an insulin injection

■Consider reducing the dose of insulin that will be acting during a period of exercise

■Have immediate access to a source of readily absorbable carbohydrate (such as glucose tablets) to treat hypoglycemia

■ at an intensity of 55–79% of maximum heart rate (40–74% of maximal oxygen uptake reserve [VO_2R] or heart rate reserve [HRR]), or rating of perceived exertion (RPE) of 12-13-14 "somewhat hard" level of effort; a lower intensity of 55–65% of maximum heart rate (40–50% of VO_2R or HRR), and RPE of 12 is appropriate for those who are unfit (Table 3.18)

Participation in aerobic exercise is safest and most effective if individuals monitor exercise intensity to ensure that they are working in an appropriate "target zone" or level of effort. Three methods that can be used to monitor exercise intensity are heart rate or pulse count monitoring, RPE, and the "talk test" (Table 3.18). Individuals with known coronary artery disease should be informed about symptoms of myocardial ischemia. Exercise-related chest pain or discomfort, excessive shortness of breath, lightheadedness, or nausea are all indicators that an individual should immediately stop an activity. Any discomfort or worrisome symptoms associated with exercise should be reported to an individual's physician.

Each session of aerobic exercise should include a 5- to 10-min warm-up and a 5- to 10-min cool-down period. The warm-up should include light general muscle movement, e.g., slow walking or stationary cycling, followed by stretching.

Table 3.18 Methods of Determining and Monitoring Exercise Intensity with Exercise

Target Heart Rate	Rating of Perceived Exertion	"Talk Test"
Monitor 10-s pulse count by palpating carotid or radial pulse or use heart rate monitor	Determine perception of effort required or level of difficulty associated with exercising at a given workload	Assess ability to talk or carry on a conversation while exercising as an indicator of staying within/not exceeding an aerobic training level
Target heart rate: 55–79% of HR_{max} or 40–74% VO_2R or HRR*	Target: rating of perceived exertion of 12-13-14 "somewhat hard" level of effort	Target: Maintaining ability to talk during an exercise session; avoid extreme shortness of breath

*HR_{max} = 220 – age (or maximal heart rate achieved on exercise stress test)
$VO_2R = VO_{2max}$ – resting VO_2 (maximal oxygen uptake reserve; can be calculated if VO_{2max} is measured during exercise stress test). HRR = ($HR_{max} - HR_{rest}$) + HR_{rest} (heart rate reserve; formula accounts for true resting as well as maximal heart rate)

The warm-up should be followed by the more vigorous aerobic training period during which the exercise "target zone" should be achieved. At the end of an exercise session, a cool-down period should include light general muscle movement and stretching. Calisthenics or other light resistance activities can be incorporated into the cool down. The heart rate should approach a resting level (<100 beats/min) before the cool down is completed.

When prescribing exercise, it is important to start each individual at a level that can reasonably be achieved. This may require that an individual who is very deconditioned begin by doing short, 5- to 10-min exercise sessions two to three times per day. The duration of each session can gradually be increased as a person becomes more fit. As the duration of each exercise session increases, the number of daily sessions can be reduced. It is important not to overlook the considerable health benefits that can be gained even if exercise is performed at an intensity below an optimal target range for improving cardiorespiratory fitness. Promoting all types of physical activity, even forms that require a low-to-moderate level of effort, is important. For individuals who dislike vigorous exercise, a physical activity program that focuses on weekly energy expenditure rather than on intensity of exercise may support improved adherence and better exercise outcomes.

Resistance exercises such as weight lifting or calisthenics can improve body composition, increase muscle strength and endurance, improve flexibility, increase insulin sensitivity and glucose tolerance, and decrease cardiovascular risk factors. Individuals who are interested in resistance exercise should be carefully screened for diabetes complications, especially proliferative retinopathy, so that a program can be safely adapted to minimize risk of aggravating existing complications. All individuals should be taught proper technique at the onset of a training program to minimize the risk of injury.

If a diabetes clinician does not feel knowledgeable enough about principles of exercise to prescribe and supervise an aerobic exercise program, a referral should be made. Hospital-based cardiac rehabilitation or wellness programs, YMCA programs, and programs offered through college and university physical education departments can be excellent and appropriate options for exercise referral. A well-qualified exercise physiologist or exercise specialist who has clinical experience and is knowledgeable about diabetes can also be a valuable resource.

STRATEGIES FOR MAINTAINING OPTIMAL GLYCEMIC CONTROL WITH EXERCISE

Based on results of SMBG, CGM, record keeping, uploads, and identification of exercise-related blood glucose patterns, individuals with type 1 diabetes can learn to make adjustments in their diabetes management to maintain optimal glycemic control with exercise. Adjustments can be made in the meal plan, insulin dosage, or both in combination. Diligence with glucose monitoring either by SMBG or CGM (before, during, and after exercise), careful record-keeping, and uploading data to retrospectively determine glucose response patterns are crucial for success with making sound exercise-related adjustment decisions.

Adjusting Carbohydrate Intake

The decision to adjust carbohydrate intake for exercise should be based on a number of factors. These include pre-exercise blood glucose level, planned exercise intensity and duration, the time of day of the planned activity and time in relation to previous food intake, an individual's level of training, and previous glycemic response to exercise. Additional carbohydrate may be necessary to prevent hypoglycemia, treat hypoglycemia if it occurs, or fuel muscle and delay fatigue during periods of prolonged activity.

When an activity session is of short duration or is unplanned, consuming additional carbohydrate is useful. For moderate activity lasting <30 min, insulin adjustment is rarely necessary, but a small snack that provides ~15 g carbohydrate may be needed. Consuming additional carbohydrate is certainly indicated if the pre-exercise blood glucose is <100 mg/dL (<5.6 mmol/L). During periods of prolonged or intense exercise when energy expenditure is high, additional carbohydrate is often necessary. Intake of 15 g carbohydrate every 30–60 min of activity is a general, safe starting guideline. Extra carbohydrate may also be needed in the postexercise period when insulin sensitivity is increased and glycogen storage is enhanced. Intake of additional carbohydrate at this time can reduce risk of hypoglycemia and enhance glycogen storage. For individuals who exercise in the late afternoon or evening, it is particularly important to be alert to the possibility of nocturnal hypoglycemia and adjust the evening snack as needed to prevent its occurrence.

The rigid recommendation to consume extra carbohydrate based only on the planned intensity and duration of exercise and without regard to the glycemic level at the start of exercise, previous metabolic response to exercise, and insulin therapy is no longer appropriate. Such an approach can easily neutralize the beneficial blood glucose–lowering effect and energy deficit that results from exercise. The amount of carbohydrate required to prevent hypoglycemia and optimize exercise performance must be determined on an individual basis and can vary with each exercise situation.

Adjusting Insulin

The increasing use of intensive insulin therapy has provided individuals with type 1 diabetes with great flexibility and the ability to make precise insulin adjustments for various activities. In certain exercise situations, it may be necessary to reduce the insulin dosage to prevent hypoglycemia.

A reduction in the insulin dosage often is necessary when a vigorous exercise session lasts greater than or equal to 30 min. The specific adjustment that will be needed depends on the insulin dosage, the timing of exercise in relation to insulin "peak" action time, and the planned intensity and duration of an activity. For a moderate amount of exercise, a modest reduction (~20–30%) in the insulin component that is most active during the period of exercise may be sufficient to prevent hypoglycemia. However, for very prolonged, vigorous exercise such as distance running, cross-country skiing, cycling, or backpacking, a large decrease in the total daily insulin dosage (by as much as 50–80%) may be needed to prevent hypoglycemia. In this case, both short- or rapid- and longer-acting insulin may need to be decreased proportionally. The DirectNet study in children using CSII showed that during strenuous activity in children, basal insulin delivery via the insulin pump should be discontinued to avoid hypoglycemia. Care should be taken to avoid discontinuation of insulin delivery for long periods of time. In addition, DirecNet has shown that after 1 h of exercise in the afternoon, children experience significantly more hypoglycemia during the ensuing night compared to sedentary days. The nadir glucose was between midnight and 2 a.m. after an afternoon exercise session between 4 and 6 p.m. In adults, or with less strenuous activity, lowering pump basal rates rather than suspending delivery may be as effective and safer. Insulin reductions may also be necessary during the postexercise recovery period.

An elevation in the pre-exercise blood glucose level can be an indicator of an insulin-deficient state. Supplemental insulin may be necessary to correct a low insulin level and improve metabolic control before exercise is initiated.

If an exercise session is to be initiated within 30 min of an insulin injection, the injection should be administered in an area of the body that will not predominantly be used for the activity. Insulin absorption and peak action time can be accelerated if insulin is injected into an area of working muscle shortly before initiation of exercise. The abdomen is generally the site of choice.

CONCLUSION

Long recognized as a cornerstone of diabetes management, exercise is an all too often underutilized therapeutic modality. Although exercise carries potential risks for people with diabetes, with careful planning, it can provide numerous health benefits that far outweigh these risks. Using established, sound guidelines, physicians and diabetes educators can frame safe and effective exercise programs that will enhance the health and well-being of individuals with type 1 diabetes.

BIBLIOGRAPHY

American College of Sports Medicine: The recommended quantity and quality of exercise for developing and maintaining cardiorespiratory and muscular fitness and flexibility in healthy adults (Position Stand). *Med Sci Sports Exerc* 30:975–991, 1998

American Diabetes Association: *Handbook of Exercise in Diabetes.* Ruderman N, Devlin JT, Schneider SH, Kriska A, Eds. Alexandria, VA, American Diabetes Association, 2002

American Diabetes Association: Physical activity/exercise and diabetes (Position Statement). *Diabetes Care* 27 (Suppl. 1):S58–S62, 2004

Centers for Disease Control and Prevention and the American College of Sports Medicine: Physical activity and public health: a recommendation. *JAMA* 273:402–407, 1995

Colberg S: *The Diabetic Athlete.* Champaign, IL, Human Kinetics, 2001

Chu L, Hamilton J, Riddell MC: Clinical management of the physically active patient with type 1 diabetes. *Phys Sportsmed* 39:64–77, 2011

Lehmann R, Kaplan V, Bingisser R, Bloch KE, Spinas GA: Impact of physical activity on cardiovascular risk factors in IDDM. *Diabetes Care* 20:1603–1611, 1997

Taplin CE, Cobry E, Messer L, McFann K, Chase P, Fiallo-Scharer R: Preventing post-exercise nocturnal hypoglycemia in children with type 1 diabetes. *J Pediatr* 157:784–788, 2010

Tsalikian E, Mauras N, Beck RW, Tamborlane WV, Janz KF, Chase HP, Wysocki T, Weinzimer SA, Buckingham BA, Kollman C, Xing D, Ruedy KJ, the Diabetes Research in Children Network Direcnet Study Group: Impact of exercise on overnight glycemic control in children with type 1 diabetes mellitus. *J Pediatr* 147:528–534, 2005

US Department of Health and Human Services: *Physical Activity and Health: A Report of the Surgeon General.* Centers for Disease Control and Prevention, National Center for Chronic Disease Prevention and Health Promotion, Washington, DC, US Govt. Printing Office, 1996

Special Situations

Highlights
Special Situations

DIABETIC KETOACIDOSIS

■ Diabetic ketoacidosis (DKA) is a life-threatening but reversible complication characterized by severe disturbances in carbohydrate, fat, and protein metabolism.

■ DKA is always due to insulin deficiency, either absolute (e.g., a previously undiagnosed patient or omitted insulin) or relative (e.g., too little insulin injected or antagonism by stress [counterregulatory] hormones).

■ Any major stress may precipitate DKA in a patient with diabetes who lacks sufficient circulating insulin.

■ The clinical signs and symptoms of DKA are listed in Table 4.1. They usually include polyuria, polydipsia, hyperventilation, dehydration, the fruity odor of ketones, and disturbances in the conscious state from drowsiness to frank coma.

■ The initial goal of therapy should be to correct life-threatening abnormalities, i.e.,

- dehydration
- hyperglycemia
- acidosis
- potassium deficiency

■ Frequent reexamination of laboratory indices is imperative, at minimum, every hour during the first 4 h and at least every 4 h thereafter.

■ Insulin therapy and hydration will reverse acidosis, and routine bicarbonate administration is not recommended. Potassium administration is recommended for all patients once urine output and renal function are assessed.

■ The cause of DKA must be aggressively pursued. Potential complications of therapy and how to avoid them are outlined.

■ DKA often can be prevented, given appropriate patient education and prompt physician attention.

HYPOGLYCEMIA

■ Hypoglycemia is a common side effect of insulin therapy. Mild hypoglycemic reactions usually consist of autonomic (neurogenic or adrenergic) symptoms, e.g., tremors, palpitations, sweating, and excessive hunger. Moderate and severe reactions include autonomic as well as neuroglycopenic symptoms, e.g., difficulty thinking, confusion, headache, slurred speech, dizziness, seizures, or coma.

■ Mild hypoglycemic reactions may produce only minimal disruption of daily activities. Moderate and severe insulin reactions may severely harm health and morale and should be avoided.

■ Certain circumstances favor development of prolonged, incapacitating, and occasionally life-threatening hypoglycemia, i.e.,

- hypoglycemia unawareness
- antecedent hypoglycemia
- failure to notice symptoms because patient is sleeping or attention is elsewhere
- intensive glycemic control
- long duration of diabetes
- certain medications or drugs, including alcohol

■ The factors precipitating an episode of hypoglycemia can often be identified, allowing prevention of future reactions in similar circumstances.

■ Self-monitoring of blood glucose (SMBG) should be used to full advantage for detection and treatment of hypoglycemia. Those with frequent or severe episodes might consider continuous glucose monitoring. Changes in insulin injection, eating, or exercise schedules and travel call for increased frequency of monitoring.

■ Guidelines for treatment of mild, moderate, and severe reactions should be clearly understood by patient, family, and school and business associates.

■ Hypoglycemia may occasionally lead to rebound hyperglycemia and should be recognized and appropriately treated if it occurs.

PREGNANCY

■ Women with type 1 diabetes who plan their pregnancies and receive optimal care by an experienced diabetes management team can expect a pregnancy outcome similar to that of women who do not have diabetes.

■ Excellent glycemic control during pregnancy has been shown to bring unequivocally beneficial results to both mother and fetus.

■ Poor perinatal outcome is associated with poor glycemic control, ketonemia, and vasculopathy.

■ Patients should be as near to normoglycemia as possible at the time of conception and throughout the 1st trimester to decrease incidence of congenital malformations, and throughout the remainder of the pregnancy to reduce the risk of macrosomia.

■ Frequent SMBG is mandatory during pregnancy. Insulin pump therapy and continuous glucose monitoring may aid in achieving optimal glycemic control during pregnancy.

■ Most women with type 1 diabetes may be managed as outpatients throughout gestation.

■ Tests to assess fetal growth and well-being should be conducted at appropriate times. Timing of delivery, management during labor and delivery, and postpartum care are covered. Family planning and contraception must be reviewed with the patient during the postpartum period.

SURGERY

■ Given appropriate preparation and management, patients with type 1 diabetes are subject to little more than normal risk during surgery.

■ Whenever possible, the patient should be in the best possible general health and glycemic control before a surgical procedure.

■ The objectives of glycemic management before, during, and after an operation are to prevent hypoglycemia and excessive hyperglycemia and ketoacidosis.

■ Because hypoglycemia is particularly dangerous in the unconscious patient, plasma glucose should generally be kept between ~100 and 150 mg/dL (~5.6 and 8.3 mmol/L) during and after the operation.

■ Intravenous insulin delivery is preferred during surgery, although subcutaneous insulin may be used if the patient has stable glucose control, the procedure is relatively minor and of short duration, and recovery is expected to be rapid.

■ In patients with DKA who need emergency surgery, efforts should be made to delay surgery until DKA is treated.

■ Guidelines are given for
• major elective surgery
• major emergency surgery
• surgery with local anesthesia

ISLET TRANSPLANTATION

■ Significant progress has been made in human islet allotransplantation, but limitations remain and the procedure remains experimental. In a long-term clinical trial, 44% of patients achieved insulin and normalization of A1C at 1 year post-islet transplantation, although a significant proportion of patients required resumption of insulin therapy in subsequent years of follow-up. The procedure also carries risks of hepatic bleeding after the administration of islets into the portal vein and complications of long-term immunosuppression. Research is ongoing to improve these results, minimize the risks from immunotherapy and develop other potential sources of islet cells.

Special Situations

DIABETIC KETOACIDOSIS

Diabetic ketoacidosis (DKA) is a life-threatening but reversible complication characterized by severe disturbances in protein, fat, and carbohydrate metabolism that result from insulin deficiency. DKA is a medical emergency requiring treatment in a medical intensive care unit or equivalent setting.

In DKA, the arterial pH is <7.3, plasma bicarbonate is <15 mEq/L, blood glucose is generally >250 mg/dL (>13.9 mmol/L), and blood ketones are elevated. In mild DKA, the bicarbonate level is 15–18 mEq/L. DKA is always due to absolute or relative insulin deficiency. The counterregulatory or stress hormones include glucagon, catecholamines, cortisol, and growth hormone and are markedly elevated in DKA. Acting in concert with the deficiency of insulin, they augment the metabolic derangements characteristic of DKA:

- hyperglycemia secondary to increased glucose production and decreased utilization
- osmotic diuresis and dehydration secondary to hyperglycemia
- hyperlipidemia secondary to increased lipolysis
- acidosis secondary to increased production and decreased utilization of acetoacetic acid and 3-β-hydroxybutyric acid derived from fatty acids
- an increased anion gap secondary to elevated ketoacids and lactate

PRESENTATION OF DKA

The clinical diagnosis of DKA is usually apparent in a patient known to have diabetes. However, DKA may not be readily considered in new-onset diabetes, particularly in very young children, in whom a delay in diagnosis may result in life-threatening complications. Those at higher risk are children <5 years and/or who, due to social or economic hardships, do not have access to regular medical care. A blood glucose concentration <250 mg/dL (<13.9 mmol/L) usually excludes DKA unless the patient has been partially treated with insulin and fluids before presentation and has severely restricted his or her calorie intake.

For patients who already have diabetes, the chances of developing DKA are 1–10% each year; however, unbalanced familial relationships, poor metabolic control, psychiatric diagnosis, eating disorders, limited medical care, and insulin pump use can cause patients to be at a higher risk of DKA development.

Table 4.1 Common Presenting Symptoms and Signs in DKA

Symptoms	Signs
Nausea and vomiting	Dehydration
Thirst and polyuria	Hyperpnea or Kussmaul breathing
Abdominal pain	Impaired consciousness and/or coma
Somnolence	Fruity odor

Clinical Signs and Symptoms

The clinical signs and symptoms of DKA include polyuria, polydipsia, hyperventilation, and dehydration (Table 4.1). The fruity odor of ketones may be apparent, especially on the breath, and disturbances in consciousness may vary from drowsiness to frank coma. Abdominal pain in association with an elevated white blood cell count and serum amylase may occur but resolves with therapy. If severe abdominal pain persists, a surgical consultation should be obtained, because an acute condition such as appendicitis, bowel perforation, pancreatitis, or infarction may coexist and may have been the DKA precipitant.

Precipitating Factors

Any major stress may precipitate DKA in a patient with diabetes. Infections such as pneumonia, meningitis, gastroenteritis, and influenza are some of the many heterogeneous causes, as are trauma or myocardial infarction. In most patients, it is possible to identify a specific precipitating cause. Among the most common are deliberate or inadvertent omission of insulin. The latter is particularly common following interruption of insulin pump delivery because of the limited available depot insulin when only rapid-acting insulin is being used. Another common cause of DKA is secondary to mismanagement of sick days, i.e., withholding insulin from a patient who is vomiting and unable to eat and mistakenly believes this situation may result in hypoglycemia (Table 4.2).

Table 4.2 Points to Consider in Treating DKA

■A precipitating cause can be identified in most patients.

■An ECG is indicated in all adult patients.

■Isotonic saline is initially preferred to rehydrate patients.

■Intravenous insulin is the preferred route of delivery.

■DKA patients are deplete in total-body potassium.

■Administration of glucose is necessary to clear ketosis.

■Bicarbonate is rarely needed.

■Cautious replacement of phosphate is sometimes used.

■Preventing DKA is a long-term goal of sound diabetes management.

ACUTE PATIENT CARE

The initial goal of therapy should be to correct life-threatening abnormalities, i.e., dehydration, insulin deficiency, and potassium deficiency. Fully correcting all biochemical abnormalities will take several days. During the first 12 h of therapy, the condition must be reevaluated frequently. Particular attention should be paid to the plasma potassium concentration as well as frequent assessment of neurologic changes (headache, mood shifts) or other symptoms of cerebral edema. A flow sheet tabulating successive changes in the patient's condition must be maintained for all patients (Table 4.3). The degree of hyperglycemia, acidosis, dehydration, and conscious state is variable. If the patient's clinical condition deteriorates after initial therapy has begun, help from an appropriate specialist is needed.

Therapy, laboratory data, and clinical assessment should be monitored at frequent intervals for the first 12–24 h. Patients are generally best followed in an intensive care setting. For a treatment schedule, see Tables 4.4 and 4.5.

Rehydration Process

Significant dehydration is present in all patients with DKA. There are many routes of water and/or electrolyte loss, including *1*) polyuria, *2*) hyperventilation, and *3*) vomiting and diarrhea. The best index of the degree of dehydration

Table 4.3 Ketoacidosis Flow Sheet

	Monitoring Interval
Clinical	
Mental status	1 h
Vital signs (T, P, R, BP)	1 h
ECG	Initially and as indicated
Weight	Initially and daily
Therapy	
Fluid intake and output (ml/h)	4 h
Insulin (units/h)	1 h
Potassium (mEq/h)	4 h
Glucose (g/h)	4 h
Bicarbonate and phosphate (if indicated) (mEq/h)	4 h
Laboratory	
Glucose (bedside)	1 h
Potassium, pH	2 h
Sodium, chloride, bicarbonate	4 h
Phosphate, magnesium	4 h
BUN and creatinine	4 h

is the magnitude of acute weight loss, which may be determined if the patient's baseline weight is known. Other clinical indices include orthostatic hypotension, dry mucous membranes, prolonged capillary refill, decreased tissue turgor, and thirst. A decrease in urine output is less reliable because of persistent osmotic diuresis with hyperglycemia. It is reasonable to assume with DKA an average water loss of 5–10% of total body weight.

Adequate rehydration is extremely important in initial therapy. Isotonic saline (0.9% normal saline [NS]) is usually the initial choice of rehydrating fluid (Table 4.4) at a rate of 10–20 mL/kg/h in the absence of shock. A patient in shock should be given isotonic saline or Ringer's lactate (crystalloid, not colloid) at a rate of 20 mL/kg/h to restore circulation. If circulation is not re-established, repeat boluses of 10 mL/kg/h can be given over 1–2 h, but likely 30–40 mL/kg total will be the maximum required. For patients who are hypertensive, hypernatremic, or at risk for congestive heart failure, a solution containing 0.45% isotonic saline may be preferable. In young children (age <10 years), calculate fluid replacement according to body surface area, not weight (e.g., a 30-kg child has ~1 m² body surface area).

Because calculations of dehydration are often over- or underestimated, IV and oral hydration should not exceed a rate of 1.5–2 times the required fluid intake for normal hydration for the age/weight/body surface of the patient.

Insulin Replacement

Because the cause of DKA in all patients includes absolute or relative insulin deficiency, insulin must be provided. Insulin is required for suppression of ketone body production and is thus necessary to correct acidosis. Insulin also inhibits glycogenolysis and gluconeogenesis, suppresses lipolysis, and facilitates the conservation of sodium and other electrolytes by the kidney.

Table 4.4 Fluid Replacement

Hour 1–2

Provide 10–15 ml/kg isotonic saline (0.9% normal saline [NS]) or 500 ml/m²/h; if patient has heart disease, administer fluid cautiously, e.g., according to central venous pressure.

Hour 3–4

Reduce fluid rate to 7.5 ml/kg/h in adults or 2,500 ml/m²/24 h in children.
Adjust fluid rate to meet clinical need. Do not consider rate of urine output in fluid replacement calculation, except in rare occasions. Fluid replacement should be administered evenly over 48 h after initial resuscitation.

When blood glucose reaches 250 mg/dL (<13.9 mmol/L), change fluid to 5% dextrose in 0.45% NS at 150–250 ml/h.

Continue intravenous fluids, including insulin, until acidosis is corrected. Then change to short- or rapid-acting insulin subcutaneously every 4 h, giving the first dose 2 h before discontinuing intravenous insulin.

Figure 4.1 Protocol for the management of patients with DKA. *After the initial history and physical examination, obtain blood glucose, venous blood gasses, electrolytes, BUN, creatinine, calcium, phosphorous, and urine analysis STAT. †Usually 1.5 times the 24-h maintenance requirements (~5 ml/kg/h) accomplish a smooth rehydration; do not exceed two times the requirement. ‖The potassium in solution should be 1/3 KPO_4 and 2/3 KCI or Kacetate. Adapted from Management of hyperglycemia crisis in patients with diabetes (Technical Review). *Diabetes Care* 24:131–153, 2001.

Short-acting (regular) or rapid-acting insulin should be used initially at a rate of 0.1 units/kg/h (or 0.05 units/kg/h for more sensitive patients). Replacing insulin with a continuous intravenous infusion is the most direct route and is preferred if methods are available to regulate the infusion rate. Insulin infusion should be initiated 1–2 h post fluid replacement/initial volume expansion. Replacement via the intramuscular route is an alternative, but only if unable to give IV insulin and should not be used in patients with impaired peripheral circulation. This titration method will adapt to any degree of insulin resistance and prevent severe hypoglycemia as insulin resistance wanes.

Insulin infusion must be continued until both hyperglycemia and acidosis are corrected. Treating acidosis requires higher doses of insulin than reversing hyperglycemia, and it will take longer to regulate than hyperglycemia alone. Therefore, when blood glucose levels approach <250 mg/dL (13.9 mmol/L), 5% glucose should be added to the rehydrating fluid to allow continuation of adequate doses of insulin therapy until acidosis resolves. Not giving glucose will delay clearing acidosis. Some clinicians, particularly those treating patients in the pediatric age range, recommend moderating the glycemic target to ~200-mg/dL (~11.1-mmol/L) range for 12 h, fearing that more rapid reduction in blood glucose increases the risk of cerebral edema.

Particular attention should be paid to the decrease rate of serum glucose at initial rehydration, as glucose levels will drop with fluid intake. After this initial drop, and with the administration of insulin, the rate of decrease is approximately 35–90 mg/dL per hour. The addition of 5% glucose to the saline solution can be added before the serum glucose reaches 250 mg/dL if the rate of fall is more rapid.

Potassium Replacement

Patients with DKA are depleted in total body potassium, despite a normal or even elevated serum potassium level. The reasons for this are complex and include the catabolic state, potassium wasting in urine secondary to polyuria, inability of kidney to rapidly conserve potassium, and often, the effects of vomiting and/or diarrhea.

Correct potassium replacement requires both caution and timely action. The following procedure is recommended:

- Establish urine output to be certain patient does not have renal failure.
- Send blood samples to the laboratory to measure serum potassium.
- Do an electrocardiogram (ECG) to rapidly estimate whether hypokalemia or hyperkalemia is present (high peaked T-waves in hyperkalemia; low T-waves with U-waves in hypokalemia). Patients who are hypokalemic should receive potassium at initial rehydration. Patients who are hyperkalemic should not receive potassium until after initial expansion and with insulin initiation.
- Begin potassium replacement at the suggested rate (Figure 4.1).
- When laboratory reports are available, alter rate with the goal of maintaining the plasma potassium level between 3.5 and 6.0 mEq/L at all times.

If starting potassium at initial volume expansion, a concentration of 20 mEq/L should be used. If starting at insulin initiation, a concentration of 40 mEql/L is advised and should continue through the entirety of therapy. Potassium can be a combination of potassium phosphate or potassium chloride or acetate. When combining, use a concentration of 20 mEql/L of each acetate and phosphate. IV administration should not exceed 0.5 mEq/kg/h, and if no response in levels is apparent and hypokalemia persists, reduction in insulin administration can occur until potassium levels begin to rise.

Once insulin infusion is begun, potassium replacement is particularly critical. Insulin tends to lower serum potassium by enhancing its movement back into cells, and hypokalemia-induced cardiac arrhythmia may result from insufficient replacement. If there is anuria, potassium should be infused with special caution and stringent monitoring.

Bicarbonate and Phosphate Replacement

Although it seems reasonable to administer sodium bicarbonate to the patient with DKA to correct the metabolic acidosis with alkali, it is not clear whether the potential benefits outweigh potential risks. The potential harmful effects are accelerated reduction in plasma potassium concentration and exacerbated intracellular acidosis. Randomized trials have shown no better outcomes in patients with DKA with bicarbonate therapy. For these reasons, routine bicarbonate administration is not recommended in most cases of DKA when pH is greater than or equal to 7.1. With severe acidosis (i.e., arterial pH <7.0), particularly when hypotension, shock, and arrhythmias are also present, or a patient has life-threatening hyperkalemia, bicarbonate should be given as an infusion of 1–2 mEq/kg over 60 min and then after checking plasma bicarbonate level. Repeat as needed until pH is >7.1.

Patients presenting in DKA are usually phosphate depleted and as with potassium, insulin administration enhances the movement of phosphate into cells. This can further reduce the plasma phosphate concentration.

There are pros and cons to administering phosphate, an ion important to many chemical reactions at the cellular level. One potential benefit is that hyperchloremia may be less likely to result when potassium is replaced as potassium phosphate instead of potassium chloride. However, administering too much phosphate can induce hypocalcemia. Therefore, calcium levels should be checked before phosphate is administered.

Although routine phosphate replacement has not been shown to be of benefit in the treatment of DKA, conservative potassium phosphate administration not to exceed 1.5 mEq/kg/24 h may be recommended, especially in patients with severe hypophosphatemia. The bulk of the potassium is administered as potassium chloride.

OTHER IMPORTANT CONSIDERATIONS

It is important to pursue other aspects of therapy while correcting the laboratory abnormalities. The cause of DKA must be pursued aggressively. The physician must be certain that there is no coexisting medical condition. In several reported series of adult patients admitted to the hospital with DKA, infection was the most common precipitating factor. Therefore, depending on clinical signs and symptoms, a chest X-ray and cultures of the urine, throat, sputum, or blood may be warranted.

An ECG is mandatory in adults to access potassium levels and also because myocardial infarction may precipitate DKA. The clinician should also carefully investigate all possible causes of abdominal pain.

Malfunction of the infusion system is the most likely cause of DKA in those on pumps and the most readily treatable cause of DKA. Recommendations for prevention and treatment of impending DKA in patients on pump therapy are covered more fully in Chapter 3.

In addition to determination of the cause of DKA, other supportive therapy must be considered. Ensuring an airway and inserting a nasogastric tube to drain gastric contents in comatose patients are strongly recommended to prevent aspiration pneumonia. Low-dose subcutaneous heparin (5,000 units every 12 h) is often recommended to prevent hypercoagulability, especially in elderly patients. However, data that demonstrate the benefit of heparin administration in DKA are lacking.

Be alert to complications of treatment. Potential complications directly attributable to the treatment of DKA must be anticipated.

- Generally, glucose will be normalized more quickly than acidosis. Premature discontinuation of insulin may result in persistence and worsening of ketoacidosis. Hyperchloremic acidosis can also occur as the result of excessive chloride replacement as both sodium and potassium chloride.
- Failure to give IV glucose at 5–6.25 g/h when blood glucose is <250 mg/dL (<13.9 mmol/L) will cause persistence of ketogenesis due to inability to continue high-dose insulin.
- Hypoglycemia can occur if the insulin infusion rate is not lowered after correction of acidosis, as insulin resistance improves and glucose toxicity clears.
- Nausea and vomiting from gastric atony due to hypokalemia or from feeding the patient before gastric peristalsis has returned can result in aspiration pneumonia.
- Hypokalemia from inadequate or delayed potassium replacement.

Cerebral Edema

Cerebral edema is the leading cause of death from DKA in children and youth; the incidence of cerebral edema is 0.5–0.9% and, once developed, the mortality rate is 21–24% with an almost equal percent suffering permanent neurologic impairment and 60–90% of DKA deaths are from cerebral edema compared to those with neurologic recovery. Those who have severe DKA appear to be at heightened risk to develop cerebral edema. Characteristics include young age, new-onset diabetes, and long duration of symptoms. Retrospective studies have shown that risk factors for cerebral edema include excess fluid administration, insulin administration in the first hour of treatment, a greater degree of hypocapnia, increased serum urea nitrogen, use of bicarbonate, and an attenuated rise in measured serum sodium concentrations during treatment. The pathophysiology for cerebral edema, previously thought secondary to intracerebral osmotic shifts, may be, in fact, due to cerebral ischemia and reperfusion injury. It remains critical to determine the mechanism of cerebral edema, since this may alter the approach to the initial treatment of DKA and rehydration strategy.

Clinically significant cerebral edema usually develops 4–12 h into therapy, though it can occur before, as well, and can be detected by a changing neurologic examination that may include onset of severe headache, pupillary changes, incontinence, vomiting, hypertension and bradycardia, neurogenic respiratory pattern, and decorticate or decerebrate posturing. Once diagnosed, cerebral edema is treated by the administration of mannitol 0.5–1 g/kg IV over 20 min. This is repeated if there is no initial response in 30 min to 2 h. Hypertonic saline (3%), 5–10 ml/kg over 30 min, may be an alternative to mannitol, especially if there is no initial response to mannitol. Intubation may be required. When the patient is stabilized, a cranial CT or MRI scan should be obtained to rule out other possible intracerebral causes of neurologic deterioration (~10% of cases), especially thrombosis or hemorrhage, which may benefit from additional therapy. Since there is no way to completely avert the development of cerebral edema, and approximately 50% of patients who develop cerebral edema suffer permanent neurologic deficit or die, eliminating DKA should be the goal of public and professional awareness campaigns.

INTERMEDIATE PATIENT CARE

Intravenous fluid and insulin should be continued until vital signs are normal, acidosis has been corrected, nausea and vomiting have stopped, and the DKA precipitating factor has been controlled.

When subcutaneous insulin is begun, three points should be considered.

- Because subcutaneous insulin takes effect more slowly than intravenous insulin loses its effectiveness, the first subcutaneous insulin injection should be given 1–2 h before stopping intravenous insulin infusion if using regular insulin and should be 15–30 min if using rapid-acting insulin. For basal insulin, release from IV insulin should be gradual (e.g., a reduced dose of SC basal insulin begins at night and the patient is completely suspended from IV insulin in the morning).

- Extra short- or rapid-acting insulin, every 4–6 h for the first 24–72 h, or an increase in basal insulin delivery with continuous subcutaneous insulin infusion (CSII), should be used to meet the increased insulin demands of continuing stress surrounding DKA, to overcome "glucose toxicity," and to facilitate rapid adjustment of the insulin dose to control blood glucose during this transition phase. The patient should be carefully observed to prevent recurrence of acidosis in the transition phase.

- The patient may remain mildly insulin resistant for several weeks, so the dose of subcutaneous insulin may exceed the patient's usual requirements.

PREVENTIVE CARE

Most often, DKA can be prevented, given appropriate patient education and prompt attention. All patients with type 1 diabetes should be performing self-monitoring of blood glucose (SMBG) regularly or using CGM in addition to being able to perform urine or blood ketone testing when hyperglycemic (>250 mg/dL [>13.9 mmol/L]) or sick. Patients must be taught how to give appropriate corrective doses of insulin when they develop hyperglycemia. A proven method of doing this is to use their previously prescribed correction bolus formula and repeat the dose at 2-h intervals until hyperglycemia has cleared.

Patients on insulin pumps must know to change all their disposables, i.e., infusion set, syringe, and insulin, at the first evidence of hyperglycemia (>250 mg/dL [>13.9 mmol/L]) that is associated with ketones or does not respond to an initial correction bolus.

Patients must contact their health care team as soon as they become ill or have nausea and vomiting, fever, or persistent hyperglycemia and hyperketonuria. When contacted early, the physician is often able to treat impending DKA successfully by prescribing frequent injections of short- or rapid-acting insulin and by oral administration of fluids. It may also be possible to rehydrate and adequately replace insulin in the doctor's office or emergency room, thereby preventing hospitalization.

However, when there is any doubt that the patient can be successfully treated in the home, office, or emergency room, hospitalization is indicated.

Attempts are being made to decrease the rates of DKA at the time of diagnosis, particularly in children. In children, the rate of DKA at diagnosis varies by age, with children under 2 years of age having the highest rates. Worldwide studies have shown that DKA rates vary by country. But in general, the incidence of DKA at diagnosis has been decreasing. This decrease in DKA is likely due to a number of factors, including increasing public and professional awareness about the signs and symptoms of diabetes and the need for early diagnosis. In Parma, Italy, a public awareness campaign conducted with physicians and schools, essentially eliminated DKA at diabetes onset in children. In the US, it has been shown that genetic screening combined with monitoring for signs of β-cell autoimmunity has decreased the severity of illness at diagnosis.

CONCLUSION

The pathophysiology of DKA can be understood in the context of insulin deficiency and excessive counterregulatory hormones, combining their effects to produce a severe state of life-threatening metabolic decompensation. Insulin, fluids, and electrolytes, given judiciously under appropriate guidelines in a hospital setting, form the cornerstone of treatment. A precipitating event such as infection, infarction, or accidental or deliberate omission of insulin must be identified and treated. All efforts at prevention should be employed with patients, as well as with the public, so that DKA at diagnosis and in those with known diabetes can eventually be eradicated.

BIBLIOGRAPHY

American Diabetes Association: Hyperglycemic crises in patients with diabetes mellitus (Position Statement). *Diabetes Care* 27 (Suppl. 1):S94–S102, 2004

Barker JM, Goehrig SH, Barriga K, Hoffman M, Slover R, Eisenbarth GS, Norris JM, Klingensmith GJ, Rewers M: Clinical characteristics of children diagnosed with type 1 diabetes through intensive screening and follow-up. *Diabetes Care* 27:1399–1404, 2004

Dunger DE: European society for pediatric endocrinology and the Lawson Wilkins pediatric endocrine society consensus statement on diabetic keto-acidosis. *Pediatrics* 113:33–40, 2004

Glaser N, Barnett P, McCaslin I, Nelson D, Trainor J, Louie J, Kaufman FR, Quayle K, Roback M, Malley R, Kuppermann N: Risk factors for cerebral edema in children with diabetic ketoacidosis. *N Engl J Med* 344:264–269, 2001

Glaser N: Cerebral injury and cerebral edema in children with diabetic ketoaci-dosis: could cerebral ischemia and reperfusion injury be involved? *Pediatric Diabetes* 10:534–554, 2009

Kaufman FR, Halvorson M: The treatment and prevention of diabetic keto-acidosis in children and adolescents with type 1 diabetes. *Pediatr Ann* 28:576–582, 1999

Kitabchi AE, Umpierrez GE, Murphy MB, Barrett EJ, Kreisberg RA, Malone JI, Wall BM: Management of hyperglycemic crises in patients with diabetes mellitus (Technical Review). *Diabetes Care* 24:131–153, 2001

Kraut JA, Kurtz I: Use of base in the treatment of severe acidemic states. *Am J Kidney Dis* 38:703–727, 2001

Larsson HE, Vehik K, Bell R, Dabelea D, Dolan L, Pihoker C, Knip M, Veijola R, Lindblad B, Samuelsson U, Holl R, Haller MJ, on behalf of the TEDDY Study Group, SEARCH Study Group, DVP Study Group, and Finnish Diabetes Registry Study Group: Reduced prevalence of diabetic ketoacidosis at diagnosis of type 1 diabetes in young children participating in longitudinal follow-up. *Diabetes Care* 34:2347–2352, 2011

Marcin JP, Glaser N, Barnett P, McCaslin I, Nelson D, Trainor J, Louie J, Kaufman FR, Quayle K, Roback M, Malley R, Kuppermann N: Factors associated with adverse outcomes in children with diabetic ketoacidosis-related cerebral edema. *J Pediatr* 141:793–797, 2002

Vanelli M, Chiari G, Ghizzoni L, Costi G, Giacalone T, Chiarelli F: Effective-ness of a prevention program for diabetic ketoacidosis in children: an 8-year study in schools and private practices. *Diabetes Care* 22:7–9, 1999

Viallon A, Zeni F, Lafond P, Venet C, Tardy B, Page Y, Bertrand JC: Does bicarbonate therapy improve the management of severe diabetic ketoacido-sis? *Crit Care Med* 27:2690–2693, 1999

Wolfsdorf J, Craig ME, Daneman D, Dunger D, Edge J, Lee W, Rosenbloom A, Sperling M, and Hanas R :Diabetic ketoacidosis in children and adolescents with diabetes. *Pediatric Diabetes* 10 (Suppl. 12):118–133, 2009

HYPOGLYCEMIA

The precise blood glucose level at which patients develop symptoms of hypoglycemia is difficult to define, but generally, symptoms do not occur until blood glucose is <50–60 mg/dL (<2.7–3.3 mmol/L). Clinical hypoglycemia is the occurrence of typical autonomic and/or neuroglycopenic symptoms with low blood glucose levels, and its symptoms are relieved by the administration of carbohydrate. Because of its sporadic and somewhat unpredictable nature and because of the need for rapid treatment, hypoglycemia is often self-diagnosed on the basis of predominantly autonomic symptoms and may be treated without documentation of the blood glucose level.

PATHOPHYSIOLOGY

Hypoglycemia occurs when there is an imbalance between the rate of glucose removal from the circulation (e.g., uptake into muscle) and the rate of glucose entry into the circulation (e.g., release of glucose from the liver or ingestion of nutrients). Clinically, this most often occurs when there is one of the following:

- a relative excess of insulin (which inhibits hepatic glucose production and stimulates glucose utilization by muscle and adipose tissue)
- a decrease or delay in food intake (which decreases the availability of dietary carbohydrate or gluconeogenic precursors)
- an increase in the level of exercise (which accelerates glucose utilization by muscle)

In individuals without diabetes, as the glucose level declines below normal (typically to 50–60 mg/dL [2.7–3.3 mmol/L]), a complex series of neuroendocrine events occur that raise the plasma glucose concentration back toward normal. Glucagon and epinephrine are thought to be the most important counterregulatory hormones in this process because of their prompt secretion and potent ability to stimulate the release of glucose from the liver. In addition, epinephrine can contribute to glucose recovery by reducing glucose uptake into insulin-sensitive tissues, and it is responsible for many of the autonomic warning symptoms of hypoglycemia (see below). The other major counterregulatory hormones—cortisol and growth hormone—generally are released more slowly than glucagon and epinephrine and appear to have a more permissive role in glucose recovery. Finally, endogenous insulin secretion is typically inhibited by hypoglycemia, also facilitating the rise in plasma glucose levels.

In contrast, the patient with type 1 diabetes has several abnormalities in this feedback system. First, the secretion of glucagon typically becomes deficient within the first 2–5 years of diabetes. Second, with more prolonged duration of the disease, epinephrine secretion may also be impaired as a result of the development of subclinical autonomic neuropathy. Epinephrine secretory thresholds can also be lowered by antecedent hypoglycemia or by tight glycemic control, with these effects being reversible. Finally, the rate of absorption of insulin from a subcutaneous depot is not regulated by normal homeostatic mechanisms, such as nutrient availability, and thus, it continues despite the presence of ongoing hypoglycemia. The combination of these and other factors makes the patient with type 1 diabetes particularly susceptible to the frequent development of hypoglycemia.

MILD, MODERATE, AND SEVERE HYPOGLYCEMIA

Symptoms of Mild Hypoglycemia

Mild low blood glucose reactions usually consist of tremors, palpitations, sweating, blurred vision, mood variations, difficulty with auditory processing, and excessive hunger. These symptoms are mostly mediated through the autonomic (adrenergic) nervous system. Major cognitive deficits usually do not accompany mild reactions, so patients are generally capable of self-treatment. These mild symptoms respond within 10–15 min after oral ingestion of 10–15 g carbohydrate.

Signs and Symptoms of Moderate Hypoglycemia

Moderate low blood glucose reactions include neuroglycopenic as well as autonomic signs and symptoms, e.g., headache, mood changes, irritability, decreased attentiveness, and drowsiness. Because of confusion, impaired judgment, and/or weakness, patients may require assistance in treating themselves. Moderate reactions produce longer-lasting and somewhat more severe symptoms and often require a second dose of carbohydrate.

Signs and Symptoms of Severe Hypoglycemia

Severe low blood glucose reactions are characterized by unresponsiveness, combativeness, unconsciousness, or seizures and typically require assistance from another individual for appropriate treatment. Approximately 5–10% of type 1 diabetes patients suffer at least one severe reaction each year that requires emergency measures such as parenteral glucagon or intravenous glucose. Subjects who experience a hypoglycemic seizure with severe hypoglycemia are at risk for recurrence.

Potential Effects of Hypoglycemia

Mild hypoglycemic reactions may produce only minimal disruption of daily activities. Hypoglycemia can cause hunger with consequent overeating, thus contributing to obesity or hyperglycemia. Patients may experience cognitive dysfunction and counterregulatory hormone impairment related to moderate hypoglycemia even if they never reach a critically low blood glucose level if there is a steep rate of fall. Cognitive dysfunction due to rapid rate of fall has been shown to correlate with decreased counterregulatory hormone production.

In contrast, moderate and severe reactions may be seriously disabling in many ways and their prevention is critical. Hypoglycemia that interferes with normal thinking makes taking a school examination an impossible task; riding a bicycle, driving a car, or operating dangerous machinery become potentially disastrous. Repeated or prolonged episodes may cause irreparable damage to the central nervous system in very young children. In adults, this is quite rare, and careful cognitive testing of the DCCT cohort has shown no decrement in cognitive ability in intensively treated subjects or those with severe hypoglycemia. However, despite the DCCT findings, there still remains a potential link between cognitive dysfunction and prolonged or repetitive hypoglycemic events. Severe hypoglycemia is frightening and deleterious on the morale of the patient and family members, a final reason for highlighting the need for prevention.

Some patients develop either an excessive fear of hypoglycemia or an inappropriate lack of concern. Fear of hypoglycemia can lead to chronic overeating, undertreatment with insulin, or both. Maintaining very high blood glucose levels to avoid hypoglycemia increases the risk of metabolic complications, including DKA, and of chronic complications of diabetes. In contrast, patients with a nonchalant attitude toward hypoglycemic reactions may maintain levels of blood glucose that are too low, may take inadequate preventive or treatment steps, and will consequently be at greater risk for recurrent severe hypoglycemia. These patients can sometimes be identified by glycated hemoglobin (A1C) levels in the normal range.

Antecedents of Severe Hypoglycemia

Certain circumstances favor development of prolonged, incapacitating, and occasionally life-threatening hypoglycemia. Patients with hypoglycemia unawareness are always at increased risk for severe reactions. The counterregulatory hormone response to hypoglycemia and the autonomic symptoms tend to decrease after several years of diabetes so that neuroglycopenic symptoms become the first manifestation for many patients. β-Blockers, methylxanithines, selective serotonin reuptake inhibitors (SSRIs), and certain other medications may also diminish early warning signs.

Hypoglycemia occurs more frequently at night, and it is more prolonged than realized by most adults and children with type 1 diabetes. Hypoglycemia has been described to occur during 8.5% of nights. The duration of hypoglycemia was >2 h on 23% of nights with hypoglycemia. Risk factors for nocturnal hypoglycemia are lower A1C and the occurrence of prior nocturnal hypoglycemia, but not age or insulin treatment with CSII versus MDI. The predictors of severe hypoglycemia are a prior severe episode in the preceding 6 months and being female. Studies have also shown that hypoglycemia begets hypoglycemia. In studies done with CGM, increased CGM readings <70 mg/dL and greater area under the hypoglycemic threshold increase the risk for severe hypoglycemia.

Intensive insulin therapy also increases the risk of asymptomatic hypoglycemia. Although the increased frequency of low glucose levels can be attributed partly to the more stringent treatment goals associated with intensive regimens, it is now apparent that physiologic alterations occur in the patient's ability to secrete counterregulatory hormones, and thus, the ability to recognize and recover from hypoglycemia is clearly impaired. As few as two moderate episodes of hypoglycemia can blunt counterregulatory hormones. These observations emphasize the importance of SMBG and CGM in such patients to detect and prevent these asymptomatic reactions.

Delaying treatment of mild hypoglycemia can lead to more severe hypoglycemia as glucose stores are depleted from antecedent episodes. Because early autonomic warning signs such as headache, hunger, mood or behavior changes, or weakness are not specific to hypoglycemia, they are frequently misinterpreted or overlooked. This is especially likely if the patient's attention is directed elsewhere, which may occur during strenuous activity. Hypoglycemia during sleep is particularly difficult to detect as the counterregulatory hormones are suppressed during sleep and therefore do not provide detectable symptoms. The patient should be questioned for the presence of nightmares or nocturnal diaphoresis, and family members should be alert to unusual sounds or activity during the patient's sleep.

COMMON CAUSES OF HYPOGLYCEMIA

The factors precipitating an episode of hypoglycemia can often be identified by looking back over the events of several hours preceding the reactions (Table 4.5).

Inadvertent or deliberate errors in insulin dose are a frequent cause of hypoglycemia; other causes are changes in timing or schedule of insulin administration or meals. For example, sleeping later than usual for patients on fixed regimens is potentially dangerous because it disrupts the balance and timing between insulin and food. Changing insulin type from a short- to rapid-acting preparation or changing the insulin regimen can cause hypoglycemia because of more rapid absorption or other factors.

Vigorous unexpected exercise or activity is commonly associated with hypoglycemia. Aerobic exercise of prolonged duration or increased intensity can cause hypoglycemia up to 17 h after the activity ends or even the next day.

Alcohol, marijuana, or other drugs often mask a patient's awareness of hypoglycemia in its earliest stages. By inhibiting the liver's gluconeogenic capacity, alcohol also prevents the body's normal ability to provide glucose and restore low glucose

Table 4.5 Common Causes of Hypoglycemia

Insulin errors (inadvertent or deliberate)
- Reversal of morning and evening dosage
- Reversal of short- or rapid- and intermediate- or long-acting insulin
- Improper timing of insulin in relation to food
- Excessive insulin dosage

Intensive insulin therapy

Erratic or altered absorption of insulin
- More rapid absorption from exercising limbs
- Unpredictable absorption from hypertrophied injection sites

Changing insulin preparations or regimens

Nutrition
- Omitted or inadequate amounts of food
- Timing errors: late snacks or meals

Exercise
- Unplanned activity
- Prolonged duration or increased intensity of activity

Alcohol and drugs
- Impaired hepatic gluconeogenesis associated with alcohol intake
- Impaired mentation associated with alcohol, marijuana, or other illicit drugs

levels toward normal. Some of the most severe hypoglycemic reactions occur during or after parties because the combination of physical activity and the use of alcohol or drugs can mask recognition of the problem and prevent the usual self-correction of hypoglycemia. Drugs used for treatment of depression are linked with increased risk for hypoglycemia. Several other drugs including levothyroxine (liver impairment) and ACE inhibitors are also correlated with more insulin sensitivity and hypoglycemia. Sulfonylureas, and other antihyperglycemic drugs, such as pramlintide, used in concert with insulin increase risk for hypoglycemia.

Anticipating and Preventing Hypoglycemia

Once a situation that leads to hypoglycemia is identified, adjustments can often be made to prevent future episodes.

Sleeping late. Although most patients on regimens of multiple daily injections can safely sleep an extra 30–60 min without particular adjustments, patients who oversleep more than 1 h may need to plan in advance to alter insulin or food intake. For example, if sleeping late is anticipated, a 10–15% reduction of intermediate- or long-acting insulin on the previous evening is an effective means of preventing hypoglycemia. However, it may also lead to excessive morning hyperglycemia. When the patient awakens, the entire day's schedule of insulin and meals is advanced in time. Even the next day's schedule may be affected. All patients should be cautioned against awakening and taking insulin without eating and then resuming sleep. However, awakening early, performing a blood glucose test, administering insulin, eating breakfast, and then going back to sleep is generally safe. Patients on insulin pumps, and many on long-acting analogs, may be able to sleep late without a problem if their basal insulin doses are appropriate. Before doing so, it would be wise to check the basal rate periodically by skipping or delaying breakfast and observing the glucose changes every 2 h by SMBG.

Exercise. To compensate for increased caloric needs of exercise, increased absorption of insulin from exercising muscles, and increased insulin sensitivity induced by extra activity, several strategies to prevent hypoglycemia can be employed. Most important, the exercising patient should always have a source of short-acting carbohydrate immediately available.

If early signs of hypoglycemia develop during exercise, the exercise should be halted and an appropriate amount of carbohydrate eaten (Table 2.6). If similar exercise has previously resulted in hypoglycemia, patients can anticipate and prevent it by snacking before, during, or after exercise, depending on when the episode occurred. Decisions regarding the type and time of extra food can be made based on SMBG.

Alternatively, hypoglycemia can be prevented by anticipatory adjustments of insulin. For example, if a patient usually takes short- or rapid-acting insulin before breakfast but is planning to exercise after breakfast, the insulin dose can be reduced by 10–20%. This strategy may be preferable for patients who do not want to increase the size of a meal before exercise or who are overweight. Patients on insulin pumps can remove their pumps or implement a decreased temporary basal rate, with the percentage of the decrease depending on the severity and duration of the exercise.

Role of CSII

It is recommended for patients to switch from MDI to CSII if they are unable to mitigate hypoglycemia. A meta-analysis of 22 randomized controlled trials and before/after studies confirmed that both A1C level and rate of severe hypoglycemia were significantly lower with CSII compared to MDI. The greater improvements from CSII in reducing or preventing severe hypoglycemia were in those with the highest initial rates of hypoglycemia, lower A1C values, younger age, shorter duration of diabetes and more frequent use of SMBG. Reports of nonrandomized clinic experiences have shown improved glycemic control without increased risk of severe hypoglycemia when patients are switched from MDI to CSII, and with the positive benefit sustained for up to 8 years. In addition, improvement in hypoglycemia unawareness has been reported with CSII.

Role of SMBG and Continuous Glucose Monitoring

The availability of SMBG has made the detection and treatment of hypoglycemia practical, even in the subclinical range. Therefore, the frequency of SMBG should be increased in patients with recurrent hypoglycemia. The addition of continuous glucose monitoring (CGM), with its frequent testing and alarms for low or rapidly decreasing glucose, has demonstrated the ability to further reduce hypoglycemia. Changes in insulin injection, eating or exercise schedules, travel, and other activities recognized as contributors to hypoglycemia call for increased frequency of monitoring. Patients should be instructed to treat asymptomatic hypoglycemia detected by SMBG or continuous monitors.

CGM is able to alert at hypoglycemic thresholds, with rapid rate of change and with a predictive horizon, allowing the patient to prevent or reduce the time spent in hypoglycemia. A short-term trial using CGM showed that time spent in hypoglycemia decreased by 21% in subjects using real-time CGM compared to controls. Nocturnal hypoglycemia was also significantly reduced, despite that fact that it has been shown that many people sleep through the hypoglycemia alarms. Long-term studies with CGM have shown that it results in a "relative" reduction in hypoglycemia. This occurs because it is expected that as A1C levels decrease, hypoglycemia, including severe hypoglycemia, will increase. But this has not been the case, and lower A1C levels have not been associated with increasing hypoglycemia during CGM usage.

Attempts have been made to develop algorithms to predict risk of severe hypoglycemia. These take into account the A1C, hypoglycemia unawareness, ability to mount an autonomic response as glucose levels fall, and the frequency and extent of recent low blood glucose levels on SMBG.

TREATMENT

Mild Hypoglycemic Reactions

For mild reactions, ingesting 15–20 g carbohydrate works quickly to increase the blood glucose and stop classic symptoms. Several sources of short-acting carbohydrate exist. Employing premeasured glucose products instead of juice or food is recommended because patients have a tendency to consume >15 g of juice or food when they have symptomatic hypoglycemia, and also because additional calories from fat or protein may cause weight gain.

Hypoglycemic reactions that occur during the night should be treated initially with 15–20 g carbohydrate and repeated if needed to treat hypoglycemia. People have often been instructed to combine carbohydrate with protein to prevent further hypoglycemia during the night; however, research does not show that the addition of protein in the treatment of hypoglycemia sustains blood glucose longer than carbohydrate alone. Having a larger snack does make sense, including during the day if the next planned meal is >1–2 h away.

Commercially available glucose tablets have the added benefit of being premeasured to help prevent overtreatment. Glucose gels or small tubes of cake frosting are convenient for children or patients who are uncooperative when hypoglycemic. Chocolate and ice cream should be avoided for treating acute hypoglycemia because the fat content retards absorption of available sugar and could contribute to weight gain from ingestion of unnecessary calories.

Because there is always a risk that mild hypoglycemia will progress to a more severe reaction, all episodes must be treated promptly and patients must test again in 15 min to insure that they are normoglycemic. Treatment and follow-up testing should be repeated if hypoglycemia persists. Patients should be instructed never to continue driving when they begin to experience hypoglycemia. They should stop, treat the hypoglycemia, and wait 15 min to do SMBG, repeating as needed to ensure full recovery before they resume driving. Patients with type 1 diabetes should always have with them their meter and glucose products with which to treat hypoglycemia. Evaluation of the effect of nonsevere hypoglycemia on work productivity has shown that it is associated with substantial economic consequences. Lost productivity was estimated to be 8.3–15.9 h of lost work time per month, and, therefore, strategies to reduce even mild hypoglycemia could have a major positive impact on lost work productivity for people with diabetes and their employers.

Moderate Hypoglycemia

Individuals with moderate reactions will often respond to the oral carbohydrates listed in Table 2.6 but may require more than one treatment and take longer to fully recover. These patients may be alert but will frequently be uncooperative or belligerent. Under such circumstances, if it becomes difficult to cajole the patient to take oral carbohydrate, administration of subcutaneous or intramuscular glucagon may be more appropriate.

Severe Hypoglycemia

Patients with impaired consciousness or an inability to swallow may aspirate and should not be treated with oral carbohydrate. These patients require either parenteral glucagon or intravenous glucose. If these are not available, glucose gels, applied between the patient's cheek and gum, may be of some help.

Generally, clinical improvement should occur within 10–15 min after glucagon injection and within 1–5 min of intravenous glucose administration. However, if hypoglycemia was prolonged or extremely severe, complete recovery of normal mental function may not occur for hours to days. Repeated boluses of intravenous glucose do not hasten recovery unless blood glucose measurements show persistent hypoglycemia. If the hypoglycemic event was associated with convulsions, the postictal period may be associated with severe headaches, lethargy, amnesia, or vomiting. Decreased muscle control may also be seen and requires medical evaluation if it persists.

Glucagon. The dose of glucagon needed to treat moderate or severe hypoglycemia for a child <5 years old is 0.25–0.50 mg; for an older child (age 5–10 years), 0.50–1 mg; and for those >10 years old, 1 mg. Glucagon should be given intramuscularly or subcutaneously in the deltoid or anterior thigh region. For children, parents and school or day care providers, and for adults, roommates or spouses should be taught how to mix, draw up, and administer glucagon so that they are properly prepared for emergency situations. Kits that include a syringe prefilled with diluting fluid are available. For mild or moderate hypoglycemia that is associated with nausea or vomiting, administration of a low dose of glucagon should be considered. In general, the dose is 1 unit per year of age up to about 15–20 units. This can be administered subcutaneously via normal 30–50 unit syringe, rather than the intramuscular syringe provided with the kit. Full doses of glucagon cause nausea or vomiting after recovery from hypoglycemia in some patients.

Intravenous glucose. If medical staff and equipment are available, intravenous glucose should be given as a primary treatment in preference to glucagon. The usual dose is 10–25 g administered as 50% dextrose over 1–3 min. A useful formula for giving 50% dextrose in the hospital is

cc of D50 = (100 − blood glucose mg/dL) × 0.4 ([5.5 − glucose mmol/L] × 0.4).

The dose can be titrated according to the patient's response. After the bolus injection, intravenous glucose (5–10 g/h) should be continued until the patient has fully recovered and is able to eat.

HYPOGLYCEMIA UNAWARENESS

In the Diabetes Control and Complications Trial (DCCT), about one-third of all episodes of severe hypoglycemia seen during waking hours in intensively treated patients were not accompanied by sufficient signs or symptoms so that patients could effectively prevent neuroglycopenia. In the past, hypoglycemia without warning was viewed as a rare condition associated with advanced autonomic neuropathy. This concept is incorrect. Forms of hypoglycemia without warning can occur in recently diagnosed patients, particularly in patients with repeated episodes of recent hypoglycemia and low A1C levels. Repeated episodes of hypoglycemia cause two problems. First, they blunt hormonal defense mechanisms that prevent hypoglycemia. Second, they lower the level at which early hypoglycemic symptoms are perceived.

The key clinical issue is that patients need to be reminded that the absence of symptoms of hypoglycemia when glucose level is <55 mg/dL (<3.1 mmol/L) should prompt consultation with their diabetes team and increased vigilance. Frequent blood glucose monitoring, particularly before driving and after strenuous exercise, is recommended. Evidence suggests that hypoglycemia unawareness can be reversed by intensive education and self-management training and efforts that successfully avoid hypoglycemia. These efforts may include adapting slightly higher blood glucose targets before meals and during the night (e.g., lower target to >100 mg/dL [>5.5 mmol/L]) and self-management training to help detect and respond to subtle early signs of hypoglycemia. Continuous glucose monitors with alarms that predict hypoglycemia have also been shown to help reinstate hypoglycemia awareness and the epinephrine response to subsequent hypoglycemia. This suggests that real-time CGM might be a useful tool to reverse the hypoglycemia unawareness associated with type 1 diabetes.

HYPOGLYCEMIA WITH SUBSEQUENT HYPERGLYCEMIA

Hypoglycemia followed by "rebound" hyperglycemia, also called the Somogyi effect, may complicate diabetes management in some patients. The phenomenon originates during hypoglycemia, with the secretion of counterregulatory hormones (glucagon, epinephrine, growth hormone, and cortisol). This hormonal surge, together with decreasing insulin levels, leaves counterregulatory hormones relatively unopposed. Hepatic glucose production is stimulated, thereby raising blood glucose levels. These hormones may cause some insulin resistance for a 12- to 48-h period. Moreover, excessive carbohydrate intake may be a major contributor to rebound hyperglycemia.

The frequency of this phenomenon is debated, and studies suggest that it is much less common than previously reported. It may follow nocturnal hypoglycemia, but it also may occur after hypoglycemia at any time. The hypoglycemic event that precedes the rebound may not produce sufficient symptoms to make it recognizable.

If rebound hyperglycemia goes unrecognized and insulin dosage is increased, a cycle of overinsulinization may result, i.e., more hypoglycemia, more rebound hyperglycemia, more insulin, more hypoglycemia. As a general rule, when hyperglycemia does not respond as expected to treatment adjustments, undetected hypoglycemia and rebound hyperglycemia should be considered as a possible explanation. Rather than increasing insulin dosage day after day, the clinician who suspects rebound hyperglycemia should endeavor to detect (via SMBG) and avoid the initiating hypoglycemic event.

Nocturnal hypoglycemia leading to fasting rebound hyperglycemia should be investigated by measuring blood glucose levels between 2:00 and 4:00 a.m. and again at 7:00 a.m. If blood glucose levels between 2:00 and 4:00 a.m. are <50–60 mg/dL (<2.8–3.3 mmol/L) and those at 7:00 a.m. are >180–200 mg/dL (>10.0–11.1 mmol/L), rebound hyperglycemia may have occurred. The increased blood glucose level may be exacerbated by the waning effect of the previous dose of intermediate-acting insulin or a prominent dawn phenomenon (see below). A decrease in presupper intermediate-acting insulin or its deferral to ~9:00 p.m. or a change to a basal analog (glargine) should prevent nocturnal hypoglycemia.

DAWN AND PREDAWN PHENOMENA

The amount of insulin required to normalize blood glucose during the night is less in the predawn period (1:00–3:00 a.m.) than at dawn (5:00–8:00 a.m.). The modest (20–40 mg/dL [1.1–2.2 mmol/L]) increase in plasma glucose commonly seen in patients with type 1 diabetes given enough insulin to avoid hypoglycemia in the predawn period is referred to as the dawn phenomenon. This increment can be greater if insulin levels decline between the predawn and dawn periods or if hypoglycemia occurs during the predawn period. The key clinical implication is that attempts to normalize prebreakfast glucose level (i.e., 70–115 mg/dL [3.9–6.4 mmol/L]) often result in predawn hypoglycemia.

Several strategies can be used to identify and prevent nocturnal hypoglycemia. These should include monitoring blood glucose at bedtime and at 2:00–3:00 a.m., especially when insulin doses are being adjusted to correct prebreakfast hyperglycemia or when blood glucose level is frequently in the normoglycemic range before breakfast. In the DCCT, >50% of all episodes of severe hypoglycemia occurred during the night or when patients were asleep, even with the use of long-acting insulin preparations given at night or insulin infusion pumps. As a consequence, the median blood glucose before breakfast was 140 mg/dL (7.8 mmol/L), and >75% of all prebreakfast values were over the upper target range of 120 mg/dL (6.7 mmol/L). Adding extra food at bedtime (particularly protein, which helps stimulate glucagon secretion) and giving insulin that does not "peak" between 1:00 and 3:00 a.m. should be considered. Increasing the bedtime snack is particularly important when nocturnal hypoglycemia is most likely (e.g., after sustained exercise during the day or when prebedtime glucose is <100 mg/dL (<5.6 mmol/L). Among patients taking twice-daily injections, giving the evening intermediate-acting insulin at bedtime or substituting it with long-acting insulin may be effective. Changing the regimen to an insulin pump can also help dramatically; the basal rate can be programmed to prevent nocturnal hypoglycemia as well as cover the dawn rise of glucose.

CONCLUSION

Severe hypoglycemia can be life-threatening if not treated promptly. Even mild and moderate hypoglycemia can cause both short- and long-term problems. All patients should be taught to be aware of the signs of hypoglycemia and should be encouraged to use SMBG frequently to prevent and monitor episodes. Continuous glucose monitoring may be a helpful adjunct in patients, particularly with severe episodes and hypoglycemia unawareness. Patients should be aware to change their regimen with exercise. All families, child care or school personnel, and spouses or roommates of adults, should be taught how to use glucagon and when to call for medical assistance.

BIBLIOGRAPHY

American Diabetes Association: Hypoglycemia and employment/licensure (Position Statement). *Diabetes Care* 31 (Suppl. 1):S94, 2008

Brod M, Christensen T, Thomsen TL, Bushnell DM: The impact of non-severe hypoglycemic events on work productivity and diabetes management. *Value in Health* 14:665–671; 2011

Cox DJ, Gonder-Frederick L, Ritterband L, Clarke W, Kovatchev BP: Prediction of severe hypoglycemia. *Diabetes Care* 30:1370–1373, 2007

Cryer PE: Diverse causes of hypoglycemia-associated autonomic failure in diabetes. *N Engl J Med* 350:2272–2279, 2004

Cryer PE, Davis SN, Shamoon H: Hypoglycemia in diabetes (Technical Review). *Diabetes Care* 26:1902–1912, 2003

DCCT Research Group: Hypoglycemia in the Diabetes Control and Complications Trial. *Diabetes* 46:271–286, 1997

Havlin CE, Cryer PE: Nocturnal hypoglycemia does not commonly result in major morning hyperglycemia in patients with diabetes mellitus. *Diabetes Care* 2:141–147, 1987

Juvenile Diabetes Research Foundation Continuous Glucose Monitoring Study Group: Prolonged nocturnal hypoglycemia is common during 12 months of continuous glucose monitoring in children and adults with type 1 diabetes. *Diabetes Care* 33:1004-1008; 2010

Juvenile Diabetes Research Foundation Continuous Glucose Monitoring Study Group: Factors predictive of severe hypoglycemia in type 1 diabetes. *Diabetes Care* 34:586-590; 2011

Ly TT, Hewitt J, Davey RJ, Lim EM, Davis E, Jones TW: Improving epinephrine responses in hypoglycemia unawareness with real-time continuous glucose monitoring in adolescents with type 1 diabetes. *Diabetes Care* 34:50-52, 2011

Perlmuter LC, Flanagan BP, Shah PH, Singh SP: glycemic control and hypoglycemia: is the loser the winner? *Diabetes Care* 31:2072-2076, 2008

Realsen JM, Chase HP: Recent advances in the prevention of hypoglycemia in type 1 diabetes. *Diabetes Technol Ther* 13:1177-1186; 2011

PREGNANCY

Type 1 diabetes complicates ~0.1–0.2% of all pregnancies. During the last 40 years, perinatal outcome has improved remarkably in this high-risk group. The perinatal mortality rate for women with diabetes who receive optimal care now approaches that of the general obstetric population.

Management of the patient with type 1 diabetes during pregnancy ideally involves an experienced medical management team, including the diabetologist or endocrinologist, obstetrician or maternal-fetal specialist (perinatologist), pediatrician or neonatologist, certified diabetes educator, dietitian, the patient, and her partner. Experience indicates that the outcome for both mother and baby is generally more favorable when an experienced team is responsible for management during pregnancy, delivery, and the perinatal period. When a team is not conveniently available, phone consultation with individual specialists is of paramount importance. Pregnant women are usually highly motivated; therefore, this time is ideal for teaching self-care skills they can use for the rest of their lives.

RISK FACTORS

What factors help quantify maternal and fetal risk in pregnancies complicated by diabetes? Generally, risk factors fall into two categories: those relating to diabetes and its control and those relating to vascular complications. Thus, pregnancies complicated by type 1 diabetes can be divided into two groups: women with diabetes and women with diabetes and vascular complications.

Diabetes and Its Control

No longer does the onset and duration of diabetes influence the prognosis for good perinatal outcome. Instead, the degree of glycemic control at conception and the presence or absence of secondary nephropathy, vasculopathy, microalbuminuria, and hypertension greatly influence the prognosis for a favorable outcome for the mother and the fetus. The quality of maternal glucose control throughout pregnancy is also an important consideration. Poor blood glucose control, including ketoacidosis, is associated with intrauterine death.

Vasculopathy

The greater the degree of vasculopathy, the greater the likelihood of a poor outcome for mother and child. Nephropathy, particularly if associated with hypertension, appears to bring the greatest hazards, increasing the risk of preeclampsia, fetal growth retardation, and preterm delivery. Pregnancy can contribute to a worsening of retinal disease in women with background or proliferative retinopathy, especially in the presence of hypertension; women with active proliferative retinopathy are at greatest risk for progression, but visual loss can be minimized with laser therapy. Maternal deaths have been reported in patients with coronary artery disease. Other prognostically bad signs during pregnancy include ketoacidosis, pyelonephritis, preeclampsia, and poor clinic attendance or neglect.

MATERNAL METABOLISM DURING PREGNANCY

During gestation, maternal metabolism adapts to provide the fetus with an uninterrupted supply of fuel. During the 1st trimester of a normal pregnancy, accelerated utilization of glucose by the developing fetus generally produces a decrease in maternal glucose levels. In addition, pregnancy-associated nausea and vomiting can result in a decrease in food consumption. As a result, women with diabetes are prone to hypoglycemia in the 1st trimester and insulin requirements may decrease. Later in gestation, insulin resistance produced by the changing hormonal milieu typically results in an increase in insulin requirements.

In nondiabetic pregnant women, glucose levels are typically lower than those in the nonpregnant state. In pregnancy, human placental lactogen, prolactin, and progesterone alter maternal islet cell function, producing β-cell hyperplasia and contributing to maternal hyperinsulinemia. In addition, maternal cortisol is elevated during pregnancy, which potentiates glucose intolerance. Human placental lactogen (hPL), a growth hormone–like protein synthesized by the placental syncytiotrophoblast, produces insulin resistance and augments maternal lipolysis. As placental mass enlarges during pregnancy, hPL levels rise, allowing increased maternal utilization of fats for energy and sparing of glucose for fetal consumption. In late pregnancy, the progression of overnight maternal fasting ketosis is so accelerated that delaying breakfast may result in significant ketonuria.

In pregnancy complicated by diabetes, periods of maternal hyperglycemia produce fetal hyperinsulinemia. Larger amounts of maternal amino acids and other fuels also cross to the fetus. Elevated levels of maternal glucose and other nutrients stimulate the fetal pancreas, resulting in β-cell hyperplasia and hyperinsulinemia. This combination of fetal overnutrition and fetal hyperinsulinemia contributes to macrosomia in the infant of the mother with diabetes. In a report describing a 40-year experience in women with type 1 diabetes in Scotland, despite a marked decrease in perinatal mortality from 225 per 1,000 total births after 28 weeks in the 1960s to 10 per 1,000 births in the 1990s, standardized birth weight (adjusted for gender, gestational age, and parity) did not change, indicating that intrauterine overgrowth of the fetus still occurred due to failure to completely normalize maternal glycemia.

PRECONCEPTION CARE AND COUNSELING

To prevent early pregnancy loss and very costly congenital malformations in infants of mothers with diabetes, optimal medical care and patient education and training must begin before conception. This is best accomplished through a multidisciplinary team comprised of a diabetologist, internist or family practice physician, obstetrician, diabetes educators, including a nurse and registered dietitian, and other specialists as necessary. Ultimately, the woman with diabetes must become the most active member of the team, calling on the other members for specific guidance and expertise to help her toward her goal of a healthy pregnancy and offspring.

Because treatment of the patient with type 1 diabetes must begin before gestation, any regular visit to the physician by a reproductive-age woman, from teenage to middle age, should be considered a preconception visit (Table 4.6). These

Table 4.6 Care Before Conception

■Discuss contraceptive program	■Optimize glycemic control: A1C as close to normal as possible without significant hypoglycemia

■Establish database for perinatal risk
Assess vascular status:
    Ophthalmologic examination
    ECG
    Consider exercise stress test if
      diabetes >20 year duration
    Urine albumin excretion
    Creatinine clearance
    Peripheral pulses
Assess glycemic control via A1C testing
Assess thyroid function: free T$_4$, TSH
    level, antimicrosomal antibodies
	■Refer for medical nutrition therapy
	■Determine immune status against rubella
	■Evaluate psychosocial setting
	    Caution patient against smoking or
	      excessive alcohol
	    Assess exercise program
	■Begin daily folate supplement (600 mg)

contacts provide an important opportunity to discuss the patient's contraceptive needs and her thoughts and concerns about a future pregnancy and to establish a database that can be used in assessing perinatal risk. Adolescents in particular should be encouraged to discuss these issues routinely with members of the diabetes management team.

Important periodic assessments include measurements of blood pressure, dilated eye examinations, and assessments of kidney function and urine albumin excretion. Note that preexisting cardiovascular disease significantly increases morbidity and mortality to the mother and should be considered in women of childbearing age with long duration of diabetes. A1C testing should be performed routinely and SMBG taught, if needed. Continuous glucose monitoring should be considered. The desired outcome of glycemic control in the preconception phase of care is to lower A1C (at least 6.1% to <7%, preferably as close to normal as possible without risks) so as to achieve maximum fertility and optimal embryo and fetal development. Poor glycemic control during the period of organogenesis (first 7 weeks after conception) significantly increases the risk of congenital anomalies and early pregnancy loss. Since much of this period may pass before the woman is aware she is pregnant, preconception planning and excellent glycemic control are critical.

Immune status against rubella should also be checked before conception. Consultation with a nutritionist and a review of the patient's exercise program are important. Daily folate supplementation (600 µg) should be advised. The patient must understand that smoking and alcohol are strictly prohibited during pregnancy.

Because pregnancy complicated by type 1 diabetes may cause emotional and financial stress, it is essential to evaluate the psychosocial interactions of the patient and her partner, their support network, and their financial resources.

Women with type 1 diabetes who are contemplating pregnancy often have questions regarding its impact on their health and the possible consequences for the fetus. Some of the most commonly encountered questions, along with suggested answers, are presented below.

Q. How will pregnancy affect my health and life expectancy?

A. Pregnancy is not generally life-threatening, but serious complications can occur if glycemic control is not maintained during pregnancy. There is no evidence that pregnancy shortens the lives of women with type 1 diabetes, except for some with established coronary artery disease. However, women with diabetes do face a higher risk for certain complications. If ketoacidosis occurs, there is the additional threat of fetal death. Preeclampsia and preterm delivery of the fetus by cesarean section are more common in women with diabetes.

Q. What effect will pregnancy have on diabetic nephropathy?

A. There is no evidence that pregnancy will permanently worsen diabetic nephropathy, although a temporary increase in proteinuria and decrease in creatinine clearance may occur. On the other hand, advanced nephropathy may jeopardize both mother and infant, increasing the risk for early preeclampsia requiring preterm delivery and/or a smaller-than-normal infant. Factors that point in this direction include

- proteinuria >2 g/24 h
- creatinine clearance <50 ml/min or serum creatinine >2 mg/dL
- hypertension: >130/80 mmHg despite treatment

Q. What effect will pregnancy have on diabetic retinopathy?

A. Except for women with active proliferative retinopathy, pregnancy is usually an ophthalmologically stable period. Women without diabetic retinopathy will not usually develop it during pregnancy. Very few women who have background retinopathy at the start of pregnancy experience a worsening of this condition and very rarely to a proliferative stage. Proliferative retinopathy treated by laser photocoagulation and stable before pregnancy will generally remain so. In contrast, women with active proliferative retinopathy that has not been treated with photocoagulation may experience a serious worsening of this complication during pregnancy. A dilated eye examination prior to conception or in the first trimester is advised.

Q. Will the baby develop diabetes?

A. The infant is slightly more likely to develop type 1 diabetes later in life because of maternal diabetes, but the risk is not very high, i.e., ~3–4%.

Q. Can I use birth control pills?

A. Young women without vascular complications may use a low-dose estrogen (≤35 μg)/progestin oral contraceptive. Those with hypertension or vasculopathy should use a progestin-only pill (or some other means of birth control).

Q. What effect will diabetes have on the baby?

A. The answer to this question appears to hinge largely on the mother's blood glucose control; generally, the better the diabetes control, the fewer the

Table 4.7 Techniques and Purpose of Fetal Assessments Used in Pregnant Women with Preexisting Diabetes According to Gestational Age

Testing Modality	Timing	Comments
Ultrasound, transvaginal, or transabdominal • Crown-rump length • Fetal cardiac activity • Nuchal translucency (NT) thickness at 12–13 weeks; couple with free β-hCG, PAPP-A	1st trimester	Important to confirm living fetus, establish gestational age and estimated due date as early as possible; elevated NT measurement is associated with fetal Down Syndrome, and specific congenital anomalies (cardiac defects, diaphragmatic hernia, skeletal and neurologic abnormalities) more common in women with PDM
Maternal serum marker screening	1st trimester (with or without ultrasonic NT measurement) Second trimester (triple[1] or quad[2] marker test, or MSAFP alone)	PDM is associated with an increased risk of open neural tube defects (detected by 2nd trimester triple or quad marker test, or MSAFP alone)
Ultrasound, transabdominal • Fetal biometric measurements • Fetal anatomy	2nd trimester	Important to establish gestational age when this has not been done earlier in pregnancy; detailed fetal anatomic examination and fetal echocardiography should be considered in all women with PDM, but particularly in those at highest risk for congenital anomalies[3]
Ultrasound, transabdominal • Fetal growth rate (abdominal circumference measurement reflects fetal adiposity) • Amniotic fluid volume	3rd trimester	Following fetal growth by ultrasound examinations at regular intervals may be warranted when a pregnancy is at risk for fetal growth restriction (hypertension or vascular complications) or excessive fetal growth (poor glycemic control), or in lower risk women when a fundal height dates discrepancy is noted
Non-stress test (NST)	3rd trimester	Abnormal NST and BPP tests suggest possible decreased fetal oxygenation status, but are affected by other factors. The optimal testing regimen and the ideal time to initiate testing are not known. However, women with hypertensive disorders, vascular disease, or evidence of fetal growth restriction should begin testing earlier, with a frequency of every 3–7 days
Biophysical profile (BPP)	3rd trimester	
Amniotic fluid markers of fetal lung maturity	Before delivery in indicated cases	Positive tests suggest a low risk of RDA in the newborn infant[4]

[1]Maternal serum α-fetoprotein (MSAFP), unconjugated estriol, chorionic gonadotropin
[2]All components of the triple marker test, plus inhibin
[3]Elevated 1st trimester hemoglobin A1C value, abnormal multiple marker results, abnormality suspected on basic ultrasound study, or personal history of a prior birth affected by congenital anomalies
[4]RDS, respiratory distress syndrome

complications. In the first weeks of pregnancy, poor diabetes control appears to increase the occurrence of fetal malformations. Later, high blood glucose levels may bring about other serious consequences. Because glucose crosses from the mother to the fetus but insulin does not, high maternal glucose stimulates the fetus to overproduce insulin, which may

- cause excessive fetal growth, which increases the risk of shoulder dystocia, birth injury, and need for cesarean delivery
- prevent the baby's lungs (and other organs) from maturing at a normal pace
- give the baby serious hypoglycemia after birth, when it no longer receives glucose from the mother

In addition, high glucose levels are associated with sudden unexplained fetal death late in pregnancy. The incidence of preeclampsia is lowest in women with optimal glycemic control and rises as A1C increases. Preeclampsia in women with type 1 diabetes is also correlated with the presence of microalbuminuria.

CONGENITAL MALFORMATIONS: RISK AND DETECTION

The incidence of major congenital malformations in the offspring of women with type 1 diabetes that is well controlled in the first trimester is similar to the 2–3% rate observed in the general population. However, the rate increases with poorer glycemic control to as high as 20–25% among women with markedly elevated A1C in the 1st trimester. Cardiac and neural tube defects are common classes of malformation in these cases. Elevated A1C in the beginning weeks of pregnancy and second-trimester hypertension have also been linked to early delivery (pre 34 weeks).

Much evidence links such malformations with inadequate diabetes control during embryogenesis (gestational week 3–7). The magnitude of risk for abnormalities increases proportionally to the degree of elevation of A1C during this period. For this reason, patients should have as close to normal glycemic levels as possible at conception and throughout the 1st trimester. All women of childbearing age should be made aware of these risks, and if pregnancy is considered, they should be encouraged to use contraception until excellent glycemic control is achieved (see Philosophy and Goals, page 27). The risk of fetal anomalies should be reviewed at the first prenatal visit.

Table 4.8 Target Blood Glucose Levels in Pregnancy

Time of Measurement	Blood Glucose (mg/dL [mmol/L])
Before breakfast	60–99 (3.3–5.4)
Before lunch, supper, and bedtime snack	60–99 (3.3–5.4)
1 h after meals	100–129 (5.4-7.1)
2:00–6:00 a.m.	60–99 (3.3–5.4)

A1C levels should be within the normal range for pregnancy.

Fetal anomalies associated with diabetic embryopathy can be detected pre-natally in most cases. Ultasonography for nuchal translucency (possibly with 1st trimester biochemical screening with pregnancy-associated plasma protein A and β-human chorionic gonadotropin) should be offered at 11–13 weeks. At 16 weeks, further evaluation for a potential fetal malformation should include a maternal serum β-fetoprotein level, possibly combined with unconjugated estriol and cho-rionic gonadotropin ("triple screen") or additionally with inhibin ("quadruple screen"). A detailed ultrasound examination of fetal anatomy should be done at 16–18 weeks. In women with high risk of fetal cardiac anomalies (such as those with poor 1st trimester glycemic control), assessment of fetal cardiac structure by echocardiography at 20 weeks should be considered. All of these studies require interpretation by specialists experienced in prenatal diagnosis.

MATERNAL GLUCOSE CONTROL DURING PREGNANCY

Excellent control of maternal diabetes will reduce the risks of fetal demise, excessive fetal growth, and delayed pulmonary maturation. During a nondiabetic pregnancy, maternal plasma glucose rarely exceeds 100 mg/dL (5.6 mmol/L), ranging from fasting levels of 60 mg/dL (3.3 mmol/L) to postprandial levels <120 mg/dL (<6.7 mmol/L). These values should be therapeutic objectives for preg-nancies complicated by type 1 diabetes (Table 4.8).

Maintaining maternal glucose levels in this range throughout gestation is difficult. During the 1st trimester, when morning sickness may be troublesome, the risk of hypoglycemia is increased; hypoglycemia is most likely during the night, when the mother is fasting but the fetus and placenta continue to consume glucose. Severe hypoglycemia is three times more frequent in early pregnancy (8–16 weeks) compared to the prepregnancy time period. In the 3rd trimester, hypoglycemia decreases when insulin resistance from the counterregulatory hor-mones of pregnancy is greatest. Insulin needs may rise 50–100% over the final 4–6 weeks, and the total insulin dose at the time of delivery may double or even triple that of prepregnancy.

Monitoring Control

SMBG and CGM. During pregnancy, women with type 1 diabetes must use SMBG to assess control. SMBG has been shown to decrease the need for hos-pitalization and reduce the cost of care. Patients should monitor in the fasting state, before each meal, and 1 h after meals. Testing at 2:00–3:00 a.m. is necessary for most patients, particularly for those who are likely to experience nocturnal hypoglycemia, those who have persistent fasting hyperglycemia, or those who are using continuous subcutaneous insulin infusion. Continuous glucose monitoring (CGM) can be used in pregnancy and may help diagnose high postprandial glu-cose levels and nocturnal hypoglycemia that are missed with SMBG. The patient should be instructed to self-adjust insulin and maintain a careful record of the daily glucose and insulin values with comments about calorie intake and exercise.

Available data are too limited to permit specific recommendations regarding exercise programs in pregnant women with diabetes, but in most women with type 1 diabetes, the general recommendations for all pregnant women apply.

A1C testing. A1C testing should be obtained at the patient's first prenatal visit to assess previous glycemic control. This test should be repeated every 4–6 weeks.

Ketone testing. Patients should be instructed to test for ketones any time glucose levels exceed 200 mg/dL (11.1 mmol/L).

Insulin Regimen During Pregnancy

An insulin regimen tailored to the patient's needs can be developed based on SMBG or continuous glucose monitoring system (CGM) data, the meal plan, and the exercise regimen. Almost all women will require preprandial rapid- or short-acting insulin with a basal insulin. Although the basal insulins glargine and detemir are FDA pregnancy category C, there have been reports of the use of insulin glargine in pregnancy that have shown no increase in morbidity or macrosomia. For women who are well controlled on a long-acting analog prior to pregnancy, the theoretical benefit of switching to NPH insulin (which has a long track record of safety in pregnancy) must be weighed against the risks of a deterioration in glycemic control or increased number of hypoglycemic reactions with a change in regimen. The greatest flexibility and control is provided by insulin pump therapy.

Some women may be controlled with a morning mixture of intermediate-acting and rapid- or short-acting insulins, rapid- or short-acting insulin before supper, and intermediate-acting insulin near bedtime. This regimen helps avoid glycemic irregularities overnight, decreasing the likelihood of nocturnal hypoglycemia and providing effective prophylactic treatment for the dawn phenomenon and/or the waning of the insulin effect in the early morning hours leading to prebreakfast hyperglycemia. However, postlunch glucose levels may be difficult to control without a prelunch injection of rapid- or short-acting insulin.

During pregnancy, most women prefer the flexibility of a four-injection regimen: a mixture of intermediate-acting and rapid- or short-acting insulins at breakfast, rapid- or short-acting insulin at lunch and supper, with an injection of intermediate- or long-acting insulin at bedtime.

In general, if glucose levels remain elevated pre- or postmeal, the corresponding insulin dose is increased by 10–20%. Although glycemic goals are lower, strategies for titrating insulin doses are similar in pregnant women to those used in non-pregnant adults (see Optimizing Blood Glucose Control, Chapter 3).

Insulin pump therapy. Pump therapy in pregnancy is best managed by a diabetes team with expertise in this form of therapy. Patients who have used insulin pump therapy before gestation should continue on this program. Patients who are not at goal either preconception or during pregnancy should be considered for pump therapy.

Pump therapy in pregnancy offers several advantages over multiple daily injections. Most important, quick titration of both basal insulin and bolus insulin to achieve the stringent goals of pregnancy without hypoglycemia is relatively easily accomplished. In times of morning sickness in the 1st trimester, the patient can rely on her basal infusion and take the bolus postmeal once the food is consumed. Boluses for snacks are also easily covered without the need of a separate injection. Most pregnant women use at least 2–3 basal infusion rates per 24 h, with an increased rate in the early morning hours to counteract the increased release of the counterregulatory hormones, growth hormone, and cortisol later in pregnancy. The pump also allows the nocturnal basal infusion to be decreased early in pregnancy if needed to reduce the risk of hypoglycemia.

Pump therapy is not without risks during pregnancy. Most important, should there be interruption of insulin delivery, rapid development of ketoacidosis may occur. All pregnant patients on pumps must be instructed at each visit how to troubleshoot hyperglycemia and change the infusion set and insulin reservoir if hyperglycemia (>200 mg/dL [>11.1 mmol/L]) does not respond to a correction bolus. In addition, changing of the infusion site every 2 days is often needed in addition to rotation of the sites away from the abdominal area in the 3rd trimester. Skin irritation can be more common in pregnancy, and appropriate troubleshooting must be done.

NUTRITION NEEDS

The daily nutrition needs of pregnant women with type 1 diabetes should be based on a nutrition assessment by a dietitian. SMBG results, ketone tests, appetite, and weight gain can be a guide to developing and evaluating an individualized meal plan.

For most patients, 10% of the calories should be consumed at breakfast, 30% at lunch, and 30% at supper. The remaining 30% of calories can be distributed among several snacks, particularly at bedtime snack to decrease the risk of nocturnal hypoglycemia. Additional snacks may be added if the patient anticipates an increase in physical activity. Patients with persistently elevated midmorning glucose levels should reduce the calorie and/or fat content of breakfast and redistribute the calories to lunch and supper. Fat can slow digestion, resulting in elevated blood glucose levels later than when carbohydrate alone is eaten. The presence of morning ketonuria with normal glucose levels indicates the need to increase the calorie content of the bedtime snack or to consider adding a snack around 3:00 a.m. However, there is no evidence that starvation ketosis has an effect on outcome. The calorie content of the meal plan may be reduced in women who are obese, who demonstrate early excessive weight gain, or who have a sedentary lifestyle. Guidelines for calorie needs for women who begin pregnancy at a desirable weight can be obtained from appropriate references (see also Nutrition, page 98). Attention should be paid to providing sufficient intake of folate, in the form of supplementation of 600 µg daily, calcium, other vitamins, and iron, although these vitamins and minerals are important for all pregnant women and not specific to women with diabetes.

OUTPATIENT CARE

Most women with type 1 diabetes may be managed as outpatients throughout gestation. Some may benefit from early hospitalization to evaluate cardiovascular and renal status and glucose control. Failure to maintain acceptable glucose levels, worsening hypertension, or infectious complications, such as a viral illness or pyelonephritis, may necessitate hospitalization. A urine culture should be ordered in the 1st trimester, because up to 25% of type 1 diabetic women can have asymptomatic urinary tract infections in the 1st trimester.

Clinic visits can be scheduled at monthly intervals early in pregnancy if glycemic control is good, and at 1- to 2-week intervals during the first trimester. At each visit, the patient's SMBG meter, log, or uploaded data should be reviewed, problems with hyperglycemia and/or hypoglycemia discussed, and the patient's weight gain and blood pressure checked. The patient should also be instructed to telephone the team promptly if there are any episodes of hypoglycemia (<50 mg/dL [<2.8 mmol/L]) or hyperglycemia (>200 mg/dL [>11.1 mmol/L]) so that appropriate immediate remedial action may be taken.

Throughout gestation, the physician coordinating the patient's management must communicate regularly with other members of the medical management team. If background retinopathy has been detected, repeat ophthalmologic examinations should be obtained in the 2nd or 3rd trimester; proliferative retinopathy requires more intensive follow-up. If rapid normalization of blood glucose is needed, then monthly visits to the ophthalmologist are necessary to treat any development of neovascularization. Renal function studies, including creatinine clearance and protein excretion, should be repeated in each trimester if baseline values are abnormal.

Assessment of Fetal Condition

Significant advances have been made in the ability to assess fetal growth and well-being. The detection of fetal malformations between 16 and 20 weeks is discussed above (see Congenital Malformations: Risk and Detection, page 166). In the 3rd trimester, attention should be directed toward the assessment of fetal well-being, growth, and pulmonary maturation. Several approaches should be used to assess fetal condition to prevent sudden intrauterine death, a catastrophe most likely to occur during the final 4–6 weeks of gestation.

Patient self-assessment. Maternal monitoring of fetal activity has proved to be a simple yet valuable screening approach in high-risk pregnancies. Daily assessment of fetal movement may be started at 28 weeks' gestation. The patient counts fetal activity for several 30- to 60-min periods throughout the day or records the time of day at which she has felt a total of 10 fetal movements. A significant decrease in fetal activity demands further evaluation.

Nonstress test. The nonstress test (NST) is an ideal screening technique that is easily performed in an outpatient setting and usually requires no more than 20 min. Fetal heart rate is recorded with an external heart rate monitor. A normal response is the presence of two or more accelerations of at least 15 beats and lasting at least 15 s during 20 min of observation. This "reactive" test is considered a reassuring finding. In a metabolically stable patient, a reactive NST will predict fetal survival for up to 1 week.

The NST may be performed weekly after 28 weeks' gestation and then twice weekly at 32 weeks of gestation. Because normal fetal activity and a reactive NST are rarely associated with an intra-uterine fetal death, the primary value of surveillance is to allow the clinician to delay delivery safely while the fetus gains further maturity. However, because the screening tests have significant false-positive rates, an abnormal test, e.g., as a decrease in fetal activity, must be further evaluated.

Biophysical profile. Some clinicians have turned to the biophysical profile to assess fetal condition. The biophysical profile utilizes real-time ultrasound to observe fetal activity, fetal breathing movements, amniotic fluid volume, and fetal tone. Like the NST, the biophysical profile can usually be completed in 15 min and, if normal, indicates fetal well-being.

Assessment of Fetal Growth

Fetal growth assessment with serial ultrasound examinations may be warranted during the 3rd trimester in women at risk for fetal growth restriction (maternal hypertension or vasculopathy) or excessive fetal growth (poor glycemic control), or in lower-risk women if there is a discrepancy between fundal height and pregnancy dates. Delivery by cesarean section should be considered if the ultrasound suggests excessive fetal size. In pregnancies complicated by diabetes, an infant >4,000 g increases the risk of shoulder dystocia. At 20–22 weeks, an anatomic ultrasound may help detect congenital malformations and a maternal Doppler may be a good early assessment for preeclampsia.

The techniques utilized today for antepartum fetal surveillance permit most patients to remain outside the hospital even during the final 4–6 weeks of gestation, as long as maternal control is acceptable and fetal evaluation is reassuring. Nevertheless, hospitalization may be necessary if the patient has nephropathy and/or hypertension, if she has not adhered to the regimen, or when fetal jeopardy is suspected.

TIMING OF DELIVERY

In the past, preterm delivery was often elected to avoid the risk of intrauterine fetal death. In many instances, such infants, although born alive, succumbed to respiratory distress syndrome (RDS). An increased incidence of RDS due to the combined effects of prematurity and diabetes, which may retard normal maturation of pulmonary surfactant production, was observed in infants of mothers with diabetes.

Today, delivery can be safely delayed until 38 weeks in most pregnancies complicated by type 1 diabetes. Labor may then be induced after 38 weeks without amniocentesis to confirm lung maturity, or the onset of spontaneous labor may be awaited. Patients must continue excellent glycemic control, and all parameters of antepartum fetal surveillance should remain normal.

In women who have vasculopathy, who have been in poor control, who have had a prior stillbirth, or who have not adhered to the program of care, early elective delivery to prevent a late fetal death may be planned provided that fetal pulmonary maturation has been confirmed by the analysis of amniotic fluid obtained by amniocentesis. RDS is highly unlikely when the amniotic fluid lecithin-to-sphingomyelin ratio is >2.0 and phosphatidylglycerol is present.

If the fetal lungs are immature, delivery may be postponed as long as the results of fetal assessment remain reassuring. It is essential that the obstetrician know the reliability of the analytical technique used for phospholipid analysis in the reporting laboratory, particularly in pregnancies complicated by diabetes.

Delivery despite fetal lung immaturity may be necessary when testing suggests fetal compromise or if the pregnant patient develops preeclampsia, rapidly worsening retinopathy, or renal failure. As is the case in nondiabetic pregnancies, antenatal glucocorticoids are indicated to enhance lung maturity for preterm delivery at 24–33 weeks' gestation. There are no clinical trials specifically in diabetic pregnancies or in deliveries at 33–38 weeks if indices of fetal lung maturity are abnormal. Administration of high-dose corticosteroids will cause hyperglycemia in the diabetic mother, and this should be treated aggressively.

LABOR AND DELIVERY

The timing and site of delivery must be discussed and coordinated with the neonatologists who are to be present. If delivery is anticipated and adequate maternal or neonatal care cannot be provided, the patient should be transferred to a hospital with an appropriately equipped nursery. Expert care is required to deal with the various complications that may arise in the infant of the mother with diabetes.

Intrapartum electronic monitoring of the fetal heart rate is mandatory. Labor should be allowed to progress as long as cervical dilation and descent follow the established curves for normal labor. Any evidence of an arrest pattern should alert the physician to the possibility of cephalopelvic disproportion and fetal macrosomia.

Maternal Glucose Levels During Delivery

Maintenance of normal maternal glucose levels (60–100 mg/dL [3.3–5.6 mmol/L]) during labor and delivery is important in eliminating hypoglycemia for the mother and keeping both mother and child safe. Though a more recent study shows a stronger correlation of maternal A1C during the second trimester to neonatal hypoglycemia than maternal glucose levels during labor and delivery, other studies show normal maternal glucose levels will reduce the risk of subsequent neonatal hypoglycemia. A glucose and insulin infusion can be used to maintain glucose levels in this range. Below are insulin infusion rates deemed safe and effective in maintaining maternal glucose levels during labor. They are used with a 10% dextrose solution at an 80 mL/h rate and with hourly capillary blood glucose monitoring:

- Constant 1U/h with a BG level of 3.4–7.8 mmol/L (61–140 mg/dL)
- Increase to 1.5 U/h for BG of 7.8–10.0 mmol/L (140–180 mg/dL)
- Increase to 2 U/h for BG of 10.0–12.2 mmol/L (180–220 mg/dL)
- Increase to 3 U/h for BG above 12.2 mmol/L (220 mg/dL)

During active labor in most patients, insulin requirements typically decrease substantially, with most patients requiring a reduction in their basal insulin. Glucose levels should be determined hourly with SMBG or CGM techniques at the bedside, because even small doses of insulin may produce hypoglycemia during active labor. Adjustments in the delivery of insulin and/or glucose should be made based on the glucose determinations. See *Medical Management of Pregnancy Complicated by Diabetes* (see Bibliography, page 174).

If labor is electively induced or a cesarean section is planned, the procedure should be scheduled for the early morning and the patient's usual morning rapid- or short-acting insulin dose withheld. Further glycemic control can be achieved if the patient is fasting. If using an insulin pump, the basal insulin may be continued at low rates with further decrease in the basal rate at the time of delivery to avoid maternal hypoglycemia. Epidural anesthesia is preferred in patients scheduled for cesarean section. After the operation has been completed, glucose levels should be monitored every 1–2 h, and an intravenous solution containing 5% dextrose should be continued. Because hPL and its counterregulatory actions fall rapidly after removal of the placenta, no insulin may be required for the remainder of the day if the previous injection of the long-acting insulin is still in effect.

POSTPARTUM CARE

In the immediate postpartum period, the patient's insulin requirements are usually lower than her prepregnancy needs. The antepartum objective of physiologic glycemic control is usually relaxed at this time and returned to pre-pregnancy levels (90–130 mg/dL [5.0–7.2 mmol/L]. If the patient uses an insulin pump, the basal rate should be reset at or below the prepregnancy rate. Breast-feeding is encouraged. The meal plan for the breast-feeding mother should be 30–37 kcal/kg desirable body weight.

If the patient delivered vaginally, and if glucose levels are ≥200 mg/dL, short-acting insulin should be administered as necessary as a correction bolus based on prepregnancy requirements, or an insulin infusion can be continued or started. Once eating, the insulin regimen can be resumed but lowered to or below the prepregnancy insulin requirements. The doses should be adjusted based on SMBG.

In patients who have undergone a cesarean section, minimal insulin may be required for the first 2 postoperative days because calorie intake is limited. By day 2 or 3, the prepregnancy insulin schedule may be resumed and the dose adjusted using SMBG. Further adjustment of insulin needs in the postpartum period should always be individualized based on SMBG results.

FAMILY PLANNING AND CONTRACEPTION

Family planning and contraception must be reviewed with the patient during the postpartum period. Although oral contraceptives are the most effective method available, the increased risk of thromboembolic disease and vasculopathy require that combined estrogen/progestin oral contraceptive preparations be used with caution, and then only in women who have no macrovascular diseases or diabetes for less than 20 years. For these women, only low-dose (≤35 µg) estrogen agents or intrauterine devices (IUDs) should be prescribed. Combination agents are contraindicated in women with hypertension or vasculopathy, who may be offered a progestin-only pill or nonhormonal contraception instead. After >20 years of diabetes, women, regardless of presence of macrovascular disease, retinopathy, nephropathy, or neuropathy or not, should be removed from a combination hormone treatment and placed on a nonhormone treatment or an IUD. Condoms should be encouraged in all patients as a secondary/dual form of contraception as they also help protect against sexually transmitted diseases.

Motivated patients may do well with one of the barrier methods of contraception, such as the diaphragm, although their efficacy is significantly lower than that of oral contraceptives. Sterilization of the patient or her partner should be discussed with the patient when she has completed her family or if she has serious vasculopathy. All contraception discussions should be in accordance with the patient's religious beliefs.

CONCLUSION

Advances in prenatal care and diagnosis, fetal surveillance, and perinatal care have markedly improved maternal and fetal well-being in pregnancy complicated by diabetes. Meticulous metabolic control before and during pregnancy holds the key to a successful outcome and to minimizing fetal malformations or perinatal complications. A team approach is more likely to achieve a desirable result.

BIBLIOGRAPHY

American Diabetes Association: Preconception care of women with diabetes (Position Statement). *Diabetes Care* 27 (Suppl. 1):S76–S78, 2004

American Diabetes Association: *Medical Management of Pregnancy Complicated by Diabetes.* 4th ed. Jovanovic L, Ed. Alexandria, VA, American Diabetes Association, 2008

Codner E, Soto N, Merino PM: Review of puberty, contraception, and pregnancy in adolescents with type 1 diabetes. *Pediatric Diabetes.* http://dx.doi.org/10.1111/j.1399-5448.2011.00825.x, 2011

Jensen DM, Beck-Nielsen H, Damm P, Westergaard JG, Ovesen P, Moeller M, Mølsted-Pedersen L, Mathiesen ER: Microalbumenuria, preeclampsia and preterm delivery in pregnant women with type 1 diabetes. *Diabetes Care* 33:90–94, 2010

Johnstone FD, Lindsay RS, Steel J: Type 1 diabetes and pregnancy: trends in birth weight over 40 years at a single clinic. *Obstet Gynecol* 107:1297–1302, 2006

Jovanovic L, Peterson CM, Reed GF, Metzger BE, Mills JL, Knopp RH, Aarons JH: Maternal postprandial glucose levels and infant birth weight: the Diabetes in Early Pregnancy Study. The National Institute of Child Health and Human Development—Diabetes in Early Pregnancy Study. *Am J Obstet Gynecol* 164:103–111,1991

Lepercq J, Abbou H, Agostini C, Toubas F, Francoual C, Velho G, Dubois-Laforgue D, Timsit J: A standardized protocol to achieve normoglycaemia during labour and delivery in women with type 1 diabetes. *Diabetes and Metabolism* 34:33–37, 2008

Price N, Bartlett C, Gillmer MD: Use of insulin glargine during pregnancy: a case-control pilot study. *BJOG: An International Journal of Obstetrics and Gynecology* 114:453–457, 2007

Trujillo AL: Insulin analogs and pregnancy. *Diabetes Spectrum* 20:94–99, 2007

Yogev Y, Chen R, Ben-Haroush A, Phillip M, Jovanovic L, Hod M: Continuous glucose monitoring for the evaluation of gravid women with type 1 diabetes mellitus. *Obstet Gynecol* 101:633–639, 2003

SURGERY

The physician caring for patients with type 1 diabetes must become familiar with perioperative management. With excellent glucose management, a person with diabetes can undergo surgery with little more than normal risk.

GENERAL PRINCIPLES

The objectives of glycemic management during surgery are to maintain normal glucose levels and normal metabolism. Insulin resistance and glucogenesis will increase during stress. For this reason, the customary basal insulin dosage is the minimum requirement during the perioperative period. Additional insulin also will be needed to prevent excessive hepatic glucose release and decreased peripheral utilization while maintaining normal glucose levels and normal fluid and electrolyte balance. Perioperative hyperglycemia will delay healing and increase the risk of infection and ischemia. Although one large study suggested that postoperative patients who are intubated and in the intensive care unit have lower morbidity and mortality if they are treated to normoglycemia with an insulin infusion, it is unclear whether this applies to patients with type 1 diabetes or those who do not require ventilator support. Plasma glucose levels between 100 and 150 mg/dL (5.5 and 8.3 mmol/L) during and after the operation may be a reasonable target range for patients who are less critically ill. An operative/postoperative team guided by frequent point of care glucose monitoring, using a simple and safe algorithm for intravenous insulin administration, can maintain normal glucose levels and metabolism.

MAJOR SURGERY

Elective Surgery

The patient scheduled for elective surgery should be placed on intravenous insulin and glucose several hours preoperatively and maintained at 100–150 mg/dL (5.5 to 8.3 mmol/L). Evaluation of the metabolic state, lipid profile, renal function, and myocardial function must be completed before surgery. Once these procedures are done, surgery can be performed at any time of the day based on the urgency of the surgical condition.

Intravenous infusion of insulin rather than subcutaneous insulin administration is indicated during the perioperative period. Intravenous infusion allows careful control of the amount and speed of insulin delivery and circumvents problems with subcutaneous absorption in the event of shock.

Emergency Surgery

In the event of emergency surgery requiring general anesthesia, there is usually sufficient time to optimally evaluate and stabilize the patient. In the event of

DKA in a patient who needs emergency surgery, e.g., trauma and ketoacidosis, the condition can be treated concurrently with surgery.

MINOR SURGERY

Patients undergoing elective surgery with local anesthesia (e.g., dental work) should eat only after surgery. The ideal management during these circumstances is to withhold food, withhold short-acting insulin, and continue basal insulin as insulin glargine or detemir or via insulin pump. If the person with type 1 diabetes is being managed in some other manner, they should be switched to a basal-bolus program before the elective procedure. Alternatively, the morning dose of NPH can be decreased by one-third and supplemental regular insulin or rapid-acting analogs can be used as needed.

CONCLUSION

Medical management of the patient with diabetes requiring surgery must focus on provision of glucose and insulin in amounts to normalize blood glucose levels during and after surgery. Intravenous insulin and glucose at a rate adjusted for the individual's insulin requirement titrated from frequent blood glucose values can safely keep blood glucose levels between 100 and 150 mg/dL (5.5 and 8.3 mmol/L).

BIBLIOGRAPHY

ACE/ADA Task Force on Inpatient Diabetes: American College of Endocrinology and American Diabetes Association Consensus Statement on Inpatient Glycemic Control: A Call to Action. *Diabetes Care* 29:1955–1962, 2006

Pittas AG, Siegal RD, Lau J: Insulin therapy for critically ill hospitalized patients: a meta-analysis of randomized controlled trials. *Arch Intern Med* 164:2005–2011, 2004

Van den Berghe G, Wouters P, Weekers F, Verwaest C, Bruyninckx F, Schetz M, Vlasselaers D, Ferdinande P, Lauwers P, Bouillon R: Intensive insulin therapy in critically ill patients. *N Engl J Med* 345:1359–1367, 2001

Zerr KJ, Furnary AP, Grunkemeier GL, Bookin S, Kanhere V, Starr A: Glucose control lowers the risk of wound infection in diabetics after open heart operations. *Ann Thorac Surg* 63:356–361, 1997

ISLET TRANSPLANTATION

Significant progress in the field of islet transplantation has occurred over the past years. In July 2000, a team from University of Alberta in Edmonton reported success in achieving up to 14 months of insulin independence with normalization of A1C and resolution of recurrent severe hypoglycemia in seven type 1 diabetes patients by human islet allotransplantation from cadaver pancreases. Their success was attributed to improved human islet isolation and purification procedures, along with different immunosuppression regimens that avoid the use of glucocorticoids and cyclosporine, which have in the past been shown toxic to the islets. After their initial report, hundreds of other islet allotransplantations into the portal vein of the liver have been done in designated research centers around the world using variations of the Edmonton Protocol. Individual centers reported good success; however, the 2006 results of a carefully conducted multi-center trial of the Edmonton Protocol were somewhat mixed: 44% of patients achieved insulin independence and normalization of A1C at 1 year post-islet transplantation, but the majority of patients required resumption of insulin therapy in subsequent years of follow-up. More than one cadaver pancreas was used in staged procedures in most patients, with some requiring islets from three or more cadaver pancreases.

Success in human islet allotransplantation has not occurred without risks and complications to the patients. The most significant complication has been hepatic bleeding, with two reported cases of portal vein thrombosis. Other complications include mouth ulcerations from sirolimus, transient rise in liver enzymes, the need for statin therapy, renal dysfunction, severe neutropenia, and rare cases of pneumonitis, with one death from pneumonitis reported in a European center. No cancers or infection with cytomegalovirus have been reported, but these remain theoretical risks with longer-term immunosuppression.

As a result of these risks, islet allotransplantation is only recommended in a research setting for patients where the benefits of improved metabolic control with avoidance of severe hypoglycemia are greater than the risks of the islet allotransplantation procedure and the ongoing risks of chronic immunosuppression. Most islet transplants to date have been done in patients with recurrent, refractory, severe hypoglycemia or marked glycemic instability. It is not known yet whether such transplantation will reverse or stop microvascular complications, because glucose intolerance persists.

Additional research is ongoing in multiple areas to improve the current clinical results. These areas involve:

- improvement in islet yield from cadaver pancreases
- refinements to the protocol to improve engraphment
- long-term prevention and recurrence of autoimmunity
- development of safe immunomodulation strategies
- achievement of donor-specific immune tolerance

If success is achieved in these areas, the critical challenge will be to identify sufficient and suitable sources of insulin-producing tissue to treat the large number of patients who could benefit from this therapy. For these reasons, research on xenogeneic islets, embryonic and adult stem cells, islet regeneration and proliferation, and engineering of insulin-producing cells must be continued. It is important to identify the ideal source of insulin-producing tissue that will be utilized on a large scale once the current impediments and limitations of immunosuppression are resolved.

BIBLIOGRAPHY

Shapiro AMJ, Lakey JRT, Ryan EA, Korbutt GS, Toth E, Warnock GL, Kneteman NM, Rajotte RV: Islet transplantation in seven patients with type 1 diabetes using a glucocorticoid-free immunosuppressive regimen. *N Engl J Med* 343:230–238, 2000

Shapiro AM, Ricordi C, Hering BJ, Auchincloss H, Lindblad R, Robertson RP, Secchi A, Brendel MD, Berney T, Brennan DC, Caglièro E, Alejandro R, Ryan EA, DiMercurio B, Morel P, Polonsky KS, Reems JA, Bretzel RG, Bertucci F, Froud T, Kandaswamy R, Sutherland DE, Eisenbarth G, Segal M, Preiksaitis J, Korbutt GS, Barton FB, Viviano L, Seyfert-Margolis V, Bluestone J, Lakey JR: International trial of the Edmonton Protocol for islet transplantation. *N Engl J Med* 355:1318–1330, 2006

Psychosocial Factors Affecting Adherence, Quality of Life, and Well-Being: Helping Patients Cope

Highlights

Periods of Increased Emotional Distress
Maintaining Adherence
Diabetes Complications
Developmental Considerations in Children
Developmental Considerations in Adolescents
Adults
The Elderly
Emotional and Behavioral Disorders and Diabetes
Stress and Diabetes

Highlights
Psychosocial Factors Affecting Adherence, Quality of Life, and Well-Being: Helping Patients Cope

Diabetes is a demanding chronic disease. The diabetes management team must understand the patient's daily schedule, lifestyle, developmental stage, social and financial supports, as well as preferences and values when working collaboratively to make diabetes management decisions and establish treatment goals. Maintaining quality of life is as important an outcome as good glycemic control.

PERIODS OF INCREASED EMOTIONAL DISTRESS

■ Emotional distress can be high at the time of diagnosis, when the honeymoon period is over, when planning pregnancy, and at the onset of complications. Psychological equilibrium can generally be reestablished with early identification of distress; initiation of medical, psychological, and social supports; and monitoring of intervention effects. Initiation of multidisciplinary intervention can improve adaptation and adherence and prevent deterioration in metabolic control.

■ Monitoring of emotional status, quality of life, and well-being is an ongoing component of comprehensive diabetes care.

MAINTAINING ADHERENCE

■ Over time or periodically, motivation to maintain optimal diabetes control may wane. Maintenance strategies include planning a lifestyle-based diabetes regimen, improving patient/care provider communication, addressing barriers, screening for depression, and employing research-tested educational and behavioral strategies.

DIABETES COMPLICATIONS

■ Psychosocial factors should be suspected in the case of extreme poor control and/or recurrent diabetic ketoacidosis.

■ Repeat episodes of severe hypoglycemia can have serious psychosocial consequences, which call for medical, educational, behavioral, and family intervention.

■ When chronic complications begin, feelings of anger and guilt are common. Interventions that include psychological counseling and adaptive coping strategies can help resolve these emotional reactions. Family members should be included in the intervention whenever possible.

DEVELOPMENTAL CONSIDERATIONS IN CHILDREN

■ Although a diagnosis of diabetes during childhood can be a devastating experience for parents and children, families are usually resilient and adapt to the demands of the regimen within the first year.

■ Because children and adolescents are growing, developing, acquiring new motor skills, cognitive abilities, and emotional maturity, the management priorities and self-management issues change over time. However, continued parental involvement is necessary throughout childhood and adolescence. Caution should be exercised in forcing too much self-care too soon or abandoning parental oversight during adolescence. Sharing diabetes care responsibilities produces the best glycemic outcomes and reduces individual burden.

DEVELOPMENTAL CONSIDERATIONS IN ADOLESCENTS

■ For adolescents, peer influences, together with family support and supervision, play an important role in adherence and glycemic control.

■ Many aspects of the treatment regimen are at odds with adolescents' normal drive for independence and peer acceptance. New technologies have enabled adolescents to maintain a flexible lifestyle but at the cost of increased monitoring and diabetes care tasks.

ADULTS

■ Misunderstandings about diabetes on the part of the patient or parent can interfere with young adult patients' carrying out usual developmental tasks such as developing an independent life from parents.

■ Adults with diabetes must deal with a disease and care regimen that complicates their interpersonal relationships and their attempts to establish a family and career, and presents a financial burden as well. Thorough and anticipatory education of patients, family members, and significant others can facilitate normalization of expectations.

THE ELDERLY

■ Older adults with longstanding diabetes can often benefit from re-education regarding newer technologies and care regimens.

■ The demands of the diabetes regimen may be especially burdensome for the elderly, who face other difficult life events such as retirement, loss of physical function, living on a fixed income, the death of a spouse and/or friends, and their own mortality.

■ The goal of diabetes care is to maximize physical and psychosocial functioning while respecting the patient's autonomy and independence as much as possible. Availability and maintenance of social support can be particularly difficult for the elderly, who often find themselves dependent on family and friends when physical capacities and financial resources diminish.

EMOTIONAL AND BEHAVIORAL DISORDERS AND DIABETES

■ Ongoing monitoring of the psychological status of patients will help with detection of diabetes-related distress and non–diabetes-related psychopathology. It is important to determine whether psychopathology is diabetes related or due to other causes.

■ Whenever possible, it is recommended that the care-provider team include a mental health professional familiar with diabetes and its care regimen.

■ Depression and anxiety disorders have been found to occur frequently in patients with diabetes. Some disorders, such as fear of hypoglycemia, needle phobia, and fear of complications and premature death, are specifically related to having diabetes.

■ Eating disorders should be suspected in individuals, especially young women with a history of unstable or poor metabolic control, recurrent ketoacidosis, or recurrent severe hypoglycemia, and in girls with growth retardation, pubertal delay, and/or amenorrhea.

STRESS AND DIABETES

■ Results of studies investigating the relationship between stress and blood glucose control have been inconclusive. The impact of stress on glycemia seems to be highly individualized.

■ It is important to establish a patient's stress reactivity to develop coping strategies to maintain good glycemic control up to, during, and after stressful events.

■ Stress can indirectly affect blood glucose control by undermining adherence to the diabetes treatment regimen.

Psychosocial Factors Affecting Adherence, Quality of Life, and Well-Being: Helping Patients Cope

A lthough type 1 diabetes taxes the patient's psychosocial well-being, the converse is also true: psychosocial factors can affect diabetes management. The unrelenting demands, inconveniences, frustrations of treatment, and possibilities of disability or death put tremendous emotional and financial strain on patients with diabetes and their significant others. Patients must struggle continuously to achieve a balance between the demands of their everyday lives and those of their diabetes regimen. To help patients cope successfully with diabetes in their everyday lives, the diabetes management team must consider the patient's daily schedule, lifestyle, and developmental stage, social and financial supports, and patient values and preferences when working collaboratively to make diabetes management decisions and treatment goals. Maintaining quality of life is as important an outcome as good glycemic control.

PERIODS OF INCREASED EMOTIONAL DISTRESS

Psychological and emotional distress is high at the time of diagnosis, after the honeymoon period ends, and at the onset of complications (Table 5.1). At diagnosis, initial shock, denial, and anger often give way to mild depression and anxiety. Studies of newly diagnosed children and their families have found, however, that the initial reactions of both parents and children resolve rather quickly, and psychological equilibrium is reestablished within the first year. More extreme or long-lasting psychological reactions may indicate a need for referral to a mental health professional for evaluation and treatment.

Ongoing monitoring of the emotional status of the patient is part of comprehensive diabetes care. Initiation of an intervention as soon as emotional distress is identified may improve adaptation, prevent psychosocial maladjustment, improve compliance, and prevent deterioration in metabolic control. All members of the diabetes management team can be a great help during these periods by being accessible and sensitive to the patient's and family's need for information, support, and resources. When indicated, a referral to a mental health professional who specializes in working with patients with diabetes is suggested.

The following are suggestions for intervention aimed at facilitating adjustment and enhancing metabolic control.

- It is essential that the patient and his or her significant others are involved in the initial and ongoing discussions and education regarding diabetes care behaviors and regimens, lifestyle accommodations, sharing of diabetes

Table 5.1 Factors Causing Emotional Distress

■Uncertainty about the outcome of the immediate situation
■Feelings of intense guilt and/or anger about the occurrence of diabetes, poor glycemic control, and/or complications
■Feelings of incompetence and helplessness about the responsibility of managing the illness
■Fears about future complications and early death
■Loss of valued life goals and aspirations because of illness
■Anxiety about planning for an uncertain future
■Recognition of the necessity for a permanent change in living pattern as a result of diabetes
■Fear of loss of insurance coverage

Adapted from Hamburg SA, Inoff GE: Coping with predictable crises of diabetes. *Diabetes Care* 6:409–416, 1983.

care tasks, and the need to balance family needs with diabetes care tasks. Both parents in the case of a child, the patient's spouse, the adult children in the case of an elderly patient, or any significant others should be included. This is important given the wealth of research showing significant associations between family and peer support and adherence, problem-solving, and glycemic control. Research with families of children who have diabetes has shown that sharing diabetes care tasks and responsibilities reduces burdens and can improve glycemic control.

■ A comprehensive approach to diabetes education and management can be achieved if the roles of the diabetes management team are coordinated and regular communication takes place between care providers. Led by a physician or health professional who specializes in diabetes care, involvement of a nurse educator, a dietitian, a social worker, and/or a psychologist will ensure that the patient and family receive the educational, dietary, and psychosocial support they need.

■ Self-management education with newly diagnosed children and their families in the months after diagnosis prevents deterioration in metabolic control during the first 2 years after diagnosis of type 1 diabetes. Close follow-up by the diabetes management team in the weeks after the initial education will increase, reinforce, and clarify diabetes knowledge. Furthermore, emphasis on developing self-management strategies during these weeks appears to enhance adaptation and metabolic control. Self-management education includes reinforcement of accurate glucose monitoring and recording and the use of these data to understand blood glucose fluctuations and make appropriate insulin and behavioral treatment changes. The goal is to help patients adopt a problem-solving approach to diabetes self-management. See also Patient Self-Management Education, page 37.

■ Self-management education must be ongoing and accommodate the developmental lifestyle and agreed-on treatment goals of the patient and/ or family members if the patient is a child, adolescent, or elderly person who requires assistance with care.

■ Goals of treatment, diabetes care regimen tasks, and expectations for glycemic control should be negotiated with the patient and/or supervising
adult so that unrealistic goals do not cause burnout and feelings of failure.

MAINTAINING ADHERENCE

Expectations that an individual and family will make multiple and significant
behavior changes at one time may be unrealistic and unfeasible. Focus on "survival
skills" at the time of diagnosis (self-monitoring of blood glucose [SMBG], insulin dosing, and monitoring and treatment of hypo- and hyperglycemia and ketosis) and clear communication about the expectation of working toward intensive
management of glucose control provide the foundation for success in diabetes self-
management. Explaining the importance of each of these survival skills and how
they will affect short- and long-term health is important. A step-by-step approach
to behavior change is often most successful, although highly motivated patients and
parents will attempt to implement health provider recommendations when they are
presented.

Failure to maintain self-care behaviors in diabetes management and resul-
tant poor metabolic control are frequently the result of the lack of attention to
maintenance issues. Caution is needed to monitor burnout and feelings of being
"controlled" by the disease.

Individualized Treatment Regimens

Regardless of age, a patient's treatment regimen should be individually tailored. Patients have been shown to follow complex treatment regimens when the
regimens meet the needs and requests of the patient and quality of life is maintained. Flexibility of lifestyle has become an important consideration in diabetes
care, and advances in monitoring technology, insulins, and delivery systems have
facilitated this aim. Holding a patient with diabetes to an inflexible diabetes care
routine might seem to providers to be an easier way to achieve good glycemic
control, but the negative impact on family and individual functioning should not
be underestimated and may actually undermine success.

The priorities and personality of the patient and his or her inherent organi-
zational proclivities should help shape the diabetes care regimen that is adopted.
For example, forcing a child or adult with attention-deficit hyperactivity disorder
to keep detailed glucose records may be an exercise in frustration for all involved.
Conversely, if such a patient prioritizes good glucose control, the diabetes care
regimen may provide structure by which the individual organizes his or her daily
routines. The adolescent, in particular, may be motivated to perform more frequent monitoring, take additional insulin injections, and adhere to a specific
meal plan if it is perceived that he or she can participate in desired activities or
be granted special requests. Many adolescents and young adults are attracted to
and comfortable with technology, so tools such as software for organizing SMBG
reading may facilitate adherence and self-care. Conversely, some adolescents and
adults will attain better metabolic control with more adherence to a simplified
regimen than little or no adherence to a more complex or demanding regimen
such as being placed on the insulin pump or continuous glucose monitoring.

Negotiations regarding treatment regimens should be viewed by the care provider as an accommodation of the patient's treatment within lifestyle realities and shaped by the patient's value system and preferences. Patients are people who happen to have diabetes, and these people are the ones who must carry out the vast majority of management tasks. This is a departure from the philosophy of diabetes care in the past and may present difficulties for the care provider who wishes to enforce a one-size-fits-all formula for good glycemic control. Adoption of a patient-centered point of view not only is more likely to facilitate long-term successful patient self-management, but also may help providers avoid burnout and frustration as well.

DIABETES COMPLICATIONS

Short-Term Complications

Recurrent diabetic ketoacidosis can be the consequence of underdosing or omission of insulin that occurs because of psychosocial problems, e.g., depression, psychiatric illness, financial stress, parental neglect, lack of family involvement, chronic family conflict, weight concerns, or eating disorders. Psychosocial factors should always be suspected in the case of recurrent ketoacidosis, especially after it has been established that good glycemic control can be achieved under monitored conditions. A mental health evaluation should be considered for these patients.

Severe Hypoglycemia

Most patients with well-controlled type 1 diabetes experience frequent hypoglycemia that is asymptomatic and several mildly symptomatic low blood glucose reactions each month. In general, these symptomatic mild reactions, although distracting and uncomfortable, do not pose a serious problem for the patient. Severe hypoglycemia, however, defined as an episode in which patients are unable to treat themselves, lose consciousness, and/or have seizures, can be frightening and may have serious cognitive, neurological, and psychosocial consequences. The patient may develop fear of hypoglycemia and decide to maintain blood glucose values at unacceptably high levels. The family may also become overly fearful, watchful, or angry, blaming the patient for the disturbing glycemic episodes. Patients who experience severe hypoglycemia at work may jeopardize their job or chances for advancement.

Many patients with longstanding, well-controlled type 1 diabetes fail to recognize the early warning symptoms of hypoglycemia (hypoglycemia unawareness). These patients are at risk for repeated episodes of severe hypoglycemia and attendant medical and psychosocial consequences. Efforts should be made to prevent these episodes through reeducation and adjustments in the diabetes regimen.

The health care provider should discuss the patient's attitudes regarding hypoglycemia and help to establish safe blood glucose goals. Target blood glucose levels may need to be raised to restore hypoglycemic awareness and the patient's confidence in recognition of symptoms. A program called Blood Glucose Awareness Training (BGAT) successfully reduces the incidence of severe hypoglycemia. The family or significant others should be trained to recognize early or subtle hypoglycemic signs and provide adequate prevention and treatment measures, including the administration of glucagon. If the family is angry and blames the patient, the diabetes management team will need to help the family understand the difficulty many patients have in recognizing and avoiding hypoglycemia. The family should also understand that the patient frequently cannot control his or her behavior during a severe low blood glucose reaction.

Long-Term Complications

Although most patients are aware of the possibility of long-term complications of diabetes, the detection of the first evidence of retinopathy, nephropathy, or neuropathy can be a devastating event. When the onset of a severe complication occurs, the patient and family must cope with the grief associated with the potential or actual loss of body function. Once again, the patient and family may experience feelings of shock, denial, and anger. Feelings of anger at the health care provider for "letting this happen" or guilt ("I should have taken better care of myself") are common. These feelings can be eased by emphasizing the positive steps that can still be taken to forestall or prevent serious problems. When complications cause disability and restrictions in lifestyle, the treating physician or health care provider may need to refer the patient to a rehabilitation program that includes expert care or suggest counseling by an experienced mental health professional who is familiar with the disease and its treatment. Support groups or contact with people who have successfully adapted to complications can provide useful information and role models and help patients maintain a hopeful outlook.

Care providers and patients may be hesitant to broach the issue of sexual dysfunction—a common complication of diabetes in all adults, both men and women. Though it is widely accepted that men with diabetes experience sexual dysfunction, women (especially older women) with type 1 diabetes can experience a wide range of symptoms as well. It is critical to ask patients routinely about sexual function in a straightforward manner. Patients may be more likely to confide in the physician or another member of the diabetes management team if they know that sexual problems are common in diabetes and that a variety of treatment options are available. Along with issues of sexual functioning, issues of reproductive health should be addressed with teens, young adults, and adults of childbearing age. As modern diabetes care has enabled women with diabetes to have healthy babies, misinformation about the inevitability of poor pregnancy outcomes need to be counteracted. However, tight glycemic control is necessary for a healthy pregnancy and baby. Patients with diabetes must plan pregnancies and achieve excellent glycemic control *before* conception and maintain it throughout pregnancy. This information should be incorporated into routine diabetes care so that patients can make informed decisions regarding childbearing.

DEVELOPMENTAL CONSIDERATIONS IN CHILDREN

Although a diagnosis of diabetes during childhood is a devastating experience for parents and children, families are usually resilient and adapt to the demands of the regimen within the first year. Some of those demands, viewed from a developmental and family perspective, are outlined in Table 5.2.

Table 5.2 Major Developmental Issues, Management Priorities, and Family Issues in Type 1 Diabetes in Children and Adolescents

Developmental Stages (approximate ages)	Normal Development Tasks	Type 1 Diabetes Management Priorities	Family Issues in Type 1 Diabetes Management
Infancy (0–12 months)	• Developing a trusting relationship "bonding" with primary caregiver	• Preventing and treating hypoglycemia • Avoiding extreme fluctuations in blood glucose levels	• Coping with stress • Sharing the "burden of care" to avoid parental burnout
Toddlers (13–36 months)	• Developing a sense of mastery and autonomy	• Preventing and treating hypoglycemia • Avoiding extreme fluctuations in blood glucose levels due to irregular food intake	• Establishing a schedule • Managing the "picky eater" • Setting limits and coping with toddler's lack of comprehension of regimen
Preschoolers and early elementary school (3–7 years)	• Developing initiative in activities and confidence in self	• Preventing and treating hypoglycemia • Unpredictable appetite and activity • Positive reinforcement for cooperation with regimen • Trusting caregivers with management	• Reassuring child that diabetes is no one's fault • Educating other caregivers about diabetes management
Older elementary school (8–11 years)	• Developing skills in athletic, cognitive, artistic, social areas • Consolidating self-esteem with respect to the peer group	• Making diabetes regimen flexible to allow for participation in school/peer activities • Child learning short- and long-term benefits of optimal control	• Maintaining parental involvement in insulin and blood glucose monitoring tasks while allowing for independent self-care for "special occasions" • Continue to educate school and other caregivers
Early adolescence (12–15 years)	• Managing body changes • Developing a strong sense of self-identity	• Managing increased insulin requirements during puberty • Diabetes management and blood glucose control become more difficult • Weight and body image concerns	• Renegotiating parent and teen roles in management so acceptable to both • Learning coping skills to gain ability to self-manage • Preventing and intervening with diabetes-related family conflict • Monitoring for signs of depression, eating disorders, risk-taking behaviors
Later adolescence (16–19 years)	• Establishing a sense of identity after high school (location, social issues, work, education)	• Begin discussion of transition to a new diabetes team • Integrating diabetes into new lifestyle	•Supporting the transition to independence •Learning coping skills to gain ability to self-manage •Monitoring for signs of depression, eating disorders, risk-taking behaviors

Generally, children's responsibilities for care should increase in tandem with cognitive, motor, emotional, and psychological development. Children who share responsibility for their diabetes care are generally more knowledgeable about their diabetes and are in better metabolic control. When treating a school-age child, the diabetes management team should be attuned to his or her cognitive maturity and abilities with regard to accurately interpreting results of SMBG or continuous glucose monitoring, calculating carbohydrate intake, and preparing the correct amount of insulin with a pen, syringe, or pump. If cognitive abilities are questioned, referral for testing by a psychologist familiar with the treatment of diabetes should be considered.

Self-esteem is built through mastery of the developmental tasks of childhood and the positive regard of significant others. Children feel good about themselves when they succeed in tasks children their age are expected to master—school work, sports, social relationships, etc. Having diabetes presents children with opportunities to build self-esteem when they learn to perform diabetes-related tasks. These may be as simple as setting up supplies for blood glucose tests or as advanced as calculating the correct dose and giving their own injections or wearing and/or operating an insulin pump. This is especially true if parents, the diabetes management team, and others provide positive reinforcement for their achievements. Conversely, expectations of independent functioning in diabetes care tasks without the foundation of skill mastery, parental support and monitoring, and adequate time-management skills or structure can predispose the child to feelings of failure, low self-esteem, and feeling controlled by their illness. A child's comfort with self-care tasks should be monitored, because although a skill may be mastered, the child's desire to perform the task can change over time (e.g., during adolescence).

The Family

Diabetes affects every aspect of family life and affects all family members. Research has shown that shared responsibility within the family is associated with improved adherence and metabolic control. These results underscore the importance of educating family members regarding the treatment of diabetes and defining diabetes care tasks for each family member. Facilitating open discussion of the problems encountered in day-to-day diabetes management will help prevent blaming the child for poor diabetes control and enlist family support. Siblings, who commonly feel neglected or left out because of the extra attention given to the child with diabetes, may feel more involved if they are a part of the family's diabetes management effort, especially because they may be on the front lines with regard to recognition of hypoglycemia and its treatment. Fathers may be more likely to be involved if they, too, have clearly defined tasks. Full family involvement may help prevent overinvolvement of the mother and unhealthy dependence between the mother and the child with diabetes.

Diabetes, School, and Peers

Although school-aged children begin doing more diabetes management tasks, it is important that parents and children continue to share diabetes care responsibilities. A child's early independence in diabetes management can lead to poor diabetes control. School entry can be a difficult experience for parents and children. It is often more traumatic for the parent and child with diabetes, as they must now depend on school nurses, teachers, and other school staff members (who often are not knowledgeable about diabetes) to monitor the child's well-being and potentially handle situations that could be life-threatening. The student's health management team can help by providing diabetes literature and training for school nurses, teachers and school staff, and by being advocates for the child and family. Many school districts incorporate diabetes training for school nurses into their overall training curriculum. Every effort should be made for the school nurse and the diabetes management team to be familiar with each other and to work collaboratively to manage the student/patient. There are programs that can help bring nurses, teachers, administrators, other parents, and diabetes educators together for training such as the American Diabetes Association's "Safe at School" program. Often there can be resistance with accommodating a child with diabetes from school personnel due to fear of responsibility or misunderstanding of the disease itself. Proper training can make everyone, families and faculty alike, feel more at ease that a child with diabetes will be attending school and ensure a safe and optimal learning environment for the child.

An important goal of diabetes management during childhood is to prevent the diabetes regimen from disrupting the child's school experience. Every effort should be made to ensure the child's safety at school and ability to participate in all school activities. An individualized Diabetes Medical Management Plan, developed by the student's health care team (with input from the parent/guardian), outlines what is required for diabetes management at school. Specific issues outlined in the diabetes medical management plan are insulin administration; signs, symptoms, and treatment of hypoglycemia and hyperglycemia; the timing of meals; management of exercise; where and when SMBG occurs; and which tasks need to be done by school personnel, which can be done independently, and which require supervision. The school, mainly the school nurse, should determine how to execute the plan. Federal laws such as Section 504 of the Rehabilitation Act of 1973, the Americans with Disabilities Act, and the Individuals with Disabilities Education Act prohibit schools from discriminating against children with disabilities—including diabetes. Parents should work with their child's school to document required accommodations in a written plan developed under applicable federal law such as a Section 504 Plan or an Individualized Education Program (IEP). In addition, some states have laws that provide additional legal protections to students with diabetes.

The student's health care team should work with parents, teachers, and school nurses to minimize absences and missed class time and school activities. Some children may quickly learn to use their diabetes to avoid difficult school situations. Allowing children to check blood glucose levels and treat hypoglycemia at their desks or in the classroom will help prevent missed classroom time. Children who are frequently allowed to stay home for minor diabetes problems may fall behind in school and lose motivation to return to school. Social stigmatization can also occur because of being "sick" or "different." Children and adolescents with diabetes should be able to participate in all school-sponsored activities, including field trips and sports.

During the elementary school years, peer relationships become increasingly important. This means that the student's health care team must work with parents to ensure that children attend birthday parties and slumber parties, actively participate in school and recreation league sports, and participate in other normal childhood activities. This does not mean relaxing treatment goals. Use of basal-bolus insulin injection regimens or an insulin pump make adjusting to calorie, activity, and timing changes in the child's diabetes care routine feasible and straightforward. Adequate preparation and planning can allow the child to incorporate almost any usual childhood activity, including dosing of insulin for excessive calorie consumption or consuming extra calories for high levels of exercise.

DEVELOPMENTAL CONSIDERATIONS IN ADOLESCENTS

The adolescent years are known for difficulty with glycemic control, in part because of innate insulin resistance associated with puberty, and in part because of nonadherence to self-care regimens, and increased distress on the part of clinicians, parents, and the children themselves. Research has shown, however, that these difficulties can be lessened and that strategies can be developed to maintain glycemic control during this period of transition to early adulthood.

For the young child with diabetes, successful adherence to the treatment regimen depends largely on parental interest, management skills, and other resources. For adolescents, peer influences, together with family support and supervision, play an increasingly important role in adherence and glycemic control. Many aspects of the treatment regimen are at odds with adolescents' normal drive for independence and peer acceptance. Adolescents may neglect monitoring, dietary considerations, insulin administration, and even visits to the clinic to avoid drawing attention to their illness or disturbing their daily activities. These actions can have negative short-term consequences, such as feeling sluggish and unfocused or developing ketoacidosis or severe hypoglycemia, as well as potentially negative long-term consequences in terms of future onset of chronic complications. The diabetes management team can use various strategies to help the adolescent patient and his or her family keep their diabetes control within acceptable limits.

Understand the Scope of the Challenge

Almost all adolescents display characteristic behaviors and attitudes that reflect their drive for independence. Adolescents with diabetes are no exception. They undergo the same developmental process but with the added burden of diabetes. Do not assume that major difficulties are inevitable. There is no evidence that adolescents with diabetes suffer from serious psychological problems any more frequently than their nondiabetic peers, though adults with diabetes show a higher incidence of psychological distress than adults without diabetes. There is evidence that interventions can be suggested that are acceptable to the adolescent, parents, and health care providers that preserve glucose control and the adolescent's sense of autonomy. Use of the peer group and the diabetes management team to support and monitor the health status and behaviors of adolescents holds promise for affecting the decay in glycemic control often found during these years. Inclusion of the adolescent in devising a solution for nonadherence and/or poor control is highly recommended.

Many hormonal changes occur at puberty, some of which can adversely affect blood glucose levels. Puberty is associated with decreased sensitivity to insulin, which may result in increased insulin requirements. Poor control may be due to underinsulinization, lack of adherence, depression, or other psychopathologies or poor understanding of required health care behavior on the part of the adolescent. Do not assume nonadherence to care behaviors over a physiological reason until good glycemic control has been achieved under supervised conditions utilizing the current insulin and diabetes care regimen. Blaming the adolescent for poor control can set the stage for further struggles with the adolescent and negatively affect communication, which is essential to problem-solving. Empower the adolescent as an agent of his or her own good health outcomes.

Family and Patient Factors

Because family routines overlap with the various aspects of the diabetes treatment regimen (i.e., timing and content of meals, need for monitoring and exercise), family factors and adherence to treatment are strongly interrelated. Adherence to treatment is better among adolescents if their families are characterized by lower levels of general and diabetes-related conflict, greater cohesiveness (i.e., family members interact more and are supportive of one another), and clear assignments are made among family members for diabetes care tasks.

Effective clinical interventions with adolescents with diabetes and their families should target (for change) negative family interactions, especially those that focus on adherence with the care regimen. Whenever blood glucose values are outside of a target range, rather than blaming the adolescent, it is important for the family to problem-solve regarding the source of the poor glycemic control. Parents may need guidance in setting realistic expectations for their teen's self-management behaviors and blood glucose levels. Parents face a difficult balancing act wherein they must respect their teen's growing independence but remain responsible for their child's health and well-being. Negative family interactions may have the inadvertent effect of undermining the teen's attempts at independence in diabetes care. Education and problem-solving intervention efforts with adolescents should include parents, peers, and other acceptable support people, including the diabetes care team, at least as external monitors of glycemic status. Focus on the identification and development of coping strategies that decrease diabetes-related conflicts and tensions in the family and facilitate mastery of diabetes care skills is recommended.

Diabetes Management Team Factors

In addition to acquiring an understanding of normal adolescent development, members of the diabetes management team should enjoy working with adolescents and show a genuine interest in them as individuals. Patient valuation of their health care providers has been shown to be associated with better control. It is important for the diabetes care provider to directly interact with and involve the adolescent in his or her care, not just direct communication to parents.

Try to develop rapport. The diabetes management team should work toward rapport with the teen. Clinicians should avoid being placed in a parental role and make every effort to remain nonjudgmental and supportive in encouraging mastery and success in diabetes care behavior. Recommendations that are viewed by the adolescent as parental demands may be rejected. Clinicians are advised to adopt a child advocacy stance when interacting with adolescents, only assuming an authoritarian position when the child's health is at risk or risk-taking behavior is being demonstrated.

To avoid being viewed as parental figures, members of the diabetes management team should make it clear to both the parents and the adolescent that they have responsibilities to each other. The clinician may agree or disagree with either the parents or the adolescent about different aspects of diabetes care. An attempt should be made to convince the adolescent and family that the clinician-patient relationship is not one between clinician and child, but an evolving one between clinician and young adult.

Be willing to compromise. Each member of the diabetes management team must be willing to compromise on almost all aspects of diabetes care and must clearly demonstrate respect for the adolescent's views. If a clinician becomes frustrated and angry when the adolescent does not adhere to the regimen, it will be difficult to retain the ability to influence the patient's self-care. It is not necessary to agree with the adolescent's views, but the clinician should at least listen to the patient and make an effort to accommodate the patient's wishes whenever possible.

Be consistent. An important factor known to affect adherence across all age-groups is consistency in caregiving. The adolescent whose outpatient care is provided by any one of several different diabetes management team members with different management styles is not as likely to adhere to the regimen as the patient seeing a diabetes management team with a consistent and predictable management style. Often, an adolescent will form a bond with one team member while professing to dislike another care provider. This may be face-saving when the adolescent is nonadherent with care and gives health care providers the opportunity to play "good cop–bad cop." This situation is often found in nonadherent adults as well.

Monitoring

The adolescent should receive SMBG training (see Monitoring, page 88) independent of his or her parents and demonstrate independent mastery. Adolescents will be more likely to monitor if these results are used to make management decisions and are perceived as increasing flexibility and safety while maintaining metabolic control. It is important that when an adolescent becomes independent in SMBG, a mechanism is set in place to communicate blood glucose results either to parents and health care providers independent of parental oversight. Parents and adolescents should review glucose results from SMBG using memory in the meter or by downloading at set times during the week. Using multiple meters can make this assessment more difficult. If the adolescent agrees to keep a logbook, this can be reviewed, but SMBG results should be verified from the meter. The goal is to assess the frequency of monitoring, the degree of hyperglycemia and hypoglycemia, and to review patterns and trends. This review can take place daily, weekly, or at some frequency in-between. A similar review should take place at each clinic visit with the diabetes management team. When discussing the importance of monitoring to an adolescent, the diabetes management team should emphasize that it is done primarily for the patient's benefit and not to placate or please the parents or clinician.

The same training procedures should occur if the adolescent is using continuous glucose monitoring so that they may gain independent mastery. Parents and health care providers should assess the amount of time the teen is wearing the sensor, how they are responding to glucose alarms, and if they are following calibration instructions. It is important to emphasize that treatment decisions must still be made from SMBG results, and that CGM is an adjunct and meant to show trends and patterns. Studies have confirmed that use of CGM in adolescents can be beneficial, and the more that sensors are worn, the better the glycemic outcome.

Periodically, the adolescent patient may refuse to monitor at all. The heath care team should not give up, but instead, renegotiate. If the adolescent is willing to perform one test, another can be added at a future office visit. This step-by-step approach often yields good results among adults as well as adolescents. Stress to patients that they need to resume more frequent monitoring if they become ill or are concerned about hypoglycemia.

Adolescents with diabetes can misrepresent glucose monitoring results. In the past, it was possible to manipulate the glucose meter results by reusing an old strip that had a "good" result, by diluting the blood specimen, or by using control solution. However, it has become increasingly difficult to falsify SMBG. Adolescents may choose to tell their parents a false number as they are doing a blood test when they are rushed, it is meal time, or as they are going out. If the parents suspect that they were told a false number, they should ask to see the meter and check its memory on the spot. Repeated misrepresentations should be suspected when the mean glucose values recorded or reported are much lower than would be expected from a very high glycated hemoglobin (A1C) level or when safe round numbers appear to have been neatly recorded at the same time with the same pen.

When approaching the adolescent with an A1C out of target, insufficient numbers of blood tests, or high values on SMBG, the diabetes management team should not be judgmental. Accusations should not be made, but rather a problem-solving approach will work best to engage the adolescent. Avoid discussions about non-ideal glycemic control in an accusatory manner as this may cause the patient to avoid the desired actions or change out of spite or rebellion.

This nonjudgmental approach may provide a good model for the parents, who should be encouraged not to punish the adolescent for having high glucose monitoring results and A1C. The diabetes management team should also remind parents that other adolescents with diabetes (and even adults) have problems adhering to the treatment regimen.

Parents often have great difficulty "letting go" of their role as primary manager of their child's diabetes. Parental worry for the child's well-being is to be expected, especially if parental responsibility for complications consequent to poor control have been warned against since diagnosis. Parents and teens may also be so used to interdependence in diabetes care that the child may view the parent as "not caring anymore" if they appear to withdraw from active participation in diabetes management. Unless the parent is assured that diabetes care tasks and reasonable glucose control are being maintained, they may be unable to let their adolescent proceed to independence in care. The need for communication, the method and frequency to be negotiated between parent and child, cannot be underestimated. This developmental task is probably the most difficult of the adolescent years, and diabetes exacerbates the dilemma. Keeping the issue in a developmental framework can help patients, family members, and caregivers be more tolerant of the uncertainties produced by transition in care responsibilities.

ADULTS

Marriage, family, employment, and finances are four major aspects of adulthood. Adults with diabetes must deal with a disease that often complicates their interpersonal relationships and their attempts to establish a family and career and presents a financial burden as well. Adults are often not prepared to include the diabetes care team in the most intimate aspects of their lives, even though every aspect of their lives is affected by having diabetes.

Development of intimate relationships can be burdened by the self-care regimen of the individual with diabetes or by short- and long-term complications such as hypoglycemia or erectile dysfunction. Men in particular may be hesitant to be seen in the patient role with their significant others. With the patient's agreement, the significant other can and should be incorporated into the diabetes care routine with proper education and knowledge of the treatment regimen. It is strongly advised that as a relationship becomes more important and central in a patient's life, the patient be encouraged to include the significant other in the diabetes care visits. It is especially important that the new person learn about the management of diabetes crises and methods of supporting adherence to the treatment regimen without demeaning the patient or treating him or her as disabled. Family planning counseling for couples planning a long-term commitment and the possibility of children will provide crucial information as the couple decides whether and/or when to have a child. Both partners should understand the risks of pregnancy for the woman with diabetes and the need for optimal metabolic control at the time of conception (see Pregnancy, page 161). Genetic counseling should be included with education to dispel misunderstandings about the genetic propensity to develop type 1 diabetes.

The diabetes management team should be able to provide psychosocial help in many other ways during the adult years. They can offer education and counsel when misunderstandings and conflicts arise in a marriage or other relationship because of diabetes; refer patients to community, state, and federal programs to help with financial problems; and educate and reassure children who worry about their parents' diabetes. Physicians can work with patients to match the regimen to the realities of their job and consult with employers if problems with diabetes management or employer misunderstanding of the disease and the legal rights of the employee threaten a patient's job security. The American Diabetes Association provides resources for health care providers and patients dealing with discrimination issues in the workplace.

THE ELDERLY

Because of increased survival rates, there is a growing number of older adults with type 1 diabetes, in addition to the increasing number of older patients with type 2 diabetes who require insulin. The elderly are often overlooked when new technologies and medicines are offered. The assumption is that more complex care is not feasible for this group of patients.

On the one hand, many older people are active and functional and may wish to increase rather than decrease the intensity of their diabetes care. Retired people may have more time and resources to devote to diabetes self-care skills. Because of the availability of Medicare coverage, older people may have greater access to health services and be able to afford to participate more actively in their care.

On the other hand, the demands of the diabetes regimen may be especially burdensome for some elderly, especially those who face reduction in resources due to retirement, loss of physical function and mobility, the death of a spouse and/or friends, and their own mortality. Aging leads to declines in physical capacity due to decreases in visual and auditory acuity, and diminished muscle mass, bone strength, joint flexibility, and aerobic capacity. In addition to the physiological deterioration, as many as 20% of the elderly may also have a diagnosable mental disorder, such as anxiety, severe cognitive impairment, and depression. The elderly are prone to hypoglycemia due to counterregulatory hormonal changes, the effects of concomitant medications, and alterations of appetite and the physical capacity to eat. It may be more difficult to keep physician appointments and purchase supplies because of transportation problems and financial limitations. Before assumptions are made about the needs or wishes of an elderly patient, a full current evaluation should be conducted that includes social factors such as interpersonal support, financial resources, and cognitive faculties. The diabetes management team should be aware that errors in insulin administration and blood testing may be due to failing eyesight or poor coordination, forgetfulness, or lack of understanding of new treatment modalities. It is essential for the diabetes management team to carefully assess each older patient to identify and address these potential barriers to sound diabetes care and, whenever possible, to identify a support person who is willing to monitor the elder person's health status and provide concrete assistance.

Inevitably, there are changes in social support as one ages. Those who have helped in the past may no longer be able or available to do so. Social support is important to the health and well-being of older adults, but its role will vary by gender, race, marital status, and illness characteristics. It is important to determine the type of help needed to maintain respect for and autonomy of the older person. The goal is to provide support while safeguarding the patient's autonomy and independence as much as possible. Home-care agencies and special programs, such as Meals-on-Wheels, are often helpful.

As emphasized for other age-groups, the relationship between the diabetes management team and patient will influence patient adherence. Patients who are satisfied with their team are more likely to adhere to their diabetes care plan. However, older adults are less likely than other age-groups to express dissatisfaction directly to the provider. Therefore, it is even more essential to encourage open communication with this group by asking and responding to questions and by taking time to show concern and discuss problems.

EMOTIONAL AND BEHAVIORAL DISORDERS AND DIABETES

It is important that care providers recognize emotional and behavioral disorders in patients with diabetes and refer these patients for evaluation and counseling. Some caregivers mistakenly view psychiatric symptoms, especially those of depression and anxiety, as expected or even normal in people coping with an illness as serious and difficult to treat as diabetes. Unfortunately, when psychiatric symptoms are seen as the norm, therapeutic intervention may not be recommended, and the patient will continue to suffer psychological distress. This situation is especially disturbing in light of the high prevalence of depression and anxiety disorders in individuals with diabetes and the availability of effective treatment options.

Depression. Individuals with diabetes have higher rates of diagnoses of depression than the general population of the US and of other developed countries. It is not known whether depression predisposes to diabetes, glucose toxicity predisposes to depression, or some other central mechanism is operating that affects both conditions. Depression in a patient with diabetes leads to an average increase of 0.5–1.0% in the A1C level. Regardless, depression is still underdiagnosed, especially in teens and the elderly, and nonadherence due to depression is often underrecognized. Ongoing monitoring of patients' mental status by a multidisciplinary team will help with prompt diagnosis and treatment. When depression is suspected, referral to a mental health provider is recommended. Pharmacologic and behavioral treatments have both been shown to be effective in treating depression. Incorporating the family and/or significant others into psychological care is also recommended.

Anxiety disorders. Anxiety disorders such as needle phobia and fear of hypoglycemia may be a consequence of treatment with insulin. Other disorders such as obsessive-compulsive disorder may be exacerbated by having diabetes. When symptoms are identified that suggest these disorders, referral to specialists who can initiate behavioral interventions while working with health care providers to maintain diabetes care behaviors is imperative. The goal is to prevent deterioration in metabolic control while reducing symptoms that limit the patient's ability to carry out diabetes care tasks and that negatively affect quality of life. An anxiolytic medication in concert with behavioral intervention can also be utilized to diminish symptoms. Once again, it is important not to mistake anxiety for willful noncompliance, especially when the patient expresses distress in association with specific diabetes care tasks (such as injections).

Fear of hypoglycemia may result in patients wishing to raise their glucose levels to avoid the unpleasant feelings and loss of control associated with hypoglycemia. As mentioned earlier, BGAT has been shown to improve patients' recognition of their glycemic status and reduce the incidence of severe hypoglycemia. Other forms of behavior therapy, used while temporarily raising glycemic targets, can improve glycemic awareness in those who have lost feelings of hypoglycemia. Increased blood glucose monitoring, use of continuous glucose monitoring, and compensatory external cues can be enlisted to maintain glycemic status in those with hypoglycemia unawareness.

It is important to treat the disorders in addition to looking for compensatory management strategies (such as pump use, increased SMBG, or addition of continuous glucose monitoring). Parents in particular may respond to their own anxiety by discussing "hurting" their child with insulin injections of SMBG. This inadvertently fosters anxiety and solidifies a child's fear. It is particularly important to include parents in treatment when children express anxiety over diabetes care behaviors, as the child/patient's fears may mirror the parent's fears.

Eating disorders. Eating disorders are common in (but not exclusive to) adolescent or young adult women with type 1 diabetes and are associated with poor metabolic control, poor adherence to the diabetes regimen, and more severe complications. Eating disorders are often related to the regain of and increasing weight associated with successful treatment of diabetes with insulin, and they may be exacerbated by the more intense focus on food that occurs in families of children with diabetes. Diagnostic criteria for anorexia nervosa include weight loss and maintenance of body weight 15% below norm, impaired body image, intense fear of weight gain, and absence of menses. Diagnostic criteria for bulimia nervosa include recurrent episodes of binge eating, feelings of loss of control over eating during binges, frequent self-induced vomiting and/or laxative use, and overconcern with body image and weight.

Many young people with type 1 diabetes may have eating disturbances that compromise their diabetes control yet do not meet stringent diagnostic criteria. They may lose calories by intentional glycosuria rather than vomiting or laxative use. This is accomplished by decreasing insulin doses or missing meal insulin boluses. The seriousness of these subclinical cases should not be underestimated because they can result in short- and long-term metabolic complications. Eating disorders, clinical and subclinical, should be suspected in young women with persistently unstable or poor metabolic control, recurrent ketoacidosis resulting from insulin omission to induce glycosuria and weight loss, or recurrent severe hypoglycemia resulting from food restriction while continuing insulin, anxiety or avoidance about being weighed, or binging with food or alcohol, and in girls with growth retardation and pubertal delay. It is important that members of the diabetes team routinely ask about eating behavior and insulin omission in a nonthreatening and nonjudgmental manner. These patients may require referral to an experienced mental health professional for psychological evaluation and treatment if an explanation for their problems is not found.

STRESS AND DIABETES

Although caregivers and patients have long observed a relationship between stress and blood glucose levels, the results of numerous studies attempting to define this relationship have yielded contradictory results. Some studies have shown an association between stress and hyperglycemia, whereas others have not. In some studies, this relationship has been idiosyncratic, with patients varying dramatically in their glucose response to the same or different stressors. The only way to establish an individual's stress reactivity is to monitor blood glucose before, during, and after a stressful life event. Compensatory strategies should be developed according to the patient's individual response. Parents and teachers need to be made aware of a child's stress reactivity as it applies to schoolwork and sports activities to plan a strategy to achieve glycemic targets during stressful times in the child's everyday life.

Stress can also have indirect effects on diabetes. Patients under stress may be less able to follow their diabetes regimen, may give a low priority to their diabetes care, or may respond to the stress by overeating or increasing their use of alcohol or illicit drugs. Care providers should explore possible explanations for poor metabolic control. Some patients, while others may find support through family, friends, religious community, or support groups, can learn to cope through stress management counseling or relaxation training.

BIBLIOGRAPHY

Anderson RJ, Grigsby AB, Freeland KE, De Groot M, McGill JB, Clouse RE, Lustman PJ: Anxiety and poor glycemic control: a meta-analytic review of the literature. *Int J Psychiatry Med* 32:235–247, 2002

Brod M, Kongsø JH, Lessard S, Christensen TL: Psychological insulin resistance: patient beliefs and implications for diabetes management. *Quality of Life Research* 18:23–32, 2008

DCCT Research Group: Sexual dysfunction in women with type 1 diabetes: long term findings from the DCCT/EDIC study cohort. *Diabetes Care* 32: 780–785, 2009

Kovacs J, Brent D, Steinberg TF, Paulauskas S, Reid J: Children's self-report of psychologic adjustment and coping strategies during first year of insulin-dependent diabetes mellitus. *Diabetes Care* 9:472–479, 1986

Lustman PJ, Anderson RJ, Freedland KE, de Groot M, Carney RM, Clouse RE: Depression and poor glycemic control: a meta-analytic review of the literature. *Diabetes Care* 23:934–942, 2000

Lustman PJ, Penckofer SM, Clouse RE: Recent advances in understanding depression in adults with diabetes. *Current Diabetes Reports* 7:114–122, 2007

Peyrot M, Rubin RR: Behavioral and psychosocial interventions in diabetes: a conceptual review. *Diabetes Care* 30:2433–2440, 2007

Rodin G, Olmsted M, Rydall A, Maharaj S, Colton P, Jones J, Biancucci L, Daneman D: Eating disorders in young women with type 1 diabetes mellitus. *J Psychosom Res* 53:943–949, 2002

Schmitz N, Wang J, Lesage A, Malla A, Strychar I: Psychological distress and short-term disability in people with diabetes: results from the Canadian Community Healthy Survey. *Journal of Psychosomatic Research* 65:165–172, 2008

Silverstein J, Klingensmith G, Copeland K, Plotnick L, Kaufman FR, Laffel L, Deeb L, Grey M, Anderson B, Clark N: Care of children and adolescents with type 1 diabetes mellitus: a statement of the American Diabetes Association. *Diabetes Care* 28:186–212, 2005

Complications

Highlights
Complications

RETINOPATHY

■ Significant retinopathy in patients with type 1 diabetes rarely occurs before the fifth year of the disease.

■ The clinician should assure that patients receive their initial ophthalmologic examination within 5 years of onset of type 1 diabetes (for children if >10 years of age and a diabetes duration of 3–5 years). Indications for more urgent ophthalmologic referral are described in Table 6.1.

■ High-risk characteristics of proliferative retinopathy greatly increase the risk of blindness and include

- new vessels on the optic disk (NVD) involving greater than ~25% of the optic disk area
- any NVD with preretinal or vitreous hemorrhage
- new vessels elsewhere covering an area ≥50% of the optic disk area (totaled for the entire retina) with preretinal or vitreous hemorrhage

■ When high-risk characteristics are present, photocoagulation therapy should generally be performed promptly. An eye with severe non-proliferative diabetic retinopathy, or worse, should be considered for photocoagulation.

■ Lesions typical of nonproliferative retinopathy, proliferative retinopathy, and macular edema are described in Clinical Findings in Diabetic Retinopathy (page 210).

■ Treatment for diabetic retinopathy can be highly effective in preserving vision. Treatment modalities include

- scatter (panretinal) photocoagulation
- focal/grid laser photocoagulation
- vitrectomy

■ Medical therapies are discussed under Treatment (page 214).

NEPHROPATHY

■ Past epidemiologic studies suggested that up to 20–30% of patients with type 1 diabetes will eventually develop kidney failure, although this rate may be decreasing with more effective screening and treatment.

■ Possible mechanisms by which diabetes damages the kidney are discussed in Pathogenesis. Elevated blood glucose, a genetic propensity, elevated blood pressure, and abnormal glomerular hemodynamics have been implicated.

■ Renal function and albuminuria should be monitored annually in all patients with type 1 diabetes after a diabetes duration of 5 years or more.

■ Patients with persistent micro-albuminuria are at a higher risk for developing renal insufficiency and may benefit from more intensive glycemic control and ACE inhibitor therapy.

■ The management of more advanced diabetic nephropathy includes strict blood pressure control, minimizing factors that are known to accelerate the natural progression of renal disease or that may otherwise jeopardize the kidney, and assisting patients in responding to changing insulin needs (Tables 6.3 and 6.4).

■ If kidney failure ensues, two options are available: dialysis and kidney transplantation.

NEUROPATHY

■ Diabetic neuropathy is classified into a set of discrete clinical syndromes, each with a characteristic presentation and clinical course (Table 6.5). The syndromes overlap clinically and frequently occur simultaneously.

■ Distal symmetrical polyneuropathy is the most common form of diabetic neuropathy.

■ Patients with chronic unrecognized neuropathy may present with late complications, e.g., foot ulceration, foreign objects embedded in the foot, unrecognized trauma to the extremities, or neuroarthropathy

(Charcot's joints). All of these conditions are avoidable with proper early diagnosis of neuropathy and institution of appropriate foot care.

■ Treatment for diabetic distal symmetric polyneuropathy is symptomatic, palliative, and supportive, with primary emphasis on preventing the late complications.

■ Persistent and severely painful neuropathy has been treated with various drugs, including standard analgesics and drugs normally used to treat other conditions (anti-depressants, anti-convulsants). Narcotics should be avoided.

■ Although autonomic neuropathy produces diffuse subclinical dysfunction, autonomic symptoms are usually confined to one or two organ systems, producing the discrete autonomic syndromes listed in Table 6.8.

■ Erectile dysfunction in men with diabetes is usually neuropathic but can also be psychogenic, endocrine, vascular, or drug or stress related.

■ Other dysfunctions related to autonomic neuropathy include diabetic cystopathy and hypoglycemia unawareness.

■ Mononeuropathies comprise neural deficits corresponding to the distribution of single or multiple peripheral nerves and are usually acute in onset and resolve spontaneously within weeks to months.

■ Screen for diabetic peripheral neuropathy (DPN) starting 5 years after the diagnosis of type 1 diabetes and at least annually thereafter.

MACROVASCULAR DISEASE

■ Coronary heart disease, peripheral arterial disease, and cerebrovascular disease are more common, tend to occur at an earlier age, and are more extensive and severe in people with diabetes.

■ Physicians should systematically assess patients for risk factors for atherosclerotic cardiovascular disease, question them about symptoms, and be alert for signs of atherosclerosis.

■ A program for modifying risk factors should be started if appropriate.

■ Guidelines for treatment of cerebrovascular disease, coronary heart disease, and peripheral arterial disease appear in Symptoms and Signs of Atherosclerosis.

COMPLICATIONS IN CHILDREN

■ Limited joint mobility (LJM), which is not restricted to children, now occurs less often than in the past, and is a potentially important clinical marker for diabetes complications such as retinopathy, nephropathy,

neuropathy, and other disorders. Glycation of tissue proteins may be responsible for LJM, which is painless, can cause some disability, and is marked by a scleroderma-like stiffness of the skin and joints.

■ Subtle abnormalities of growth and development affect 5–10% of youngsters with type 1 diabetes and usually result from inadequate metabolic control.

■ Signs of growth abnormalities include a lag in height or weight or a falling away from the patient's previously established growth curves.

■ Children most likely to be affected are those with the earliest onset of diabetes and the worst glycemic control. Boys are two to three times more likely to be affected than girls.

■ To detect growth abnormalities, the physician should regularly plot height and weight on standard growth charts. Other growth-impairing conditions should be considered in assessing growth abnormalities.

Complications

RETINOPATHY

Diabetic retinopathy is one of the most common causes of blindness in the US, the most common cause in those 20–74 years old, and is a major cause of visual disability. Several surveys suggest that a person with diabetes has a 5–10% chance of becoming legally blind and that this risk is greater in people with type 1 than type 2 diabetes. Thirty-year data from the DCCT/EDIC and the Pittsburgh Epidemiology of Diabetes Complications Experience (EDC) studies encompassing the years 1983–2005 showed the differential risk by conventional and intensive treatment groups for the DCCT/EDIC compared to the EDC cohort. After 30 years of diabetes, the cumulative incidences of proliferative retinopathy were 50% in the DCCT conventional treatment group, 47% in the EDC cohort, and 21% in the DCCT intensive therapy group, and with fewer than 1% legally blind.

Vision-threatening retinopathy virtually never appears in patients with type 1 diabetes in the first 3–5 years of diabetes or before puberty. Retinopathy detected by fundus photography reaches a prevalence of 50% by the 10th year. By the 15th year, up to 28% of patients have proliferative retinopathy, in which new blood vessels develop from the retinal circulation, with a substantial risk of hemorrhage and traction detachment of the retina. After 20 years' duration of diabetes, nearly all patients have some form of retinopathy. Earlier age at diagnosis, puberty, pregnancy, rapid intensification of blood glucose control, hypertension, hypercholesterolemia, anemia, use of tobacco, and presence of cataracts or cataract surgery may exert an accelerating influence on the progression of retinopathy. Limited data has suggested that vitamin D deficiency might be associated with an increased prevalence of retinopathy in young people with type 1 diabetes. To reduce the risk or slow the progression of retinopathy, optimization of glycemic control is important, and to reduce the risk or slow the progression, it is critical to optimize blood pressure control.

EYE EXAMINATION

Diabetic retinopathy appears primarily in the posterior retina and midperiphery. Many but not all lesions may occur within an area viewable by the nonophthalmologist with the monocular direct ophthalmoscope. However, this examination is not an adequate substitute for an annual retinal examination by an ophthalmologist or optometrist who is knowledgeable and experienced in the detection of diabetic retinopathy. It has been demonstrated that non–eye care professionals will miss a substantial amount of retinopathy, especially if pupils are not dilated. Although the finding of retinopathy by indirect ophthalmoscopy is well correlated with presence of disease and is important for prompt referral of the patient, lack of observed retinopathy does not obviate the need for comprehensive ophthalmologic evaluation in patients with diabetes.

CLINICAL FINDINGS IN DIABETIC RETINOPATHY

Mild to Moderate Nonproliferative Retinopathy

The earliest lesion visible through the ophthalmoscope is the microaneurysm, a pouch-like dilation of a terminal capillary. Ophthalmoscopically, microaneurysms look like tiny red dots. Dot hemorrhages may be indistinguishable from microaneurysms unless specialized techniques, such as fluorescein angiography, are used, but blot hemorrhages may be recognized because they are larger (Fig. 6.1). Hard exudates are another common feature of nonproliferative retinopathy. Early nonproliferative retinopathy does not cause visual symptoms unless it is associated with macular edema.

Severe to Very Severe Nonproliferative Retinopathy

Multiple extensive clustered blot hemorrhages throughout the retina suggest progression to the severe nonproliferative stage. At this stage, substantial portions of the capillary circulation may have become nonfunctional, and retinal tissue is nonperfused. This nonperfusion may result in retinal hypoxia, which is thought to stimulate new retinal blood vessel development.

Veins may appear dilated, tortuous, and irregular in caliber. Intraretinal microvascular abnormalities are other signs of significant nonproliferative retinopathy. These small loops of fine vessels usually extend from a major artery or vein and probably represent early new-vessel formation within the retina. Fluffy white lesions, commonly referred to as cottonwool spots, were formerly associated with this stage of retinopathy. Evidence suggests that these lesions, when they appear alone, may be poor prognostic indicators.

Proliferative Retinopathy

Proliferative diabetic retinopathy involves the formation of new blood vessels, extending from within the retinal substance onto the inner surface of the retina or into the vitreous cavity. These vessels commonly occur on the optic nerve head, where they are called new vessels on the disk (NVD) (Fig. 6.2). They may also occur elsewhere in the retina, usually extending from major vessels, where they are called new vessels elsewhere (NVE). New vessels are fragile and carry a substantial risk of rupture with hemorrhage. The vessels also eventually undergo fibrosis and contraction, capable of producing retinal detachment from the tractional forces exerted.

Certain findings were defined as high-risk characteristics (HRC) by the national Diabetic Retinopathy Study (DRS), a large-scale randomized controlled clinical trial completed in 1981. The presence of HRC increases an eye's risk of severe vision loss (<25/200 on two consecutive visits at least 3 months apart) to 30–50% within 3–5 years of detection if appropriate treatment is not provided. HRC include

- NVD greater than ~25% of the optic disk area
- any NVD with preretinal or vitreous hemorrhage
- NVE greater than or equal to 50% of the optic disk area (totaled for the entire retina) with preretinal or vitreous hemorrhage

Figure 6.1
Nonproliferative
retinopathy, with
microaneurysms,
dot and blot
hemorrhages.

Figure 6.2
Proliferative retinopa-
thy, with abnormal
new blood vessels
and scar tissue on
the surface of the
retina.

Figure 6.3
Scatter laser
photocoagulation
therapy for
proliferative diabetic
retinopathy.

When HRC are present, photocoagulation therapy (Fig. 6.3) is indicated to preserve vision.

Diabetic Macular Edema

Macular edema involves thickening of the central portion of the retina. The macula occupies an area of ~5 disk diameters just temporal to the optic nerve head (Fig. 6.4). Visual acuity can be decreased in this condition, particularly when the center of the macula (the fovea centralis) is involved. Macular edema is difficult to diagnose with the direct ophthalmoscope because this instrument does not allow the stereoscopic vision necessary to determine retinal thickening. However, the presence of hard lipid exudates—yellowish-white, often glistening, deposits of round or irregular shape lying within the retina, usually in the macular region—strongly suggests macular edema. This is particularly true if the exudates assume a ring-shape, or circinate, configuration. The features of clinically significant macular edema are

■ retinal thickening at or within 500 μm of the macular center
■ hard exudates at or within 500 μm of the macular center with adjacent retinal thickening
■ retinal thickening >1 disk diameter in size any part of which is within 1 disk diameter of the macular center

When clinically significant macular edema is present, focal laser therapy (Fig. 6.5) is indicated to preserve vision.

Glaucoma

Sometimes, in advanced (usually proliferative) diabetic retinopathy, new vessels may also form on the surface of the iris and extend into the "angle" of the anterior chamber of the eye, where the cornea and iris come together. Here, fibrous scar tissue extending from the new vessels may block the outflow of aqueous humor from the eye, causing a rise in intraocular pressure (neovascular glaucoma), severe pain, and loss of vision. Angle-closure glaucoma, a major complication, is a rare disorder in any age-group, especially before the age of 40 years.

EVALUATION

Patients with type 1 diabetes ≥10 years of age should have an annual detailed ocular examination within 3–5 years after the onset of diabetes. In general, this examination is not necessary before age 10 years. However, some evidence suggests that the prepubertal duration of diabetes may be important in the development of microvascular complications, so clinical judgment should be used when applying this recommendation to individual patients. The screening examination should be done by an experienced ophthalmologist or optometrist and should include

■ determination of visual acuity of each eye
■ refraction, especially if visual acuity is impaired
■ gross external examination of the eyes

Figure 6.4
Diabetic
macular edema.

Figure 6.5 Focal
laser photoco-
agulation therapy for
clinically significant
macular edema.

Figures 6.1-6.5 provided by National Eye Institute, Institute of Health website: http://www
.nei.nih.gov/photo/keyword.asp?conditions=Diabetic. Accessed March 2012.

- evaluation of ocular motility
- examination of the eyes by slit-lamp biomicroscopy
- examination of the retina with monocular direct and binocular indirect
  ophthalmoscopy after dilation of the pupils
- slit-lamp ophthalmoscopy to exclude macular edema
- in adult patients, measurement of intraocular pressures

Patients with any level of macular edema, severe nonproliferative retinopathy, or any proliferative retinopathy require the prompt care of an ophthalmologist who is knowledgeable and experienced in the management of diabetic retinopathy. Further examinations may be carried out for specific indications. These include retinal photography, which is used to document lesions, and intravenous fluorescein angiography. During angiography, a fluorescent dye is injected into a vein, and rapid-sequence photography of the retinal circulation is carried out. Both eyes are typically evaluated at a single injection sequence.

Fluorescein angiography is useful clinically to plan photocoagulation treatment for macular edema. Although it is more sensitive than ophthalmoscopy or color photography for detecting very early lesions of retinopathy, the minute lesions detected are rarely critical for making decisions regarding treatment. Therefore, intravenous fluorescein angiography should not be used as a screening test in the annual ocular examination of patients with diabetes. Guidelines for care and referral are described in Table 6.1.

TREATMENT

Clinicians should always refer patients for treatment of retinopathy to an ophthalmologist, preferably one who is an expert in retinal disease (a retinal specialist). If laser treatment (described below) has been recommended, the clinician should ensure that the treatment has been implemented and that the patient maintains the recommended follow-up.

Photocoagulation

Scatter (panretinal) photocoagulation. The principal method used to treat diabetic retinopathy is by laser or light photocoagulation. For patients with proliferative retinopathy and HRC, scatter photocoagulation with the laser is standard therapy, based on DRS results and subsequent results from the Early Treatment Diabetic Retinopathy Study (ETDRS), another large-scale randomized controlled clinical trial.

In this procedure, a series of 1,200–1,600 (or sometimes more) laser burns, 500 µm in diameter and spaced one-half burn diameter apart, are placed throughout the midperipheral retina, avoiding the macular region (Fig. 6.3). The DRS demonstrated that this procedure reduced the rate of progression to blindness by 50% in eyes with HRC over a 5-year follow-up. The ETDRS study suggested that >95% of severe visual loss could be prevented if all patients received scatter photocoagulation just as they exhibit HRC.

Many eyes with proliferative retinopathy but without HRC or with severe nonproliferative retinopathy also will require scatter photocoagulation. The factors determining whether such patients should receive treatment include type of diabetes, progression rate, contralateral eye status, systemic status, etc., and should be discussed with the patient by the retinal specialist.

Patients undergoing scatter photocoagulation should have a clear understanding of what to expect from the procedure in terms of their vision. Often prevention of severe visual loss is the goal, rather than improvement in vision. The procedure itself may result in some loss of peripheral and/or night vision.

Focal/grid laser photocoagulation. Diabetic macular edema is treated by focal/grid laser photocoagulation. With this technique, leaking microaneurysms and other vascular abnormalities in the macular region, determined by fluorescein angiography, are treated by direct application of small (50- to 100-µm) laser burns or laser

Table 6.1 Guidelines for Care

Routine Care by Physician

■Examine retina with direct ophthalmoscope annually and when indicated by symptoms or previous findings

Referral to Eye Care Specialist

■Examine retinas through dilated pupils once a year (this need not be done before puberty unless the patient has eye symptoms or other complications of diabetes)

Referral to Ophthalmologist

■At the beginning of pregnancy or if planning pregnancy within 12 months

■Moderate nonproliferative diabetic retinopathy, or worse

■Any level of macular edema (suggested by hard exudates within the macula)

■Immediate referral is mandatory (preferably to an ophthalmologist specializing in retinal disease) if any of the following are present:
  • NVD greater than ~25% of the optic disk area
  • any NVD with preretinal or vitreous hemorrhage
  • NVE greater than or equal to 50% of the disk area with preretinal or vitreous hemorrhage

■Reduced vision from any cause

■Immediate referral is strongly urged when the following are present:
  • proliferative retinopathy without HRC
  • severe nonproliferative retinopathy, which includes
    – dilated irregular veins
    – multiple dot and blot hemorrhages
    – intraretinal microvascular abnormalities

burns placed in a grid-like pattern (Fig. 6.5). The ETDRS showed that this treatment reduced the rate of visual loss from diabetic macular edema by 50% over a 3-year follow-up.

Vitrectomy

Vitrectomy is a surgical procedure used primarily to *1*) remove vitreous humor filled with blood, *2*) cut fibrous traction bands, *3*) peel contractile fibrous membranes from the inner retinal surface, and *4*) repair some types of complex retinal detachments. Vitrectomy is particularly effective in certain cases of advanced proliferative diabetic retinopathy. Although it can restore useful vision to eyes that would otherwise have severe visual impairment, vitrectomy is usually used only in more diseased eyes, as there are significant potential surgical complications.

Medical Therapy

It is important to maintain normal blood pressure levels and near-normal blood glucose levels in patients with retinopathy because diabetic retinopathy progresses more rapidly in patients with uncontrolled hypertension and hyperglycemia than in those whose blood pressure and blood glucose are controlled.

Control of systemic lipid levels is also important, as dyslipidemia is associated with increased risk of hard exudates in the macula.

Therapies Under Evaluation

Other medical treatments for diabetic retinopathy have been evaluated.

■ Aspirin (650 mg/day) was tested in the ETDRS because it inhibits platelet aggregation. Platelet microthrombi have been proposed as a factor in the cause of diabetic retinopathy. Aspirin was shown to be of no benefit or risk for retinopathy in this study.
■ Two experimental classes of drugs, both targeting pathways involved in the pathogenesis of microvascular complications, may be useful in preventing or reducing the progression of diabetic retinopathy: aldose reductase inhibitors, inhibitors of protein kinase C and inhibitors of vascular endothelial growth factors (VEGFs). Aldose reductase inhibitors have shown promise in animal studies but have not yet shown good efficacy or safety in human retinopathy trials. Although VEGF is implicated in the pathology of NV, permeability and inflammation, it also has a beneficial role in ocular health. Side effects of therapy with VEGF inhibitors are potentially significant and studies continue to determine its role in diabetic eye disease.

CONCLUSION

Diabetic retinopathy is a common complication of long-term diabetes that ranks as a leading cause of blindness and visual disability. Appropriate care includes optimization of blood glucose, blood pressure, and serum lipid levels and routine, life-long ophthalmic examinations. Although treatment strategies cannot totally prevent or cure this complication, there is clear evidence that they can substantially retard its progression if used appropriately and provided promptly when indicated. Accordingly, careful optimization of glycemic control early and persistently and other risk factors by the primary care physician, together with annual screening by an eye care professional and referral of patients with significant retinopathy to an ophthalmologist who is knowledgeable and experienced in the management of diabetic retinopathy, is a standard of care for all patients with diabetes.

BIBLIOGRAPHY

Aiello LM: Perspectives on diabetic retinopathy. *Am J Ophthalmol* 136:122–135, 2003

Aiello LP, Cahill MT, Wong JS: Systemic considerations in the management of diabetic retinopathy. *Am J Ophthalmol* 132:760–766, 2001

American Diabetes Association: Diabetic retinopathy (Position Statement). *Diabetes Care* 27 (Suppl. 1):S84–S87, 2004

DCCT Research Group: The effect of intensive treatment of diabetes on the development and progression of long-term complications in insulin-dependent diabetes mellitus. *N Engl J Med* 329:977–986, 1993

DCCT Research Group: The relationship of glycemic exposure (HbA1c) to the risk of development and progression of retinopathy in the Diabetes Control and Complications Trial. *Diabetes* 44:968–983, 1995

Diabetes Control and Complications Trial/Epidemiology of Diabetes Interventions and Complications Research Group: Retinopathy and nephropathy in patients with type 1 diabetes four years after a trial of intensive therapy. *N Engl J Med* 342:381–389, 2000

Diabetes Control and Complications Trial/Epidemiology of Diabetes Interventions and Complications Research Group: The modern-day clinical course of type 1 diabetes mellitus after 30 years' duration: the diabetes control and complications trial/epidemiology of diabetes interventions and complications and Pittsburgh epidemiology of diabetes complications experience (1983–2005). *Arch Intern Med* 169:1307–1316, 2009

Early Treatment Diabetic Retinopathy Study Research Group: Early photocoagulation for diabetic retinopathy: report number 9. *Ophthalmology* 98 (Suppl. 5):766–785, 1991

Early Treatment Diabetic Retinopathy Study Research Group: Photocoagulation for diabetic macular edema: report number 1. *Arch Ophthalmol* 103:1796–1806, 1985

Fong DS, Aiello LP, Ferris FL, Klein R: Diabetic retinopathy (Technical Review). *Diabetes Care* 27:2540–2553, 2004

Hietala K, Harjutsalo V, Forsblom C, Summanen P, Groop P-H, on behalf of the FinnDiane Study Group: Age at onset and the risk of proliferative retinopathy in type 1 diabetes. *Diabetes Care* 33:1315–1319, 2010

Frank RN: Diabetic retinopathy. *N Engl J Med* 350:48–58, 2004

Kaur H, Donaghue KC, Chan AK, Benitez-Aguirre P, Hing S, Lloyd M, Cusumano J, Pryke A, Craig ME: Vitamin D deficiency is associated with retinopathy in children and adolescents with type 1 diabetes. *Diabetes Care* 34:1400–1402, 2011

Klein R, Klein BE, Moss SE, Cruickshanks KJ: The Wisconsin Epidemiology Study of Diabetic Retinopathy. XIV. Ten-year incidence and progression of diabetic retinopathy. *Arch Ophthalmol* 112:1217–1228, 1994

Klein R, Klein BEK, Moss SE, Davis MD, DeMets DL: The Wisconsin Epidemiology Study of Diabetic Retinopathy. II. Prevalence and risk of diabetic retinopathy when age at diagnosis is less than 30 years. *Arch Ophthalmol* 102:520–526, 1984

Klein R, Lee KE, Gangnon RE, Klein BE: The 25-year incidence of visual impairment in type 1 diabetes mellitus: the Wisconsin epidemiologic study of diabetic retinopathy. *Ophthalmology* 117:63–70, 2010

Sheetz MJ, Aiello LP, Shahri N, Davis MD, Kles KA, Danis RP, Mbdv Study Group: Effect of ruboxistaurin (RBX) on visual acuity decline over a 6-year period with cessation and reinstitution of therapy: results of an open-label extension of the protein kinase C diabetic retinopathy study 2 (PKC-DRS2). *Retina* 6:1053–1059, 2011

Tayyeba AK, El-Remessy AB: Diabetic retinopathy: current management and experimental therapeutic targets. *Pharmacotherapy* 29:182–192, 2009

UK Prospective Diabetes Study Group: Intensive blood-glucose control with sulphonylureas or insulin compared with conventional treatment and risk of complications in patients with type 2 diabetes (UKPDS 33). *Lancet* 352:837–853, 1998

White NH, Sun W, Cleary PA, Tamborlane WV, Danis RP, Hainsworth DP, Davis MD for the DCCT-EDIC Research Group: Effect of the prior intensive therapy in type 1 diabetes on 10-year progression of retinopathy in the DCCT/EDIC: comparison of adults and adolescents. *Diabetes* 59:1244–1253, 2010

NEPHROPATHY

About 40% of individuals starting dialysis in the US have diabetes, and almost half of these have type 1 diabetes. In the past, epidemiological studies suggested that 20–30% of patients affected with type 1 diabetes would eventually develop kidney failure and require dialysis. More recent evidence suggests that the frequency of nephropathy may be decreasing in the type 1 population with increased implementation of intensive glycemic control and wide application of early screening and effective preventive measures. Thirty-year data from the DCCT/EDIC and the Pittsburgh Epidemiology of Diabetes Complications Experience (EDC) studies encompassing the years 1983-2005 showed the differential risk by conventional and intensive treatment groups for the DCCT/EDIC compared to the EDC cohort. After 30 years of diabetes, the cumulative incidences of nephropathy were 25% in the DCCT conventional treatment group, 17% in the EDC cohort, and 9% in the DCCT intensive therapy group and with fewer than 1% requiring kidney replacement therapy.

CLINICAL SYNDROME

In its fully established form, diabetic nephropathy is a distinct clinical entity characterized by proteinuria, hypertension, edema, and renal insufficiency; in its most severe forms, nephrotic syndrome can be present. Diabetic nephropathy occurs in type 1 diabetes patients with longstanding diabetes (usually over 10 years).

Histopathological Changes

Three classes of renal histopathological changes characterize diabetic nephropathy: 1) glomerulosclerosis; 2) structural vascular changes, particularly in the small arterioles; and 3) tubulointerstitial disease. Glomerular damage, e.g., mesangial expansion and basement membrane thickening, is the most characteristic feature of diabetic nephropathy and most often takes the form of diffuse scarring of entire glomeruli. The tubulointerstitial changes interfere with potassium ion and hydrogen ion secretion and may be at least partly responsible for the hyperkalemia and metabolic acidosis that accompany diabetic kidney disease.

NATURAL HISTORY

Shortly after diabetes is diagnosed, the glomerular filtration rate (GFR) and renal blood flow are characteristically elevated, and there is typically a corresponding increase in kidney weight and size. The increased GFR is related to the degree of hyperglycemia, and the GFR and renal hypertrophy can be normalized by improved glycemic control. The serum creatinine and urea nitrogen concentrations are slightly reduced when the renal hyperfiltration is present. Although a slight increase in urine protein is common when a patient initially presents in diabetic ketoacidosis, once glycemia is well regulated by insulin therapy, proteinuria disappears and remains absent for many years.

Early in the course of diabetes, the renal histology is normal despite renal hypertrophy. However, within 2–3 years, many kidneys demonstrate some histological evidence of mesangial expansion and basement membrane thickening. Despite these histological changes, GFR and renal blood flow may remain elevated, and proteinuria is not detectable. The earliest clinical evidence of nephropathy is the appearance of low but abnormal levels (>30 mg/day or 30 µg/mg creatinine) of albumin in the urine. This subclinical range of increased albumin excretion goes undetected with routine urine dipstick testing, but is detectable with more sensitive techniques, and is sometimes referred to as microalbuminuria. Several factors can induce microalbuminuria, including poor glycemic control, infection, and vigorous exercise. The presence of even microscopic hematuria (or contamination by menstrual fluid) is sufficient to invalidate tests for microalbuminuria. Albuminuria results vary widely from day to day, and abnormal results should be confirmed by repeat testing.

Patients with confirmed microalbuminuria are referred to as having incipient nephropathy and are at a higher risk for developing progressive kidney disease. Without specific interventions, ~80% of subjects with type 1 diabetes who develop sustained microalbuminuria have their urinary albumin excretion increase at a rate of ~10–20%/year to the stage of overt nephropathy or clinical albuminuria (>300 mg/24 h or ~300 µg/mg creatinine) over 10–15 years, with hypertension also developing. In addition to being the earliest manifestation of nephropathy, microalbuminuria is a marker of greatly increased cardiovascular risk for patients with either type 1 or type 2 diabetes. Thus, the finding of microalbuminuria is an indication for screening for possible vascular disease and aggressive intervention to reduce all cardiovascular risk factors (e.g., lowering of LDL cholesterol, antihypertensive therapy, smoking cessation, increased physical activity). In addition, some preliminary evidence suggests that lowering cholesterol may also reduce the level of proteinuria.

Once overt nephropathy occurs, without specific interventions, the GFR gradually falls over several years at a rate that is highly variable from individual to individual (2–20 ml/min/year). Kidney failure develops in 50% of patients with type 1 diabetes with overt nephropathy within 10 years and in >75% by 20 years.

Although the GFR may still be elevated at the onset of proteinuria, it usually declines by ~50% within 3 years, and the serum creatinine and urea nitrogen concentrations become frankly elevated (>2.0 and >30 mg/dL, respectively). Hypertension usually becomes manifest and become progressively more difficult to treat. Within a mean of 2 years after the serum creatinine becomes elevated, 50% of the individuals will progress to kidney failure. The mean duration of type 1 diabetes when ESRD develops is 23 years. With this, the uremic symptoms, e.g., drowsiness, lethargy, and nausea, appear and become progressively more pronounced. Most patients receive treatment before reaching this stage, and cardiovascular disease is now the most common cause of death in patients with nephropathy.

Traditionally, it has been considered unusual in type 1 diabetes to observe diabetic nephropathy in the absence of retinopathy, neuropathy, and hypertension. However, the correlation is close only in advanced kidney disease. As kidney failure progresses, the incidence and severity of all three disorders increases markedly, generally in parallel with renal status.

PATHOGENESIS

Considerable evidence suggests that diabetic nephropathy is related primarily to the hyperglycemia induced by the diabetic state. First, renal changes are absent initially in people biopsied around the time of onset of diabetes. Second, typical changes of diabetic nephropathy occur in all types of diabetes. Third, diabetic nephropathy appears in various animal models regardless of whether the diabetes is induced or spontaneous, and the damage occurs in both original and transplanted kidneys. Fourth, in these diabetic animals, intensive insulin therapy or islet cell transplantation completely prevents renal histopathologic changes and may reverse early histopathologic abnormalities. Last, improved glucose control can substantially delay the initial appearance of persistent microalbuminuria and clinical grade albuminuria in type 1 diabetes.

Possible Mechanisms of Damage

The mechanisms by which diabetes damages the kidney are not completely understood. Podocyte injury and depletion appear to play a role in the pathogenesis of diabetic kidney disease, and there is a strong correlation between podocyte density, albuminuria, and renal function decline. Understanding of the regulatory and signaling pathways involved in glomerular injury, including VEGF, Notch signaling, and others, might lead to novel therapies for prevention and treatment in the future. How these pathways might be triggered by elevated glucose *per se* or by some metabolic event that occurs as a consequence of hyperglycemia remains unknown.

A genetic propensity to diabetic nephropathy has been noted. Thus, it is possible that metabolic disturbances initiate the processes responsible for diabetic nephropathy but that these processes operate on a genetic background that predisposes to diabetic glomerulosclerosis. Some studies suggest the genetic predisposition relates to an increased familial incidence of essential hypertension.

One explanation for renal damage may involve the typical increases in GFR and renal blood flow that occur early in the course of diabetes. In animals, these alterations in renal hemodynamics are associated with increased intraglomerular pressures. Although it has not been possible to measure intraglomerular pressure in humans, it has been suggested that glomerular hypertension is the ultimate mediator of kidney damage in diabetic nephropathy. Measures aimed at reversing the resulting hemodynamic changes have proved useful in slowing the progression of kidney disease in human diabetes.

TESTING FOR NEPHROPATHY

Because microalbuminuria rarely occurs with short duration of type 1 diabetes or before puberty, screening in individuals with type 1 diabetes should begin with puberty after disease duration of 5 years. Evidence suggests that the prepubertal duration of diabetes may be important in the development of microvascular complications, so clinical judgment should be used when applying this recommendation to individual patients.

Screening for microalbuminuria can be performed by three methods: *1*) measurement of the albumin-to-creatinine ratio in a random spot collection, *2*) 24-h collection, and *3*) timed (e.g., 4-h or overnight) collection. The first method is the easiest to carry out in an office setting and generally provides accurate information. First-void or other morning collections are preferred because of the known diurnal variation in albumin excretion, but if this timing cannot be used, uniformity of timing for different collections in the same individual should be employed. Specific assays are needed to detect microalbuminuria, because both standard dipsticks and standard hospital laboratory assays for urinary protein are not sufficiently sensitive to measure such levels. Microalbuminuria is defined as in Table 6.2.

In addition to annual assessment of urinary albumin, serum creatinine should be measured at least annually and used to estimate GFR and to stage the level of CKD, if present. GFR can be estimated using formulae such as the Cockroft-Gault equation or a prediction formula using data from the Modification of Diet and Renal Disease study. GFR calculators are available at *http://www.nkdep.nih.gov*. Many clinical laboratories now report estimated GFR (eGFR) in addition to serum creatinine. Although in the DCCT/EDIC albuminuria was a strong predictor of eGFR loss and risk of developing sustained eGFR <60 ml/min/1.73 m², it is estimated that albumin excretion rate alone would have missed 24% of cases of sustained impaired eGFR. Therefore, it is recommended that serum creatinine be measured annually in adults regardless of the degree of urine albumin excretion.

MANAGEMENT OF NEPHROPATHY

Incipient nephropathy: Confirmation of microalbuminuria should trigger increased attention to improved glycemic control and the institution of angiotensin converting enzyme (ACE) inhibitor therapy, both of which have been shown to decrease the progression of nephropathy. The DCCT demonstrated conclusively that intensive glycemic control reduces the development and progression of early kidney disease. In the DCCT/EDIC follow-up study at 22 years, there remained a 50% risk reduction in the intensive therapy group. However, there is no evidence that tight glycemic control through intensive insulin therapy can reverse or even slow the progression of severely advanced kidney disease.

ACE inhibitor therapy is discussed more fully in the section on hypertension, but is indicated for patients with macroalbuminuria as well as those with

Table 6.2 Definitions in Abnormalities of Albumin Excretion

Category	24-h Collection (mg/24 h)	Timed Collection (µg/min)	Spot Collection (µg/mg creatinine)
Normal	<30	<20	<30
Microalbuminuria	30–299	20–199	<30–299
Clinical albuminuria	≥300	≥200	≥300

more advanced disease. Patients with type 1 diabetes often develop incipient nephropathy prior to developing hypertension, so the dosage of the ACE inhibitor may need to be low to avoid symptomatic hypotension. Angiotensin II receptor blockers (ARBs) have been shown to reduce the rate of progression from micro to macroalbuminuria, and combination therapy with an ACE inhibitor and an ARB have been shown to provide additional lowering of albuminuria.

Overt nephropathy: Once overt proteinuria or decreased GFR are detected, renal function should be monitored at least two to three times per year. Hypertension should be aggressively treated with blockers of the rennin-angiotensin system and usually with adjunctive medications, as discussed below. Other interventions in the management of advanced diabetic nephropathy include *1*) minimizing factors that are known to accelerate the natural progression of kidney disease or that may otherwise jeopardize the kidney, *2*) assessing for anemia and secondary hyperparathyroidism, and *3*) appropriately responding to decreasing insulin needs (Tables 6.3 and 6.4). The development of renal insufficiency may initially be associated with insulin resistance, resulting in an increase in insulin requirements. However, because insulin is cleared by the kidney, as kidney disease becomes more advanced, it is common to see a decrease in the daily insulin dose and/or an increase in hypoglycemic episodes, particularly in patients with a glomerular filtration rate <20 ml/min. For this reason, self-monitoring of blood glucose and use of the results to adjust the insulin dose are critical.

If the nephropathy is progressive, consultation with a nephrologist is indicated to plot a long-term therapeutic strategy and to discuss the possibility and implications of kidney failure with the patient. The patient should understand the two

---

Table 6.3 Treatment of Diabetic Nephropathy

The following are factors influencing diabetic nephropathy and should be addressed:

■**Hypertension.** This is the most important factor shown to accelerate progression of renal failure. Goal blood pressure is <130 mmHg systolic and <80 mmHg diastolic. Angiotensin-converting enzyme (ACE) inhibitors and angiotensin II receptor blockers (ARBs) have specific effects to preserve renal function.

■**Hyperglycemia.** Control of blood glucose is extremely important in preventing and stopping the progression of microalbuminuria and proteinuria. The recommended glycemic goals are as close to normal as possible (Table 2.1). Note that uremia may be associated with insulin resistance and increased insulin requirements. With advanced uremia (GFR 15–20 ml/min), insulin requirements may fall because the kidney removes 25% of daily injected insulin, and hepatic degradation of insulin is inhibited by uremia.

■**Hyperlipidemia.** Control of lipids (LDL <100 mg/dL) is essential in preventing cardiovascular disease and may aid in slowing the progression of nephropathy.

■**Proteinuria.** Reduction of proteinuria with ACE inhibitors, ARBs, and nondihydropyridine calcium antagonists have additive effects to preserve renal function.

■**Protein restriction.** A low-protein diet (<0.8 g/kg body wt/day) slows progression of renal disease in patients with diabetes with advanced renal insufficiency.

Table 6.4 Other Threats to Diabetic Kidneys

Several conditions can endanger the kidneys of individuals with diabetes, even if renal insufficiency has not yet come into play. Among them are the following:

■**Urinary tract infection.** Older individuals with diabetes generally have an increased incidence of urinary tract infection. Therefore, for these patients, it is important that a urinalysis be performed at each clinic visit. If leukocytes or bacteriuria are detected, a urine culture should be obtained. Positive cultures should be treated with an appropriate bactericidal antibiotic.

■**Neurogenic bladder.** The development of a neurogenic bladder is common in patients with diabetes, especially if other evidence of autonomic neuropathy is present, and may predispose to infection. Symptoms, e.g., frequent voiding, nocturia, incontinence, and recurrent urinary tract infections, may be minimal or may mimic those of prostatic hypertrophy. Once suspected, the diagnosis is easily established if a cystometrogram demonstrates a large atonic bladder with low-pressure recordings. If the presence of a neurogenic bladder is confirmed, the patient should receive instruction in Credé's manual voiding maneuver, which should be performed every ~8 h. Often this will be sufficient to prevent postvoid residual and will decompress the upper urinary tract. If not, parasympathetic agents such as bethanechol chloride may be tried. In some people with diabetes, β-adrenergic–blocking agents, such as phenoxybenzamine, have proved useful. If pharmacologic therapy proves unsuccessful, intermittent straight catheterization should be performed 2–3 times daily.

■**Intravenous pyelography and other dye studies.** Patients with diabetes are at increased risk for acute renal failure after any radiocontrast (intravenous and retrograde pyelography, arteriography, cholangiography, computed tomography scanning) procedure. With the judicious use of echography, radionuclide studies, magnetic resonance imaging, and noncontrast computed tomography scanning, studies employing iodinated radiocontrast dye are rarely necessary. If contrast media must be used, a minimum amount of dye should be given, and adequate hydration with half-normal or normal saline should be ensured before the dye study. Use of iso-osmolar, dimeric, nonionic iodinated contrast agents such as iodixanol should be considered in high-risk patients with nephropathy or serum creatinine concentrations >1.5 mg/dL. General recommendations cannot yet be made regarding the routine administration of specific agents to prevent contrast-induced reductions in renal function, such as acetylcysteine or fenoldopam, as they are still under intensive investigation. Serum creatinine concentration should be checked daily for 2–3 days after the contrast study.

options available for renal replacement therapy, dialysis and kidney transplantation, and have adequate medical and psychological preparation for renal replacement therapy.

Stages of CKD

Stage	Description	GFR (ml/min/1.73 m^2)
1	Kidney damage with normal or increased GFR	>90
2	Kidney damage with mildly decreased GFR	60–89
3	Moderately decreased GFR	30–59
4	Severely decreased GFR	15–29
5	Kidney failure	<15 or dialysis

HYPERTENSION

In type 1 diabetes, hypertension typically is secondary to the onset of more advance kidney disease; long-term survivors of diabetes without nephropathy rarely have hypertension. Hypertension is the single most important factor accelerating the progression of established diabetic nephropathy and contributes to other causes of diabetes-related morbidity and mortality, such as retinopathy and heart disease. Aggressive treatment of hypertension is the only therapeutic intervention definitively shown to slow the progression of established kidney disease.

The diagnosis of hypertension should be based on multiple blood pressure determinations before beginning treatment. Orthostatic hypotension is frequent in patients with diabetic nephropathy; therefore, both supine and standing blood pressure should be measured. Ambulatory blood pressure monitoring is used in some centers to monitor patients during treatment.

Ideally, the patient with diabetes should have blood pressure treated to below <130/80 mmHg, and those with overt nephropathy, below 120/80. For patients (generally older) with isolated systolic hypertension with a systolic pressure of >180 mmHg, the initial goal of treatment is to reduce the systolic blood pressure in stages. If these initial goals are met and well tolerated, further lowering should be pursued.

Antihypertensive Therapy

ACE inhibitors. Many studies have shown that in hypertensive patients with type 1 diabetes, ACE inhibitors reduce the level of albuminuria and reduce the rate of progression of kidney disease to a greater degree than other antihypertensive agents that lower blood pressure by an equal amount. ACE inhibitors are recommended as the primary treatment of all hypertensive type 1 diabetes patients with microalbuminuria or overt nephropathy.

ACE inhibitors have few adverse effects and may even have modest beneficial effects on lipid metabolism and insulin sensitivity. The major serious side effect of ACE inhibitors is hyperkalemia, which is of particular concern in patients with more advanced nephropathy, who may have the syndrome of hyporeninemic hypoaldosteronism. In the presence of low renin, circulating aldosterone levels are decreased and the renal tubular secretion of potassium is impaired. Any drug that further impairs aldosterone secretion or action may lead to clinically significant hyperkalemia.

Some patients may experience a precipitous rise in serum creatinine when initiating therapy with ACE inhibitors, especially those with bilateral renal artery stenosis or advanced kidney disease. In patients with impaired kidney function or suspected renovascular hypertension, the physician should determine serum creatinine and potassium levels ~1 week after therapy begins. An excessive increase in either level warrants discontinuation of the drug. Cough may also occur. Finally, ACE inhibitors are contraindicated in pregnancy and therefore should be used with caution in women of childbearing potential.

Angiotensin II receptor blockers (ARBs). ARBs also slow the progression of kidney disease. Studies have shown a slowing of the rate of transition from microalbuminuria to clinical albuminuria in hypertensive type 2 diabetes patients. Furthermore, in type 2 diabetes with hypertension, albuminuria, and elevated creatinine levels, ARBs clearly slow the progression of diabetic nephropathy compared with other antihypertensive agents. If ACE inhibitors cannot be tolerated because of side effects such as cough, substitution of an ARB should be considered.

Diuretics. Because hypertension in the patient with diabetic nephropathy is often volume sensitive, therapy with a low-sodium diet and addition of a diuretic, especially when edema is present, may be needed to reach blood pressure treatment goals. Because many hypertensive individuals with type 1 diabetes have some degree of renal insufficiency, a loop diuretic is usually necessary. Thiazide diuretics do not promote natriuresis once the serum creatinine level has risen to levels of ~2 mg/dL. In patients with renal insufficiency, diuretics that inhibit potassium secretion (e.g., spironolactone, triamterene) should be used with caution because of concern for inducing hyperkalemia.

β-Adrenergic–blocking agents. β-Adrenergic–blocking agents have also proven successful in treating the hypertensive patient with diabetes. However, this class of drugs may mask many of the warning symptoms of hypoglycemia (although sweating is not affected). β-Blocking agents also predispose the development of hyperkalemia by inhibiting renin synthesis and impairing potassium uptake by extrarenal tissues and may aggravate hypertriglyceridema. Specific $β_1$-antagonists are the preferred β-blocking agents in patients with diabetes because they are less likely to cause hypoglycemia and hyperkalemia.

Calcium antagonists. Studies have shown that nondihydropyridine calcium antagonists reduce microalbuminuria and proteinuria; however, they have not been shown to have specific renal-protective effects, so should be used as adjunctive rather than primary agents. This class of drugs is relatively free of harmful side effects and does not cause significant alterations in glucose or lipid metabolism.

OTHER ASPECTS OF TREATMENT

Low-Protein Diet

Over the last several years, there has been renewed interest in the use of low-protein diets to prevent the progression of chronic kidney failure (see Nutrition, page 98). Animal studies have shown that restriction of dietary protein intake reduces hyperfiltration and intraglomerular pressure and retards the progression of several models of kidney disease, including diabetic glomerulopathy. A meta-analysis of several small studies in humans with diabetic nephropathy indicated that protein-restricted diets reduce proteinuria and retard the rate of fall of GFR modestly. The general consensus is to prescribe a protein intake of approximately the adult recommended dietary allowance of 0.8–1.0 g/kg/day in early stages of CKD and 0.8 g/kg/day (~10% of daily calories) in patients with overt nephropathy.

A low-protein diet must be high in carbohydrate and/or fat to maintain adequate caloric intake; however, the long-term effects of such a diet on atherosclerotic complications and glycemic control are unknown. Nutrition deficiency may occur in some individuals and may be associated with muscle weakness. Low-protein diets may be difficult for the patient to maintain, and a modest restriction in dietary protein combined with the other treatment measures may be more reasonable. Protein-restricted meal plans should be designed by a registered dietitian familiar with all components of the dietary management of diabetes and chronic kidney disease.

DIALYSIS AND KIDNEY TRANSPLANTATION

Once kidney disease progresses to stage 5 (kidney failure), prolonging life requires dialysis or a functioning kidney transplant. The latter provides the uremic patient with diabetes a greater survival with greater rehabilitation than does either continuous ambulatory peritoneal dialysis (CAPD) or maintenance hemodialysis. Therapy should be individualized to the patient's specific medical and family circumstances. The pros and cons of these procedures should be discussed with patients and their families well in advance of kidney failure. The prospect of needing such measures should never be a surprise. The ultimate choice among alternatives requires input from the patient, the patient's family, a nephrologist, and the primary care physician. In patients with diabetes, the absolute indications for dialysis or transplantation occur earlier than with other causes of kidney failure, i.e., at serum creatinine >6 mg/dL or creatinine clearance ≤20 ml/min, as well as urgent uremic symptoms, e.g., seizures, uremic pericarditis, unresponsive hypertension, and muscle deterioration. More subjective criteria include worsening lethargy, nausea or vomiting, and progressive retinopathy and neuropathy. It is important not to delay the start of dialysis in patients with diabetes. No matter which renal replacement therapy has been elected, optimal rehabilitation in patients with kidney failure requires that effort be devoted to recognition and management of comorbid conditions.

Renal Dialysis

Of the various forms of renal dialysis, hemodialysis is the most frequently used in patients with diabetes, although peritoneal dialysis is also used with success. Some patients using peritoneal dialysis have insulin included with the dialysate. This procedure may help with the problematic blood glucose control that may occur due to high concentrations of dextrose in the dialysate; peritoneal insulin delivery is more physiologic than subcutaneous delivery. Peritoneal dialysis affords a motivated patient the greatest mobility. Treatment of anemia with erythropoietin or its analogs improves the general well-being both of patients on dialysis and of patients before the initiation of dialysis therapy. Dialysis may be associated with wide swings of glycemia, suggesting a role for increasing the number of glucose measurements in the peri-dialysis period or using CGM. In addition, A1C levels may significantly underestimate glycemia because of shortened red cell survival, use of erythropoetin, anemia, and uremia, while glycated albumin may be a more valid reflection of glucose control.

Kidney Transplantation

When the success rate of kidney transplantation in patients with diabetes approached the excellent success rate achieved in patients without diabetes, this procedure became the treatment of choice in patients with diabetic kidney failure. Living-donor kidneys (from first-degree relatives or, increasingly, from living unrelated donors) have higher organ survival than cadaveric kidneys, although the gap continues to narrow. The decision of whether to opt for a transplant is still not one to be taken lightly, and a patient must be well briefed on the chances of failure, the risks of immunosuppression, and the possibility that the new kidney will develop diabetic nephropathy in the future. This risk means that the patient should be committed to a program of intensive glycemic control posttransplantation. Serious consideration should be devoted to a combined kidney and pancreas transplant to control hyperglycemia in type 1 diabetes patients. Combined transplantation increases short-term morbidity, but properly selected patients may have better long-term rehabilitation.

CONCLUSION

Nephropathy is a major cause of morbidity and mortality in patients with type 1 diabetes of >15 years duration. Vigilant monitoring of evolving proteinuria and in particular its early detection with microalbuminuria testing, striving for excellent glycemic control as early as possible post diagnosis and within patient-acceptable goals, early institution of ACE inhibitor or ARB therapy, aggressive therapy of hypertension, and anticipating the need for dialysis or transplantation form the cornerstones of management. The primary care provider is pivotal in integrating available resources, including referral to a nephrologist. The options available in the event of kidney failure offer greater possibilities for salvaging quality of life and increasing longevity than were available in the past. When possible, renal transplantation is advised, as the treatment is more likely to enhance both quality and quantity of life.

BIBLIOGRAPHY

Ahn S-R, Susztak K: Getting a notch closer to understanding diabetic kidney disease. *Diabetes* 59:1865, 2010

American Diabetes Association: Diabetic nephropathy (Position Statement). *Diabetes Care* 27 (Suppl. 1):S79–S83, 2004

American Diabetes Association: Hypertension management in adults with diabetes (Position Statement). *Diabetes Care* 27 (Suppl. 1):S65–S67, 2004

Brenner BM, Cooper ME, de Zeeuw D, Keane WF, Mitch WE, Parving H-H, Remuzzi G, Snapinn SM, Zhang Z, Shahinfar S, for the RENAAL Study Investigators: Effects of losartan on renal and cardiovascular outcomes in patients with type 2 diabetes and nephropathy. *N Engl J Med* 345:861–869, 2001

Burnier M, Zanchi A: Blockade of the renin-angiotensin system: a key therapeutic strategy to reduce renal and cardiovascular events in patients with diabetes. *J Hypertens* 24:11–25, 2006

DCCT Research Group: The effect of intensive treatment of diabetes on the development and progression of long-term complications in insulin-dependent diabetes mellitus. *N Engl J Med* 329:977–986, 1993

DCCT Research Group: Retinopathy and nephropathy in patients with type 1 diabetes four years after a trial of intensive therapy. *N Engl J Med* 342:381–389, 2000

DCCT/EDIC Research Group: Intensive diabetes therapy and glomerular filtration rate in type 1 diabetes. *N Engl J Med* 365:2366–2376, 2011

Diabetes Control and Complications Trial/Epidemiology of Diabetes Interventions and Complications Research Group: The modern-day clinical course of type 1 diabetes mellitus after 30 years' duration: the diabetes control and complications trial/epidemiology of diabetes interventions and complications and Pittsburgh epidemiology of diabetes complications experience (1983-2005). *Arch Intern Med* 169:1307-1316, 2009

Gross JL, de Azevedo MJ, Silveiro SP, Canani LH, Caramori ML, Zelmanovitz T: Diabetic nephropathy: diagnosis, prevention, and treatment. *Diabetes Care* 28:164–176, 2005

La Rocca E, Fiorina P, di Carlo V, Astorri E, Rossetti C, Lucignani G, Fazio F, Giudici D, Cristallo M, Bianchi G, Pozza G, Secchi A: Cardiovascular outcomes after kidney-pancreas and kidney-alone transplantation. *Kidney Int* 60:1964–1971, 2001

Lewis JL, Hunsicker LG, Bain RP: The effect of angiotensin-converting enzyme inhibition on diabetic nephropathy. *N Engl J Med* 329:1456–1462, 1993

Microalbuminuria Captopril Study Group: Captopril reduces the risk of nephropathy in IDDM patients with microalbuminuria. *Diabetologia* 39:587–593, 1996

Molitch ME, Steffes M, Sun W, Rutledge B, Cleary P, de Boer IH, Zinman B, Lachin J, the EDIC Study Group: Development and progression of renal insufficiency with and without albuminuria in adults with type 1 diabetes and the Diabetes and Control and Complications Trial and the Epidemiology of Diabetes Interventions and Complications Study. *Diabetes Care* 33:1536–1543, 2010

Peacock TP, Shihabi ZK, Bleyer AJ, Dolbare EL, Byers JR, Knovich MA, Calles-Escandon J, Russell GB, Freedman BI: Comparison of glycated albumin and hemoglobin A_{1c} levels in diabetic subjects on hemodialysis. *Kidney Int* 73:1062–1068, 2008

Pedrini MT, Levey AS, Lau J, Chalmers TC, Wang PH: The effect of dietary protein restriction on the progression of diabetic and nondiabetic renal diseases: a meta-analysis. *Ann Intern Med* 124:627–632, 1996

Remuzzi G, Ruggenenti P, Perico N: Chronic renal diseases: renoprotective benefits of renin-angiotensin system inhibition. *Ann Intern Med* 136:604–615, 2002

NEUROPATHY

Neuropathy is one of the most common and troubling chronic complications of diabetes, potentially affecting virtually all regions of the body and producing significant impairments, alone or in concert with other conditions. Most notably, neuropathic loss of sensation in the foot regularly conspires with infection and/or vascular insufficiency (more common in people with diabetes) to make diabetes the most common cause of nontraumatic lower-limb amputations in the US. The frequency of diabetic neuropathy parallels duration and severity of hyperglycemia in both type 1 and type 2 diabetes. In patients with type 1 diabetes, it rarely occurs within the first 5 years after diagnosis. The prevalence of neuropathy in the DCCT cohort showed an increase from 9% to 25% from baseline to 13–14 years post-DCCT closeout in the intensive arm and from 17% to 35% in the former conventional group, and the evidence of the durable effect of prior intensive treatment on neuropathy.

OVERVIEW OF NEUROPATHIES

Histological Findings and Pathophysiology

Histologically, there is loss of both large and small myelinated nerve fibers, accompanied by varying degrees of paranodal and segmental demyelination, connective tissue proliferation, and thickening and reduplication of capillary basement membranes with capillary closure. Pathways by which hyperglycemia (perhaps aided by other metabolic derangements of diabetes) may cause such changes include overactivity of the polyol pathway, protein glycation, and altered intracellular oxidation-reduction potential.

Treatment of Neuropathies

There is no known direct treatment for established neuropathy, and the most effective strategies are preventive. The DCCT demonstrated that intensive glycemic control reduced by 60% the development and progression of early neuropathy. Aldose reductase inhibitors block the rate-limiting enzyme in the polyol pathway, which is activated in hyperglycemic states, and have appeared promising in animal studies but as yet disappointing in human clinical trials. Clinical trials with protein kinase C inhibitor are ongoing. Treatment strategies for established neuropathies are directed at the symptoms and dysfunction that result.

Clinical Syndromes

Diabetic neuropathy is classified into a set of discrete clinical syndromes, each with a characteristic presentation and clinical course (Table 6.5). Because the syndromes overlap clinically and frequently occur simultaneously, rigid classification of individual cases is often difficult. Identical neurological syndromes occur in other diseases and other conditions, such as alcoholic neuropathy and inflammatory neuropathies. Diabetic neuropathy is a diagnosis of exclusion (Table 6.6).

Table 6.5 Syndromes of Diabetic Neuropathy

Diffuse neuropathies (common, insidious onset, usually progressive)	**Focal neuropathies** (sudden onset, usually improve over time)
■Distal symmetrical sensorimotor polyneuropathy ■Autonomic neuropathy	■Cranial neuropathy ■Radiculopathy ■Plexopathy ■Mononeuropathy/mononeuropathy multiplex ■Other mononeuropathies

DISTAL SYMMETRIC SENSORIMOTOR POLYNEUROPATHY

Distal symmetric polyneuropathy is the most common form of diabetic neuropathy. Sensory signs and symptoms generally predominate over motor involvement and vary depending on the classes of nerve fibers. Loss of large fibers produces diminished proprioception and light touch, resulting in ataxic gait, unsteadiness, and weakness of intrinsic muscles in the hands and feet. Involvement of small fibers causes diminished pain and temperature sensation, resulting in unrecognized trauma (especially to the feet), accidental burning of the hands, etc.

Typical neuropathic paresthesia (spontaneous uncomfortable sensations) or dysesthesia (contact paresthesia) may accompany both large- and small-fiber involvement. Sensory deficits first appear in the most distal portions of the extremities and spread proximally with disease progression in a "stocking-glove" distribution. In the most advanced cases, vertical bands of sensory deficit may develop on the chest or abdomen when the tips of the shorter truncal nerves become involved (Fig. 6.6).

Occasionally, patients complain of exquisite hypersensitivity to light touch, superficial burning or stabbing pain, or bone-deep aching or tearing pain, usually most troublesome at night. Sometimes, neuropathic pain may become the overriding and disabling feature, especially in small-fiber neuropathy. Both neuropathic pain and paresthesia are thought to reflect spontaneous depolarization of newly regenerating nerve fibers.

Patients should be screened annually for distal polyneuropathy using the following tests: pinprick sensation, vibration perception using a 1,280Hz tuning fork, 10-g monofilament pressure sensation at the distal plantar aspect of both great toes and metatarsal joints, and assessment of ankle reflexes. More than one abnormal finding has >87% sensitivity in detecting polyneuropathy. Loss of 10-g monofilament perception and reduced vibration perception predict foot ulcers.

Heat shock protein 27, shown to be associated with diabetic neuropathy, and other circulating markers, as well as dermal markers, such as skin intrinsic fluorescence, maybe used in the future to indicate the presence of diabetic neuropathy.

Asymptomatic Neuropathy

Many patients with distal symmetrical polyneuropathy remain free of troubling, subjective symptoms. In these cases, it may take careful questioning to

Table 6.6 Common Conditions Resembling Various Forms of Diabetic Neuropathy

Distal symmetrical neuropathy
- Inflammatory neuropathies (vasculitic, i.e., systemic lupus erythematosus, polyarteritis, and other connective tissue diseases; sarcoidosis; leprosy)
- Metabolic neuropathies (hypothyroidism, uremic; nutritional; acute intermittent porphyria)
- Toxic neuropathies (alcohol; drugs; heavy metals, e.g., lead, mercury, and arsenic; industrial hydrocarbons)
- Other neuropathies (paraneoplastic; dys-proteinemic, amyloid, hereditary)

Autonomic neuropathy
- Pure autonomic failure (idiopathic ortho-static hypotension, Bradbury-Eggleston syndrome)
- Autoimmune autonomic neuropathy

Cranial neuropathy
- Carotid aneurysm
- Intracranial mass
- Elevated intracranial pressure

Radiculopathy
- Spinal cord/root compression
- Transverse myelitis
- Coagulopathies
- Shingles

Plexopathy
- Mass lesions
- Coagulopathies
- Cauda equina lesions (femoral neuropathy)

Mononeuropathy/mononeuropathy multiplex
- Compression neuropathies
- Inflammatory (vasculitic) neuropathies
- Hypothyroidism, acromegaly

learn of a patient's subtle feelings of numbness or cold or "dead" feet. Diminished or absent deep-tendon reflexes, especially the Achilles tendon reflex, or loss of ability to sense a 10-gram monofilament, may be early indications of otherwise asymptomatic neuropathy. However, in the absence of pain or paresthesia, diabetic neuropathy may go unrecognized unless the physician routinely tests foot sensation during office visits.

LATE COMPLICATIONS OF POLYNEUROPATHY

Patients with chronic unrecognized neuropathy may present with late complications, e.g., foot ulceration, foreign objects embedded in the foot, unrecognized trauma to the extremities, or neuroarthropathy (Charcot foot). All of these conditions are avoidable with proper early diagnosis of neuropathy and institution of appropriate foot care.

Foot Ulcerations and Infections

Acute foot ulcerations and resulting infections can occur when an individual cannot feel the pain caused by poorly fitting shoes (a source of blisters or penetrating abrasions), a retained foreign body, or accidental trauma (often unintentionally self-inflicted during nail trimming) because of neuropathy. Plantar ulcers, which form at the calloused sites of maximal walking pressure, can result from a combination of motor, sensory, and proprioceptive deficits.

Patients with longstanding diabetes and neuropathy are also predisposed to vascular ulcers due to macrovascular and microvascular insufficiency and ischemic gangrene.

In a typical sequence of events, imbalance of extensor and flexor muscles in the feet, resulting from impaired proprioception and atrophy of intrinsic extensor muscles, leads to tendon shortening and chronic toe flexion (claw toe or hammer-toe deformity). This, in turn, shifts weight bearing from the padded ball of the foot to the unprotected metatarsal heads. With pain insensitivity, trauma to the overlying skin goes undetected, producing thick calluses that further concentrate weight bearing over the bony prominences. Splitting and fissuring of the thick callus or underlying pressure necrosis initiates ulcer formation, further aggravated by infection and vascular insufficiency.

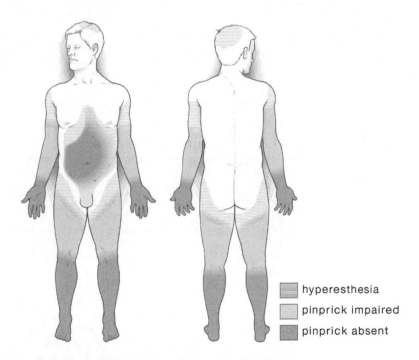

hyperesthesia

pinprick impaired

pinprick absent

Figure 6.6 Distribution of sensory loss in patient with severe chronic diabetic sensory polyneuropathy. Loss is maximal distally in limbs but also affects anterior trunk and vertex of head.

Neuroarthropathy

Neuropathy impairs normal protective proprioceptive and nociceptive functions, which normally lead patients to recognize injury and protect the foot. Neuroarthropathy, or Charcot foot, refers to the joint erosions, unrecognized fractures, demineralization, and devitalization of bones in the foot resulting from unawareness of the minor injuries that occur during routine daily weight-bearing activities. The foot may be swollen and red but it is not painful. The problem may be misdiagnosed as cellulitis despite a normal leukocyte count and differential and the absence of fever. The patient may report relatively painless trauma, and initial radiographic examination may be unrevealing, whereas follow-up X rays several days or weeks later may reveal clear traumatic changes. In more advanced cases, devitalization of bone may mimic osteomyelitis, and in the most advanced stages, the foot may look like a "bag of bones."

MANAGEMENT OF DISTAL SYMMETRIC POLYNEUROPATHY AND COMPLICATIONS

Treatment for diabetic distal symmetric polyneuropathy is symptomatic, palliative, and supportive, with primary emphasis on preventing the neuropathy and vasculopathy by near-normalization of glucose and lipids and smoking cessation. In most cases, the primary neuropathic symptoms consist of mild intermittent pain or paresthesia. Even severely painful symptoms generally remit spontaneously within a few months in most but not all patients.

Management of Pain

Persistent and severely painful neuropathy has been treated with various drugs, including standard analgesics and drugs normally used to treat pain in other conditions. Narcotics should generally be avoided. The tricyclic drugs are the first-line drugs for the relief of painful neuropathic symptoms. Their efficacy, which has been proven in controlled trials, is related to plasma drug levels, and the onset of symptomatic relief is faster than their antidepressive effects. Numerous other antidepressants have been reported to be useful in the relief of painful or paresthetic neuropathic symptoms. The antidepressant duloxetine, a serotonin and norepinephrine uptake inhibitor, is the only drug in this class to have an FDA indication for treatment of painful diabetic neuropathy. It is a viable option for patients with anxiety and depression, fibromyalgia, and other chronic pain, but it is not recommended for patients with existing renal disease or hepatic impairment. A number of anticonvulsants have been used to treat painful neuropathy, but pregabalin has undergone the most rigorous testing and is the only anticonvulsant with an FDA indication for neuropathic pain. Topical capsaicin applied frequently to the hypersensitive areas may be useful in some cases, especially those with more localized pain. Transcutaneous electrical nerve stimulation has also been used for refractory painful neuropathy.

Because early diagnosis of asymptomatic neuropathy is essential for preventing the late complications, every routine physician visit should include a thorough examination of the feet if the patient has preexisting risk factors or any foot symptoms. A list of neurologic and related symptoms to watch for is given in Table 6.7. In the absence of risk factors or symptoms, neuropathy screening is part of the annual comprehensive foot examination recommended for all patients with diabetes.

Callus Formation and Plantar Ulcers

Callus formation over weight-bearing areas indicates the need to consult an orthopedist and/or podiatrist for prescription of corrective footwear to redistribute weight bearing. Plantar ulcers should be managed by eliminating weight bearing either by special walking casts or by bed rest. Local debridement and application of growth factors may speed healing. Refractory and/or recurrent ulcers may be managed by surgical removal of the involved metatarsal. If there is evidence of impaired macrovascular circulation, vascular studies should be obtained and revascularization attempted when indicated. Neuroarthropathy is managed by reduced ambulation and weight bearing, as well as cushioned footwear.

Treatment of Infection

Infection must be treated aggressively with appropriate consultation from infectious disease specialists. Antibiotics effective against aerobic and anaerobic organisms should be included in the treatment regimen. Deep-wound cultures are necessary to direct antibiotic therapy properly. Vascular bypass surgery or percutaneous angioplasty should be considered if arterial insufficiency is a major contributing factor. Localized osteomyelitis may require a limited amputation.

AUTONOMIC NEUROPATHY

Neuropathy can affect virtually any autonomic function in patients with diabetes. Although autonomic neuropathy produces diffuse subclinical dysfunction, autonomic symptoms are usually confined to one or two organ systems, producing the discrete autonomic syndromes listed in Table 6.8.

Cardiovascular Autonomic Neuropathy

The earliest clinical signs of cardiovascular autonomic neuropathy are absence of the normal sleep bradycardia and diminished variation of the pulse rate with inspiration-expiration or Valsalva (reduced sinus tachycardia), both due to early vagal involvement.

Later, sympathetic denervation interferes with normal cardiovascular reflexes thereby diminishing exercise tolerance, possibly hypersensitizing the heart to circulating catecholamines, tachyarrhythmias, and sudden death. It also predisposes to painless myocardial infarction.

Orthostatic hypotension. Orthostatic hypotension is managed by correcting hypovolemia with fluid replacement and improved diabetes control, elastic stockings, increased salt intake, mineralocorticoids, or vasoconstrictors. Midodrine, a specific α_1-agonist, has been shown to produce arteriolar constriction and decrease in venous pooling via a constriction of venous capacitance vessels. It may

Table 6.7 Warning Symptoms and Signs of Diabetic Foot Problems

Symptoms

Vascular	Cold feet
	Intermittent claudication involving calf or foot
	Pain at rest, especially nocturnal, relieved by dependency
Neurologic	Sensory: burning, tingling, or crawling sensations; pain and hypersensitivity; complaints of cold or "dead" feet
	Motor weakness (drop foot)
	Autonomic: diminished sweating
Musculoskeletal	Gradual change in foot shape
	Sudden painless change in foot shape, with swelling, without history of trauma
Dermatologic	Exquisitely painful or painless wounds
	Slow-healing or nonhealing wounds, necrosis
	Skin color changes (cyanosis, redness)
	Chronic scaling, cracking, itching, or dry feet
	Recurrent infections (e.g., paronychia, athlete's foot)

Signs

Absent pedal, popliteal, or femoral pulses

Femoral bruits

Dependent rubor, plantar pallor on elevation

Prolonged capillary filling time (>3–4 s)

Decreased skin temperature

Sensory: deficits (vibratory and proprioperceptive, then pain and temperature perception), hyperesthesia

Motor: diminished to absent deep-tendon reflexes (Achilles then patellar), weakness

Autonomic: diminished to absent sweating

Cavus feet with claw toes

Drop foot

"Rockerbottom" foot (Charcot foot)

Neuropathic arthropathy

Skin
- Abnormal dryness
- Chronic Tinea infections
- Keratic lesions with or without hemorrhage (plantar or digital)
- Trophic ulcer

Hair
- Diminished to absent

Nails
- Trophic changes
- Onychomycosis
- Subungual ulceration or abscess
- Ingrown nails with paronychia

From Scardina RJ: Diabetic foot problems: assessment and prevention. *Clinical Diabetes* 1:1–7, 1983.

Table 6.8 Syndromes of Autonomic Neuropathy

Cardiovascular Autonomic Neuropathy
- Resting sinus tachycardia without sinus arrhythmia (fixed heart rate)
- Exercise intolerance
- Painless myocardial infarction
- Orthostatic hypotension
- Sudden death

Gastrointestinal Autonomic Neuropathy
- Esophageal dysfunction
- Autonomic gastropathy and delayed gastric emptying (gastroparesis)
- Diabetic diarrhea
- Constipation
- Fecal incontinence
- Gallbladder atony

Genitourinary Autonomic Neuropathy
- Erectile dysfunction
- Retrograde ejaculation with infertility
- Bladder dysfunction

Hypoglycemia Unawareness

Sudomotor Neuropathy
- Distal hyperhidrosis or anhidrosis
- Facial sweating
- Heat intolerance
- "Gustatory" sweating

exacerbate supine hypertension, which often coexists with orthostatic hypotension in patients with diabetes.

Gastrointestinal (GI) Autonomic Neuropathy

Nonspecific GI symptoms in patients with diabetes often reflect diffuse but subtle GI autonomic dysfunction. Esophageal dysmotility can cause dysphagia, retrosternal discomfort, and heartburn. Delayed gastric emptying (gastroparesis) causes anorexia, nausea, vomiting, early satiety, and postprandial bloating and fullness. Delayed nutrient absorption can greatly complicate glycemic control, producing otherwise unexplained swings between severe hyperglycemia and hypoglycemia. Diagnosis of upper GI symptoms may be facilitated by liquid and solid-phase radionuclide gastric-emptying studies, although results do not correlate well with symptomatology nor with response to therapy. Management of esophageal dysmotility and delayed gastric emptying includes normalization of glucose, since hyperglycemia itself acutely decreases gastric emptying, and frequent small and/or primarily liquid feedings. High-fiber diets should be avoided, because they delay gastric emptying and may result in bezoar formation. The dopamine antagonist, metoclopramide or domperidone, may be helpful, but can cause acute or chronic dyskinesia. Liquid erythromycin also sometimes improves symptoms. For patients suffering from constipation and lower GI motor issues, polyethylene glycol 3350 may be helpful. Newer therapeutic strategies for gastroparesis include drugs that target the underlying defects, prokinetic agents such as 5-hydroxytryptamine agonists that do not appear to have cardiac or vascular effects and ghrelin agonists. Refractory cases may need gastric pacing or a feeding jejunostomy tube.

Diabetic diarrhea is classically painless, nocturnal, associated with fecal incontinence, and alternates with periods of constipation. Diagnostic studies of lower GI problems are necessary to define the multiple contributing factors that stem from widespread intestinal autonomic dysfunction to determine appropriate treatment. A therapeutic trial of broad-spectrum antibiotics may also be helpful, whereas evidence of bile salt malabsorption would argue in favor of bile salt–sequestering agents, both of which are effective in properly selected patients. Hypermotility is managed with diphenoxylate hydrochloride.

Fecal incontinence, which is also usually nocturnal, reflects impaired sensation of rectal distention, and in one small series of patients, it was effectively managed with biofeedback techniques. Clonidine may also be useful.

Sexual Dysfunction

Erectile dysfunction. Erectile dysfunction in men with diabetes is usually neuropathic. In 2003, an ancillary study to the DCCT/EDIC was conducted to assess erectile dysfunction in 571 men in both the primary and secondary cohorts. The prevalence of reported erectile dysfunction was 23%; it was significantly lower in the intensive compared to the conventional treatment groups in the secondary cohort (12.8% vs 30.8%) but not in the primary cohort (17.0% vs 20.3%). The risk of erectile dysfunction in the primary and secondary cohorts was directly associated with mean A1C during both the DCCT and EDIC trials combined; age, peripheral neuropathy and lower urinary tract symptoms were additional risk factors for erectile dysfunction. In addition to neuropathy, erectile dysfunction can be psychogenic, endocrine, vascular, drug, or stress related. A normal erection on awakening or impotence only with a certain partner suggests a psychogenic cause. A band-type turgidity gauge or nocturnal penile tumescence monitoring at a sleep research facility can help clarify ambiguous situations.

Sex steroid imbalances, hypogonadotrophism, and hyperprolactinemia should be excluded by appropriate endocrine studies. Proximal vascular insufficiency is usually evident on examination of the femoral pulses, although localized obstruction of the penile artery has been reported and can be excluded only by measurement of the brachial-penile blood pressure ratio with Doppler-flow studies. Proximal or localized vascular obstruction has been managed surgically, but the success rate is low.

Drugs known to produce erectile dysfunction include various antihypertensives, anticholinergics, antipsychotics, antidepressants, narcotics, barbiturates, alcohol, and amphetamines. Drug-induced impotence is managed by altering the treatment regimen when possible. Neuropathic impotence is generally but not always accompanied by other manifestations of diabetic neuropathy.

The main therapy for erectile dysfunction of neuropathic etiology is drugs that increase nitric oxide (sildenafil, vardenafil, tadalfil), oral inhibitors of the phosphodiesterase type 5 enzyme, the predominant isoenzyme in human corpus cavernosum. The intracorporeal injection of vasoactive substances such as papaverine and prostaglandins are also effective in treating nonvascular erectile dysfunction. Patients who do not respond to pharmacologic therapy may opt for implantation of a penile prosthesis.

Retrograde ejaculation. Retrograde ejaculation, which may or may not occur in conjunction with erectile dysfunction, reflects loss of the coordinated closure of the internal and relaxation of the external vesicle sphincter during ejaculation. Presentation is usually infertility, and diagnosis is confirmed by documenting ejaculate azoospermia and the presence of motile sperm in postcoital urine. Such sperm have been successfully used for artificial insemination.

Other Autonomic Syndromes

Diabetic cystopathy. Cystopathy initially diminishes sensation of bladder fullness, reducing urinary frequency. Later, efferent involvement produces incomplete urination, poor stream, dribbling, and overflow incontinence. Patients with cystopathy are predisposed to urinary tract infections.

Conservative management involves scheduled voluntary urination with or without Credé's maneuver. Cholinergic-stimulating drugs, sphincter relaxants, periodic catheterization, and bladder-neck resection of the internal sphincter may be used in more advanced cases.

Hypoglycemia unawareness. Hypoglycemia unawareness may be related to autonomic neuropathy, which can blunt the usual adrenergic response to hypoglycemia. The condition predisposes to future episodes, and conversely is worsened by antecedent episodes of severe hypoglycemia. Hypoglycemia awareness has been shown to be improved by strict avoidance of hypoglycemia. Some relaxation of glycemic targets is indicated for patients who have one or more episodes of severe hypoglycemia or who have hypoglycemia unawareness. Insulin pump therapy and use of CGM, as well as the use of the low glucose suspend feature, minimizes or prevents recurrent spells of severe hypoglycemia.

Autonomic sudomotor dysfunction. Autonomic sudomotor dysfunction produces both asymptomatic anhydrosis of the extremities and central hyperhidrosis; the latter may be triggered by eating (gustatory sweating). Sudomotor dysfunction diminishes thermoregulatory reserve and predisposes to heat stroke and hyperthermia. Management includes avoidance of heat stress. Topical glycopyrrolate, an antimuscarinic compound, results in a marked reduction in sweating while eating a meal.

FOCAL NEUROPATHIES

Neural deficits corresponding to the distribution of single or multiple peripheral nerves (mononeuropathy and mononeuropathy multiplex), cranial nerves, areas of the brachial or lumbosacral plexuses (plexopathy), or the nerve roots (radiculopathy) are of sudden onset and generally but not always self-limiting in patients with diabetes.

The third cranial nerve may be affected, presenting with unilateral pain, diplopia, and ptosis but with pupillary sparing. Differential diagnosis includes an aneurysm of the internal carotid artery and myasthenia gravis. Spontaneous remission usually occurs within a few months.

Radiculopathy presents as band-like thoracic or abdominal pain, often misdiagnosed as an acute intrathoracic or intra-abdominal emergency.

Femoral neuropathy in patients with diabetes often involves motor and sensory deficits at the level of the sacral plexus as well as the femoral nerve, with the relative excess of motor versus sensory involvement differentiating diabetic femoral neuropathy from that seen in other conditions. When bilateral, this is sometimes termed amyotrophy. Management of focal neuropathies includes exclusion of other causes, e.g., nerve entrapment or compression and symptomatic palliation pending spontaneous resolution, which occurs generally but not always over periods of months to years.

CONCLUSION

Diabetic neuropathy is an extremely common complication of diabetes that becomes more prevalent with increasing duration and severity of hyperglycemia. Manifestations include diffuse and focal painful and painless neurological deficits in the peripheral nervous system and widespread autonomic dysfunction. Prompt and proper diagnosis is essential to effective management and avoidance of serious secondary musculoskeletal and visceral complications.

BIBLIOGRAPHY

Albers AW, Herman WH, Pop-Busui R, Feldman EL, Martin CL, Cleary PA, Waberski BH, Lachin JM, for the DCCT/EDIC Research Group: Effect of prior intensive insulin treatment during the Diabetes Control and Complications Trial on peripheral neuropathy in type 1 diabetes during the Epidemiology of Diabetes Interventions and Complications Study. *Diabetes Care* 33:1090–1096, 2010

American Diabetes Association: Preventive foot care in people with diabetes (Position Statement). *Diabetes Care* 27 (Suppl. 1):S63–S64, 2004

Camilleri M, Bharucha AE, Farrigia G: Epidemiology, mechanisms and management of diabetic gastroparesis. *Clin Gastroenterol Hepatol* 9:5–12, 2011.

Conway BN, Aroda VR, Maynard JD, Matter N, Fernandez S, Ratner RE, Orchard TJ: Skin intrinsic fluorescence correlates with autonomic and distal symmetrical polyneuropathy in individuals with type 1 diabetes. *Diabetes Care* 34:1000–1005, 2011

DCCT Research Group: The effect of intensive treatment of diabetes on the development and progression of long-term complications in insulin-dependent diabetes mellitus. *N Engl J Med* 329:977–986, 1993

Gries FA, Cameron NE, Low PA, Ziegler D (Eds): *Textbook of Diabetic Neuropathy*. New York, Thieme, 2003

Gruden G, Bruno G, Chaturvedi N, Burt D, Schalkwijk C, Pinach S, Stehouwer CD, Witte DR, Fuller JH, Perin PC, the EURODIAB Prospective Complications Study Group: Serum heat shock protein 27 and diabetes complications in the EURODIAB prospective complications study: a novel circulating marker for diabetic neuropathy. *Diabetes* 57:1966–1970, 2008

Maser RE, Mitchell BD, Vinik AI, Freeman R: The association between cardio-vascular autonomic neuropathy and mortality in individuals with diabetes: a meta-analysis. *Diabetes Care* 26:1895–1901, 2003

Ormseth MJ, Scholz BA, Boomershine CS: duloxetine in the management of diabetic peripheral neuropathic pain. *Patient Prefer Adherence* 5:343–356, 2011

Shaw JE, Abbott CA, Tindle K, Hollis S, Boulton AJ: A randomized controlled trial of topical glycopyrrolate, the first specific treatment for diabetic gusta-tory sweating. *Diabetologia* 40:299–301, 1997

Simmons Z, Feldman EL: Update on diabetic neuropathy. *Curr Opin Neurol* 15:595–603, 2002

Vinik AI, Maser RE, Mitchell BD, Freeman R: Diabetic autonomic neuropathy. *Diabetes Care* 26:1553–1579, 2003

Wessells H, Penson DF, Cleary P, Rutledge BN, Lachin JM, McVary KT, Schade DS, Sarma AV, and the DCCT/EDIC Research Groups: Effect of intensive glycemic therapy on erectile function in men with type 1 diabetes. *J Urology* 185:1828–1834, 2011

MACROVASCULAR DISEASE

Coronary heart disease, peripheral arterial disease, and cerebrovascular disease all occur more commonly, at an earlier age, with a more diffuse distribution and with greater severity and mortality in people with diabetes compared to patients without diabetes. Diabetes itself has been elevated in status from a risk factor for cardiovascular disease, to a coronary heart disease (CHD) risk equivalent in the National Cholesterol Education Panel Adult Treatment Program III (NCEP ATP III) guidelines. These guidelines focus on the necessity of aggressive preventive strategies for all patients with diabetes.

The ATP III and other recommendations are based on evidence from populations with type 2 diabetes. The American Diabetes Association recommends applying the same preventive and treatment strategies to patients with type 1 diabetes, who have high lifetime cardiovascular risk. The American Heart Association considers children and adolescents with type 1 diabetes to be in the highest cardiovascular disease (CVD) risk group. Although the prevalence of hypercholesterolemia is the same in patients with and without type 1 diabetes, the high absolute risk of heart disease in patients with type 1 diabetes creates an opportunity of substantial benefit to prevent events when lipid treatment guidelines are followed. Other risk factors, including hypertension, which is more prevalent in people with type 1 diabetes than in the general population, as well as cigarette smoking, which is as common among people with diabetes as in the general population, must also receive attention.

PREVALENCE AND RISK FACTORS

Although cardiovascular deaths are less common in patients with type 1 diabetes than in generally older patients with type 2 diabetes, mortality rates among individuals with type 1 diabetes are excessive. Patients with type 1 diabetes have at least a 10-fold increase in mortality compared to individuals of the same age without diabetes. Overall, CVD accounts for ~25% of the deaths among patients with the onset of diabetes before age 20 years. Premature CHD and stroke cause 27% and 6%, respectively, of the deaths among patients with diabetes age <45 years. Many of these deaths occur in patients with diabetic nephropathy, and a large percentage of them result from the unfavorable and avoidable interactions of diabetes, hypertension, and cigarette smoking.

Diabetes is an independent risk factor for CVD, increasing risk two- to three-fold in men and even more in women. Women with diabetes are at equivalent CHD risk to men with diabetes. They lose the normally assumed "protection" of the female gender, and their cardiovascular disease rates parallel those of men with diabetes, even before menopause. In general, A1C and mean glucose levels are associated with CVD risk factors; it is controversial as to the strength of the relationship of CVD risk factors and postprandial glycemia and glucose variability.

The prevalence of lipid abnormalities varies significantly, depending on the characteristics of the study population such as age, gender, type of diabetes, severity of obesity, glycemic control, nondiabetes drugs, and thyroid and renal status. In patients with type 1 diabetes and good glycemic control, lipid levels are no different from an age- and sex-matched control population. In fact, with excellent glycemic control, the lipid profile may show lower total cholesterol and higher HDL cholesterol levels than in control subjects. Levels of cholesterol, ratios of total cholesterol to HDL cholesterol, and triglyceride levels are generally higher in patients with type 1 diabetes during periods of poor glycemic control and then become powerful risk factors for cardiovascular disease. Diabetic ketoacidosis may be associated with a profound temporary hypertriglyceridemia. Although improved glycemic control corrects elevated triglyceride levels and may help to raise HDL cholesterol slightly, a lower A1C will usually not improve LDL cholesterol levels. Separate treatment for LDL cholesterol will be required.

Even minimal microalbuminuria becomes a potent risk factor for CHD and stroke events. When proteinuria reaches the level of early diabetic nephropathy (300–1,000 mg/24 h), the lipid levels may begin to reveal a more atherogenic pattern: decreased HDL cholesterol, increased triglyceride levels, and a shift toward larger numbers of smaller, more dense LDL particles without necessarily raising LDL cholesterol levels. The most extreme example is with the nephrotic syndrome. Even when the lipid levels are acceptable by standard lipid profile measures, glycation of lipoproteins and other lipoprotein compositional abnormalities, including oxidation of the LDL particles induced by diabetes and/or hyperglycemia, may make those lipid levels more atherogenic. The precise role of advanced lipid testing for patients with diabetes remains under investigation. It may be rational to test patients who had reached NCEP ATP III goals but were still believed to be at increased risk or those who had failed to respond clinically to treatment based on standard lipid testing.

Hypertension and cigarette smoking are major cardiovascular risk factors. In health surveys of people age 20–44 years, 29% of those with diabetes (compared with only 8% of those without diabetes) report having hypertension. Hypertension is especially seen in men, those with microangiopathy, those with overweight/obesity, those who are older, and those with longer diabetes duration. Hypertension also increases in prevalence with the degree of renal impairment. Fortunately, the percentage of smokers is decreasing, but young patients with diabetes should always be reminded not to begin this habit and reminded of effects of tobacco on the many complications of diabetes.

In the DCCT, subjects with intensively treated type 1 diabetes and lower A1C levels had trends toward lower levels of LDL cholesterol and fewer myocardial infarctions and peripheral vascular events. Long-term follow-up of the intensively treated group revealed a significant reduction in CVD events and mortality in this group. Thirty-year data from the DCCT/EDIC and the Pittsburgh Epidemiology of Diabetes Complications Experience (EDC) studies encompassing the years 1983–2005 showed the differential risk by conventional and intensive treatment groups for the DCCT/EDIC compared to the EDC cohort. After 30 years of diabetes, the cumulative incidences of cardiovascular disease were 14% in the DCCT conventional treatment group, 14% in the EDC cohort, and 9% in the DCCT intensive therapy group.

ASSESSMENT AND TREATMENT

Because of the high prevalence of cardiovascular risk factors in patients with diabetes and the effect of hyperglycemia to magnify the impact of these risk factors, physicians should consider all patients with type 1 diabetes to be at risk for developing macrovascular disease. They should systematically assess patients for risk factors for CVD (those mentioned above plus a family history of CVD), question them about symptoms of CVD, and be alert for signs of atherosclerosis. Lifestyle and pharmacologic treatments for modifying specific risk factors should be started. All patients with type 1 diabetes need to understand the critical importance of following a healthy lifestyle from childhood onward.

Although assessment of CVD can be done with non-invasive tests, for example with CT angiography, and novel blood markers, such as inflammatory cytokines, it has not been determined how these tests add to risk stratification.

Dyslipidemia

Dyslipidemia in a patient with diabetes may result from poor metabolic control; use of certain drugs, including high-dose β-blockers (other than carvedilol), high-dose diuretics, systemic corticosteroids or other immunosuppressants, protease inhibitor antiviral agents, androgens, progestins (other than micronized progesterone or despironone), or estrogens; obesity; associated conditions such as hypothyroidism, the frequency of which is increased in type 1 diabetes; or inherited dyslipidemia. Each cause must be considered in assessing patients with diabetes and abnormal blood lipid levels.

The American Diabetes Association recommends that adult patients with diabetes undergo at least annual testing of the lipoprotein profile. In adults with low-risk lipid values (LDL <100 mg/dL, HDL >50 mg/dL, triglycerides <150 mg/dL), repeat lipid assessments may be done every 2 years. In children >2 years of age, lipid assessment should be done after the diagnosis of diabetes once glucose control has been established. If values are of low risk and there is no family history of dyslipidemia, assessments should be repeated every 5 year until age 21, then every 2 years. If abnormalities are identified, more frequent testing is warranted. The SEARCH study has shown that the mean LDL-C is 100 mg/dL, HDL-C 55 mg/dL, and triglycerides 64 mg/dL, and 18% of youth with type 1 diabetes have high triglycerides, 10% have low HDL-C, and 21% have the metabolic syndrome. Children with a family history of dyslipidemia should be assessed annually.

If dyslipidemia is present, the patient should be assessed for factors that aggravate dyslipidemia. Insulin treatment should be intensified in poorly controlled patients, but retesting will be necessary to be sure that additional therapy will be provided if abnormalities persist. Any drugs that might exacerbate hyperlipidemia should be discontinued or reduced where possible. The patient should be evaluated for renal disease and alcohol abuse. Genetic hyperlipidemia, separate from the diabetes, is often the cause of moderate to marked hypercholesterolemia, and the treatment should be based on the etiology of the disorder and not limited to intensified insulin therapy.

The physician should be cognizant of American Diabetes Association guidelines regarding dyslipidemia. Optimal LDL cholesterol levels for adults with diabetes are <100 mg/dL (<2.6 mmol/L), acceptable HDL cholesterol levels are >40 mg/dL (>1.0 mmol/L) for men and >50 mg/dL (>1.3 mmol/L) for women, and desirable triglyceride levels are <150 mg/dL (<1.7 mmol/L). Patients with diabetes with non-optimal values should institute medical nutrition therapy (MNT) and exercise. Regarding pharmacological therapy, it is suggested that subjects with type 1 diabetes with clinical CVD or an LDL cholesterol level >100 mg/dL (>2.6 mmol/L) after lifestyle interventions, be treated. In addition, statin therapy is recommended in patients with diabetes who are over age 40 and have other CVD risk factors, even if LDL-cholesterol levels are below 100 mg/dL.

Statin therapy is the initial treatment of choice for most patients requiring statin therapy, because of the robust evidence for their benefits in terms of CVD events and mortality. Based on results of the Heart Protection Study and other trials, current recommendations also include statin therapy for most diabetic patients over the age of 40 years, regardless of baseline LDL level. For children with type 1 diabetes, both the American Diabetes Association and American Heart Association recommend lifestyle modification for children with LDL cholesterol >100 mg/dL. For children over the age of 10, statin therapy should be considered for those with LDL-cholesterol over 160 mg/dL on lifestyle therapy, or over 130 mg/dL in the presence of other CVD risk factors such as family history of premature CVD.

Hypertension

Blood pressure should be measured in all patients with type 1 diabetes, including children and adolescents, at each physical examination, or at least every 6 months. If hypertension develops, treatment should be initiated to reduce the risk of macrovascular and microvascular disease. To the extent possible, blood pressure should be maintained at levels <130/80 mmHg in adults or below the 90th percentile for age- and sex-adjusted norms. Patients with systolic blood pressure 130–139 mmHg and diastolic blood pressure 80–89 mmHg receive maximal lifestyle intervention first for 3 months before considering pharmacotherapy. When prescribing pharmacologic therapy, the clinician should consider the adverse effects of various antihypertensive drugs on hyperglycemia and hypoglycemia, electrolyte balance, renal function, lipid metabolism, CVD status, and neuropathic symptoms including orthostatic hypotension and impotence (Table 6.9). Overall, first-line therapy should include an ACE inhibitor or an ARB, with the addition of a second agent if blood pressure targets are not reached. Kidney function and potassium should be monitored if blockers of the renin-angiotensin system are used. Studies have shown that renal protection ensues even if creatinine levels rise on a drug in this class. Ultimately, lowering of blood pressure may require multiple agents including ACE inhibitors, ARBs, β-blockers, diuretics, and calcium-channel blockers.

Cigarette Smoking

Each patient's smoking history should also be determined. Nonsmokers, particularly children and adolescents, should be encouraged not to begin, and smokers should be strongly urged to stop. The physician's advice not to smoke has an impact and represents time well spent. Advice should be reinforced with educational materials, medications, and referral to a smoking-cessation program.

Table 6.9 Potential Interactions of Antihypertensive Medications in Type 1 Diabetes

Medication	Impact on Glycemia	Advantages	Disadvantages
Diuretics	None (unlike type 2 diabetes, where hypo-kalemia reduces β-cell function)		
Calcium-channel blockers	None		Edema, increased GI symptoms in patients with neuropathy
β-Blockers	Decreased hypoglycemic awareness		
ACE inhibitors	None	Proven to reduce risk of nephropathy	
ARBs	None	ARBs, like ACE inhibitors, can slow the progression of nephropathy	
α-Blockers	None		Increased risk of orthostasis in patients with neuropathy

Advantages and disadvantages are meant to be specific to type 1 diabetes and not to focus on generally appreciated attributes of the drugs.

SYMPTOMS AND SIGNS OF ATHEROSCLEROSIS

The physician should be particularly alert to the symptoms and signs of atherosclerosis in all patients with diabetes.

Cerebrovascular Disease

Symptoms of cerebrovascular disease include intermittent dizziness, transient loss of vision, slurring of speech, and paresthesia or weakness of one arm or leg. Vascular bruits may be heard over the carotid arteries. Noninvasive procedures, including Doppler and carotid ultrasound studies, may be helpful to confirm the diagnosis or detect earlier disease that can still be associated with symptoms.

Aspirin at a dose of 325 mg/day may prevent a recurrence of symptoms, and use of anticoagulant medications after a transient ischemic attack may help some patients. For many patients, 81 mg aspirin/day appears to provide comparable benefit with reduced risk of bleeding. Clopidogrel may be considered in aspirin-intolerant patients or patients who fail to respond to aspirin. Use of aspirin has not been studied in people with diabetes age <30 years.

Coronary Heart Disease

As in people without diabetes, CHD may be associated with chest pain, arm pain, or nausea. However, in people with diabetes, ischemia may occur in the absence of chest pain, particularly in women and those with cardiac autonomic neuropathy. Atypical symptoms such as fatigue, unexplained onset of congestive heart failure, and deterioration of glycemic control to the point of diabetic keto-acidosis may indicate silent myocardial ischemia. Myocardial infarction should be considered in the differential diagnosis of these conditions. Noninvasive procedures, including exercise tolerance tests, exercise thallium studies, and gated blood pool scans, may help establish the diagnosis of silent ischemia and/or myocardial perfusion defects. The utility, frequency, and cost-benefit ratios of these studies in older asymptomatic patients to screen for CHD have not been determined. However, a plan to substantially increase physical activity in a previously inactive patient with longstanding type 1 diabetes should include consideration of stress test evaluation.

Therapy for CHD may be medical or surgical. Medical treatments include aspirin, nitrates, calcium-channel blockers, and cardioselective β-adrenergic blockers and agents that modify the renin-angiotensin system. Coronary angiography is necessary if bypass surgery or angioplasty is being considered. Bypass surgery is recommended for left main coronary artery disease and is generally indicated for triple-vessel disease, particularly in the presence of left ventricular dysfunction. Aggressive treatment of CVD risk factors, such as hypertension and dyslipidemia, is warranted in all patients with diabetes and CHD, and has been shown to have equal efficacy to aggressive risk factor treatment plus percutaneous procedures in patients with stable angina (including those with diabetes).

Peripheral Arterial Disease

Peripheral arterial disease should be suspected in patients who complain of buttock, calf, or thigh pain that occurs during exercise and is relieved with rest (intermittent claudication) and/or who exhibit decreased pulses in the lower extremities. The diagnosis can be confirmed with noninvasive Doppler studies. Simple office screens for an abnormal ankle-brachial index (<0.9) can help to detect early disease.

An expert panel of the American Heart Association has recommended regular determination of ankle-brachial index in patients with type 1 diabetes age >35 years. Sclerotic vessels can lead to falsely elevated systolic blood pressure and invalid results. Otherwise, a decreased index not only indicates a patient with peripheral arterial disease but is also a strong indicator of possible coronary artery disease and future cardiac mortality.

Aspirin, exercise, and smoking cessation are critical components of treatment. Treatment with either cilostazol or pentoxifylline may improve symptoms. If pain is incapacitating or persists at rest, or if a foot infection results from impaired blood flow through the major leg arteries, angioplasty or surgery to bypass the diseased vessels may be indicated. Treatment with either cilostazol or pentoxifylline may improve symptoms. Aspirin and exercise are important adjuvants to treatment.

Aspirin Therapy in Type 1 Diabetes

Aspirin therapy (75–162 mg/day) is recommended for primary prevention in type 1 diabetes in patients with an increased risk of CVD defined as a 10-year risk >10%. This includes men >50 years of age and women >60 years of age who have >1 additional major risk factor including family history of CVD, hypertension, smoking, dyslipidemia, or albuminuria. There is not sufficient evidence to recommend aspirin for primary prevention in lower-risk individuals such as men <50 years of age and women <60 years of age without other major risk factors. Aspirin is used as a secondary prevention strategy for those with diabetes with a history of CVD.

CONCLUSION

Patients with type 1 diabetes should be aware of their increased risk of CVD and advised of the importance of modifying risk factors such as hypertension, hyperlipidemia, and cigarette smoking. Clinicians should systematically assess patients for risk factors for CVD and attempt to modify them. They should question patients about symptoms of CVD, examine them for signs of atherosclerosis, and seek the expertise of appropriate specialists when needed.

BIBLIOGRAPHY

American Diabetes Association: Standards of medical care in diabetes—2008 (Position Statement). *Diabetes Care* 31 (Suppl. 1):S12–S54, 2008

Bax JJ, Young LH, Frye RL, Bonow RO, Steinberg HO, Barrett EJ: Screening for coronary artery disease in patients with diabetes (Consensus Statement). *Diabetes Care* 30:2729–2736, 2007

Borg R, Kuenen JC, Cartensen B, Zheng H, Nathan DM, Heine RJ, Nerup J, Borch-Johnsen K, Witte DR on behalf of the ADAG Study Group: HbA1C and mean blood glucose show stronger associations with cardiovascular disease risk factors than do postprandial glycaemia or glucose variability in persons with diabetes: the A1C-Derived Average Glucose (ADAG) study. *Diabetologia* 54:69–72, 2011

Campos H, Moye LA, Glasser SP, Stampfer MJ, Sacks FM: Low-density lipoprotein size, pravastatin treatment, and coronary events. *JAMA* 286:1468–1474, 2001

DCCT Research Group: The effect of intensive treatment of diabetes on the development and progression of long-term complications on insulin-dependent diabetes mellitus. *N Engl J Med* 329:977–986, 1993

Diabetes Control and Complications Trial/Epidemiology of Diabetes Interventions and Complications Research Group: The modern-day clinical course of type 1 diabetes mellitus after 30 years' duration: the diabetes control and complications trial/epidemiology of diabetes interventions and complications and Pittsburgh epidemiology of diabetes complications experience (1983-2005). *Arch Intern Med* 169:1307–1316, 2009

Eeg-Olofsson K, Cederholm J, Nilsson PM, Zethelius B, Svensson A-M, Gudbjornsdottir S, Eliasson B: Glycemic control and cardiovascular disease in 7454 patients with type 1 diabetes: an observational study for the Swedish National Diabetes Register. *Diabetes Care* 33:1640–1646, 2010

Heart Protection Study Collaborative Group: MRC/BHF Heart Protection Study of cholesterol lowering with simvastatin in 20536 high-risk individuals: a randomised placebo-controlled study. *Lancet* 360:7–22, 2002

Kavey RE, Allada V, Daniels SR, Hayman LL, McCrindle BW, Newburger JW, Parekh RS, Steinberger J: Cardiovascular risk reduction in high-risk pediatric patients: a scientific statement from the American Heart Association Expert Panel on Population and Prevention Science; the Councils on Cardiovascular Disease in the Young, Epidemiology and Prevention, Nutrition, Physical Activity and Metabolism, High Blood Pressure Research, Cardiovascular Nursing, and the Kidney in Heart Disease; and the Interdisciplinary Working Group on Quality of Care and Outcomes Research. Endorsed by the American Academy of Pediatrics. *Circulation* 114:2710–2738, 2006

Nathan DM, Cleary PA, Backlund JY, Genuth SM, Lachin JM, Orchard TJ, Raskin P, Zinman B: Intensive diabetes treatment and cardiovascular disease in patients with type 1 diabetes. *N Engl J Med* 353:2643–2653, 2005

Polak JF, Backlund J-Y C, Cleary PA, Harrington AP, O'Leary DH, Lachin JM, Nathan DM for the DCCT/EDIC Research Group: Progression of carotid artery intima-media thickness during 12 years in the Diabetes Control and Complications Trial/Epidemiology of Diabetes Interventions and Complications (DCCT/EDIC) Study. *Diabetes* 60:607–613, 2011

Rodriguez BL, Fujimoto WY, Mayer-David EJ, Imperatore G, Williams DE, Bell RA, Wadwa RP, Palla SL, Liu LL, Kershnar A, Daniels SR, Linder B for the SEARCH for Diabetes in Youth Study Group: Prevalence of cardiovascular disease risk factors in U.S. children and adolescents with diabetes. *Diabetes Care* 29:1891–1896, 2006

Selvin E, Marinopoulos S, Berkenblit G, Rami T, Brancati FL, Powe NR, Golden SH: Meta-analysis: glycosylated hemoglobin and cardiovascular disease in diabetes mellitus. *Ann Intern Med* 141:421–431, 2004

Turner RC, Millns H, Neil HA, Stratton IM, Manley SE, Mathews DR, Holman DR: Risk factor for coronary artery disease in non-insulin dependent diabetes mellitus (UKPDS 23). *Br Med J* 316:823–828, 1998

UKPDS: Effect of intensive blood-glucose control with metformin on complications in overweight patients with type 2 diabetes (UKPDS 34): UK Prospective Diabetes Study (UKPDS) Group. *Lancet* 352:854–865, 1998

UKPDS: Intensive blood-glucose control with sulphonylureas or insulin compared with conventional treatment and risk of complications in patients with type 2 diabetes (UKPDS 33): UK Prospective Diabetes Study (UKPDS) Group. *Lancet* 352:837–853, 1998

Wadwa RP, Urbina EM, Anderson AM, Hamman RF, Dolan LM, Rodriguez BL, Daniels SR, Dabelea D for the SEARCH Study Group: Measures of arterial stiffness in youth with type 1 and type 2 diabetes. *Diabetes Care* 33:881–886, 2010

LIMITED JOINT MOBILITY

Limited joint mobility (LJM) used to be one of the earliest and most common clinical complications seen in type 1 diabetes. However, since the Diabetes Control and Complications Trial, there has been a marked decrease in prevalence of LJM in both children and adults. If LJM is present, it is a potentially important clinical marker for diabetes complications such as retinopathy, nephropathy, neuropathy, and statural growth abnormalities. LJM is strongly associated with duration of diabetes. Glycation of tissue proteins associated with chronic hyperglycemia may be responsible for many long-term complications, including LJM.

DETECTION AND EVALUATION

LJM may occur in children or adults, is painless, and may cause little disability. Thus, it is unlikely to be brought to the attention of family members or health professionals. The only way to detect LJM is to examine hands and joints as part of routine physical examinations.

To evaluate for LJM, the following should be included. Observe and shake both hands of the patient, noting any scleroderma-like stiffness of the skin. The patient should then be asked to place the hands in a clapping or "prayer" position with forearms as parallel to the floor as possible (Fig. 6.7). Any inability to oppose the joints of the fingers and any limitation of flexion or extension of wrist, elbow, neck, or spine should be documented.

If pain or neuromuscular findings (e.g., atrophy, paresthesia) are present, other disorders, such as tenosynovitis or carpal tunnel syndrome, should be

Figure 6.7 LJM of increasing severity.
A: Normal joint mobility.
B: Bilateral contracture of 5th fingers.
C: Bilateral contracture of more than fifth fingers.
D: Bilateral wrist involvement.

considered. In adults, another possibility is Dupuytren's contracture, which is painless and characterized by palmar nodules and involvement of the third and fourth fingers.

Because there is a relationship between the severity of LJM and the microvascular complications of diabetes, patients found to have LJM at an office visit should be carefully examined for clinical evidence of retinopathy via ophthalmoscopy; for nephropathy by a quantitative determination of urinary microalbumin excretion; and for hypertension, hepatomegaly, and neuropathy by careful clinical examination.

CONCLUSION

The prevalence of LJM, which used to be a common complication, has markedly decreased in children and adults due to improved glycemic control. The presence of LJM remains an important clinical marker of coexistant microvascular disease.

BIBLIOGRAPHY

Aljahlan M, Lee KC, Toth E: Limited joint mobility in diabetes. *Postgrad Med* 105:99–101, 105–106, 1999

Duffin AC, Conaghue KC, Potter M, McInnes A, Chan AK, King J, Howard NJ, Silink M: Limited joint mobility in the hands and feet of adolescents with type 1 diabetes mellitus. *Diabet Med* 16:125–130, 1999

Frost D, Beischer W: Limited joint mobility in type 1 diabetic patients: associations with microangiopathy and subclinical macroangiopathy are different in men and women. *Diabetes Care* 24:95–99, 2001

Lindsay JR, Kennedy L, Atkinson AB, Bell PM, Carson DJ, McCance DR, Hunter SJ: Reduced prevalence of limited joint mobility in type 1 diabetes in a U.K. clinic population over a 20-year period. *Diabetes Care* 28:658–661, 2005

ABNORMAL LINEAR GROWTH

A bnormalities of height (absolute short stature as well as decreased growth velocity) are known consequences of insulin deficiency. Although the classic example occurs in the extreme and relatively rare Mauriac syndrome (diabetic dwarfism), subtle abnormalities of growth and development are not uncommon among youngsters with type 1 diabetes. Patients with poorly controlled diabetes have decreased insulin-like growth factor-1 levels and paradoxical increments in growth hormone levels during the night and in response to provocative stimuli. These abnormalities can be prevented or corrected with better glycemic control.

SUBTLE GROWTH ABNORMALITIES

Growth abnormalities become apparent when large patient populations are studied and subtle growth changes are sought, including a lag in height or weight or a deviation from previously established growth curves (Figs. 6.8 and 6.9). Defined in this fashion, 5–10% of youngsters with type 1 diabetes will not grow well. Children most likely to be affected are those with the earliest onset of diabetes and those who have the worst day-to-day glycemic control and the highest A1C levels. Boys are two or three times more likely to have a growth abnormality than girls.

DETERMINING GROWTH RATE

The only way to determine whether growth is adequate is to measure height and weight at each office visit and to plot data on standardized growth charts.

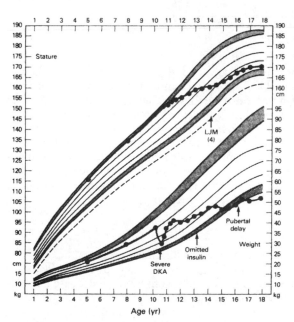

Figure 6.8 Inadequate diabetes control and growth abnormalities. Growth deceleration solely from uncontrolled diabetes. Patient refused to take two shots of insulin each day. Most of the time, patient omitted morning insulin and refused to follow any type of meal plan. The family refused psychiatric consultation.

Figure 6.9 Catch-up growth phenomenon with adequate insulin. Growth data from child with type 1 diabetes treated with one shot of morning insulin, showing growth deceleration and catch-up growth phenomenon after twice-daily insulin was started.

Ideally, data should be recorded at least every 3–4 months; at minimum, height and weight should be measured and recorded annually. Growth data obtained from other family members may be extremely valuable in placing an individual youngster's growth in perspective. Bone age determination (single radiograph of left wrist and hand compared with standard radiographs) coupled with other hormonal measurements may help assess the need for further evaluation. If growth abnormalities are found, the child should be evaluated for the presence of hypothyroidism and celiac disease. If no comorbidity is found, metabolic status should be carefully evaluated and appropriate recommendation for improvement made, such as changing to an intensified insulin treatment program.

CONCLUSION

Although mild growth retardation may not be totally preventable, evidence strongly indicates that major alterations in growth rate can be avoided by better blood glucose control in children. Therefore, the definition of adequate diabetes control must include the attainment and maintenance of normal growth and development.

BIBLIOGRAPHY

Silverstein J, Klingensmith G, Copeland K, Plotnick L, Kaufman FR, Laffel L, Deeb L, Grey M, Anderson B, Clark N: Care of children and adolescents with type 1 diabetes mellitus: a statement of the American Diabetes Association. *Diabetes Care* 28:186–212, 2005

Index